AF183579

Dental Trauma and Adverse Oral Conditions - Practice and Management Techniques

Edited by Aneesa Moolla

Published in London, United Kingdom

Dental Trauma and Adverse Oral Conditions - Practice and Management Techniques
http://dx.doi.org/10.5772/intechopen.100797
Edited by Aneesa Moolla

Contributors
Saurabh R. Nagar, Gabriela Fernandes, Shivani Bansal, Rajiv S. Desai, Diya Jayanth Kamdar, Shaimaa H Rafat Hussein Kotb, Álvaro Zubizarreta Macho, Blanca del Carmen Migueláñez Medrán, Nuria Delgado Castro, Elena Riad Deglow, Yousry Nagib Eldek, Heba Sleem, Mohamad Katamesh, Fahmy Hasanin, Prashanth Shetty, Shubham Chelkar, Shweta Hegde, Rahul Chaturvedi, Dudala Lakshmi, Shreya Mukherjee, Pankaj Bajaj, Shruti Pochhi, Aakanksha Shrivastava, Shahzada Asif Raza, Khairul Bariah Chi Adam, Nor Adilah Harun, Haszelini Hassan, Naziyah Shaban Mustafa, Pram Kumar Subramaniam, Izzati Nabilah Ismail, Desy Fidyawati, Adrianus Wicaksono, Veronica Septnina Primasari, Suci Amalia, Aneesa Moolla, Navneet Kaur, Eswari Ramassamy, Yolanda Malele-Kolisa, Nazia Khan, Mpho Primrose Molete, Maphefo Desiree Thekiso, Mzubanzi Mabongo, Sura Dakhil Jassim, Ali Abbas Abdulkareem, Manal Abdalla Eltahir, Randa Fath Elrahman Ibrahim, Hanan Alharbi, Santo Grace Umesh, Lakshmi Ramachandran, Janani Karthikeyan, Sindhuja M. Shankar

© The Editor(s) and the Author(s) 2023
The rights of the editor(s) and the author(s) have been asserted in accordance with the Copyright, Designs and Patents Act 1988. All rights to the book as a whole are reserved by INTECHOPEN LIMITED. The book as a whole (compilation) cannot be reproduced, distributed or used for commercial or non-commercial purposes without INTECHOPEN LIMITED's written permission. Enquiries concerning the use of the book should be directed to INTECHOPEN LIMITED rights and permissions department (permissions@intechopen.com).
Violations are liable to prosecution under the governing Copyright Law.

Individual chapters of this publication are distributed under the terms of the Creative Commons Attribution 3.0 Unported License which permits commercial use, distribution and reproduction of the individual chapters, provided the original author(s) and source publication are appropriately acknowledged. If so indicated, certain images may not be included under the Creative Commons license. In such cases users will need to obtain permission from the license holder to reproduce the material. More details and guidelines concerning content reuse and adaptation can be found at http://www.intechopen.com/copyright-policy.html.

Notice
Statements and opinions expressed in the chapters are these of the individual contributors and not necessarily those of the editors or publisher. No responsibility is accepted for the accuracy of information contained in the published chapters. The publisher assumes no responsibility for any damage or injury to persons or property arising out of the use of any materials, instructions, methods or ideas contained in the book.

First published in London, United Kingdom, 2023 by IntechOpen
IntechOpen is the global imprint of INTECHOPEN LIMITED, registered in England and Wales, registration number: 11086078, 5 Princes Gate Court, London, SW7 2QJ, United Kingdom
Printed in Croatia

British Library Cataloguing-in-Publication Data
A catalogue record for this book is available from the British Library

Additional hard and PDF copies can be obtained from orders@intechopen.com

Dental Trauma and Adverse Oral Conditions - Practice and Management Techniques
Edited by Aneesa Moolla
p. cm.

This title is part of the Dentistry Book Series, Volume 14
Topic: Prosthodontics and Implant Dentistry
Series Editor: Sergio Alexandre Gehrke
Topic Editor: Wen Lin Chai
Associate Topic Editor: Ghee Seong Lim

Print ISBN 978-1-80355-636-9
Online ISBN 978-1-80355-637-6
eBook (PDF) ISBN 978-1-80355-638-3
ISSN 2631-6218

We are IntechOpen, the world's leading publisher of Open Access books

Built by scientists, for scientists

6,400+
Open access books available

174,000+
International authors and editors

190M+
Downloads

156
Countries delivered to

Our authors are among the
Top 1%
most cited scientists

12.2%
Contributors from top 500 universities

CLARIVATE ANALYTICS BOOK CITATION INDEX INDEXED

WEB OF SCIENCE™

Selection of our books indexed in the Book Citation Index
in Web of Science™ Core Collection (BKCI)

Interested in publishing with us?
Contact book.department@intechopen.com

Numbers displayed above are based on latest data collected.
For more information visit www.intechopen.com

For EU product safety concerns:
IN TECH d.o.o., Prolaz Marije Krucifikse Kozulić 3, 51000 Rijeka, Croatia,
info@intechopen.com or visit our website at intechopen.com.

IntechOpen Book Series

Dentistry

Volume 14

Aims and Scope of the Series

This book series will offer a comprehensive overview of recent research trends as well as clinical applications within different specialties of dentistry. Topics will include overviews of the health of the oral cavity, from prevention and care to different treatments for the rehabilitation of problems that may affect the organs and/or tissues present. The different areas of dentistry will be explored, with the aim of disseminating knowledge and providing readers with new tools for the comprehensive treatment of their patients with greater safety and with current techniques. Ongoing issues, recent advances, and future diagnostic approaches and therapeutic strategies will also be discussed. This series of books will focus on various aspects of the properties and results obtained by the various treatments available, whether preventive or curative.

Meet the Series Editor

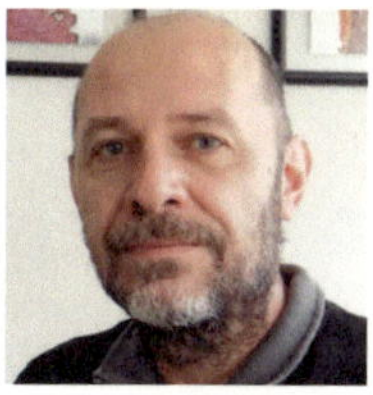

Dr. Sergio Alexandre Gehrke is a doctorate holder in two fields. The first is a Ph.D. in Cellular and Molecular Biology from the Pontificia Catholic University, Porto Alegre, Brazil, in 2010 and the other is an International Ph.D. in Bioengineering from the Universidad Miguel Hernandez, Elche/Alicante, Spain, obtained in 2020. In 2018, he completed a postdoctoral fellowship in Materials Engineering in the NUCLEMAT of the Pontificia Catholic University, Porto Alegre, Brazil. He is currently the Director of the Postgraduate Program in Implantology of the Bioface/UCAM/PgO (Montevideo, Uruguay), Director of the Cathedra of Biotechnology of the Catholic University of Murcia (Murcia, Spain), an Extraordinary Full Professor of the Catholic University of Murcia (Murcia, Spain) as well as the Director of the private center of research Biotecnos – Technology and Science (Montevideo, Uruguay). Applied biomaterials, cellular and molecular biology, and dental implants are among his research interests. He has published several original papers in renowned journals. In addition, he is also a Collaborating Professor in several Postgraduate programs at different universities all over the world.

Meet the Volume Editor

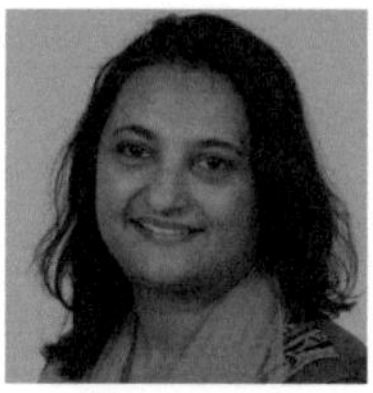

Dr. Aneesa Moolla is a lecturer at the University of Witwatersrand and a principal researcher at the Health Economics and Epidemiology Research Office (HE2RO) in South Africa. She holds a Ph.D. in psychology, her research is focused on oral health, mental health and resilience. Dr. Moolla has extensive experience in diverse healthcare fields and has worked in dental private practice, with the Red Cross Flying Doctor service, and in corporate healthcare. During her career, her research has further broadened into the fields of early childhood development, mental health, the HIV and TB care cascades and COVID. She is also a UNESCO-trained International Bioethics Facilitator.

Contents

Preface

This book focuses on dental trauma and oral conditions that significantly impact patients' well-being if not treated effectively and efficiently, including, for example, chronic periodontal disease and cysts. It is written by renowned global dental specialists with vast experience and high levels of expertise in their own areas. Concepts of dental trauma and other oral conditions are reviewed, with management techniques providing practical support for clinicians. Dental emergencies and accompanying dental trauma, with the issues associated with their management, are covered. The importance of teledentistry in the current climate of digital technologies is also highlighted.

The book opens with a chapter on dental emergencies and conditions that need prompt treatment. Dental emergencies such as injury to the hard tissue and soft tissues (teeth or gingiva) are potentially serious and should not be ignored. Ignoring a dental problem may increase the risk of permanent damage to the hard and soft tissue structures, as well as more extensive and expensive treatment to correct the problem at a later stage.

Chapter 2 covers the early management of dental trauma during COVID-19, noting how the lack of guidelines potentially promoted the spread of nosocomial COVID-19 through oral healthcare facilities, whilst simultaneously denying people in need of immediate treatment. Moreover, the cessation of dental care provision during this period actually increased the burden on hospital emergency departments that were already struggling with the pandemic. The chapter combines local guidelines and experience with a proposed algorithm for the early management of dental trauma during a pandemic.

Chapter 3 focuses on decision-making in dental traumatology when there are fractures involved, highlighting the need for detailed examinations in all such cases. A complete radiographic examination is essential in order to assess the state of the pulp, the degree of root development and the existence of any pathologies affecting the supporting tissues. This will serve to ensure that the patient receives comprehensive and holistic treatment and management.

Chapter 4 on teeth avulsion describes the significant amount of force that is required for the avulsion of a tooth. Replantation is the treatment of choice, and time management and appropriate storage of the avulsed tooth is crucial to a good prognosis. The chapter highlights the importance of a proper diagnosis and treatment strategy for a successful outcome.

In Chapter 5, there is a discussion of the splinting of traumatized teeth and other management techniques that favour the patient in terms of acceptance of the long procedures that accompany dental trauma and other chronic oral conditions. The full dental team is key in dental trauma situations, as they are often the first point of care.

Dental hygienists are key members of the emergency treatment team, contributing to the success of subsequent endodontic or restorative procedures in cases of dental trauma.

Orbital trauma entailing diverse mechanisms of injury and subsequent fracture patterns which may result in both functional and aesthetic problems is covered in Chapter 6. The suggested surgical approaches to the orbit show that regardless of how complex the fracture is, the principles of anatomic reduction, atraumatic technique and stable fixation apply to all cases. The chapter discusses the use of titanium mesh as an appropriate reconstructive material and compares this method with conventional reconstruction techniques.

Chapter 7 describes trauma from occlusion and its management. Occlusal instability is a clinical finding often ignored by general dentists; however, establishing the cause is key, since treatment is often only directed towards the effects. Thorough evaluation and occlusal analysis will lead to a definitive diagnosis that will help better anticipate the damage.

The impact of dental and orofacial trauma on oral health-related quality of life (OHRQoL) in children and adolescents is the subject of Chapter 8. OHRQoL is described in the literature as an essential part of a person's general health and overall well-being.

Chapter 9 examines new instruments that can be used to assess dental trauma impacts in young children. The psycho-social impacts of dental trauma cannot be underestimated and are an important aspect of patient management. The negative psychological effect of traumatic dental injuries is specific to an individual, and as such it is suggested that each patient should be treated holistically with all factors being taken into account.

Chapter 10 discusses injury to the periodontal tissues which includes microbial, physical, thermal, chemical, mechanical, occlusal and habitual injury which may impact the harmony of the periodontal attachment apparatus, altering the entire functioning of the dentition. When trauma is unintentional and iatrogenic, the type of tissue damage is described as acute and self-limiting. The chapter reviews the various forms of non-microbial trauma to the periodontal tissues, their clinical manifestations and appropriate management.

Antioxidants, increasingly needed as adjuncts to periodontal therapy to maintain the balance with reactive oxygen species, are discussed in detail in Chapter 11. The chapter presents new possibilities based on recent studies that have used different antioxidants as supplements to conventional periodontal therapy.

In Chapter 12, we discuss the management of periodontal emergencies during the COVID-19 pandemic. Most periodontal treatment is more dangerous work than other dental procedures due to bioaerosol generation. Transmission can occur through direct doctor-patient contact, as well as through contamination from instruments or surfaces in the dentist's surgery. This chapter offers advice for clinicians on how to approach such situations.

Salivary duct cysts, discussed in Chapter 13, are described as true cysts caused by obstruction of salivary ducts. They are rarely found in minor salivary glands. Intraoral salivary duct cysts and mucoceles represent clinically salivary gland neoplasms, making diagnosis difficult and subject to errors in treatment. It is further shown within this chapter why it is important for oral surgeons to include salivary duct cysts in the differential diagnosis of swelling affecting the buccal mucosa.

The pandemic has had a significant impact on dentistry and pushed us to the forefront of the digital era. An aspect of telehealth, teledentistry involves the exchange of clinical details and relevant imaging over remote distances for consultation and treatment planning. An innovative approach, it can reach more people who may lack access to care. Chapter 14, on teledentistry, highlights important points for both current and future consideration and research.

We hope this book will provide the reader with much useful knowledge.

Aneesa Moolla
Lecturer,
University of Witwatersrand,
Johannesburg, South Africa

Principal Researcher,
Health Economics and Epidemiology Research Office,
Johannesburg, South Africa

Section 1

Dental Trauma

Chapter 1

Perspective Chapter: Dental Emergency and Conditions

Navneet Kaur

Abstract

Dental emergencies are related to dental pain, bleeding and orofacial trauma-like conditions should be attended by dental practitioners. Even the jaw fracture requires the attention of oral and maxillofacial surgeons. Dental pain may be of odontogenic or non-odontogenic in origin, and in some cases, it may be idiopathic in nature. Bleeding in the soft tissues of the oral cavity may occur due to the infection from the microbial flora or inflammation and trauma. The management of these conditions should be based on the cause of the condition that may require the antibiotic prophylaxis along with root canal treatment or extraction of the tooth. Most of the dental conditions can be prevented by visiting to the dentists regularly and minimize the risk of oral trauma.

Keywords: management, emergencies, trauma, pulpitis, inflammation

1. Introduction

Any dental emergency such as an injury to the hard tissue and soft tissues (teeth or gingiva) can be potentially serious and should not be ignored. Ignoring a dental problem may enhance the risk of permanent damage of the hard and soft tissue structures and also more extensive and expensive treatment is required to correct the problem later on.

An acute oral disorder requiring dental and/or medical care, including fractured, loose, or avulsed teeth caused by traumas, any pathology (infections and inflammation) of the soft tissues of the oral cavity; and complications of oral surgery, such as dry tooth socket, fracture jaw and swelling in the jaw.

A dental emergency is basically determined by health care staff which includes any dental condition that require immediate diagnostic evaluation and treatment which is necessary to prevent severe or long-term illness, or to reduce or lessen severe pain. Some of the examples of dental emergencies are acute oral and maxillofacial conditions such as trauma, infection, pain, swelling, or bleeding that are likely to remain acute or will worsen if not provided with immediate intervention and treatment.

Some of the conditions that always require dental emergencies include, but are not limited to like Airway/breathing difficulties occurring mostly from oral infection, A swift spread of oral infection, such as Ludwig's angina, cellulitis which is characterized by severe swelling on the floor of the mouth, with elevation of the tongue and acute abscess which includes an abscess at root end or a gingival abscess.

Maxillofacial injury or trauma to the jaws or dentition that put on to decrease the loss of airway.

By presuming the shock due to oral infection or trauma, Uncontrolled or spontaneous severe bleeding from the oral cavity, Head injuries (including stabbing or gunshot wounds) that involve maxillary or mandibular jaw along with its dentition, Moderate to severe dehydration associated with altered response in masticatory function due to any infection or trauma, Clear signs of physical distress, (e.g., respiratory distress), related to infection or injury to the jaws or dentition, Suspected or known fractures involving the nasal bones, mandible, zygomatic arch, maxilla and zygoma, Acute Temporomandibular Joint (TMJ) pain, "closed-lock" TMJ, or dislocation of the TMJ, Aspiration or swallowing of a tooth/teeth or foreign object that threatens loss of airway, Acute, severe, debilitating pain due to suspected oral infection, oral trauma, bleeding disorders of oral mucosa, oral ulceration or other dental-related conditions. Infections, including infected third molars, (Pericoronitis) and acute infections with a fever of 101° F or above, infections not responsive to antibiotic therapy, and acute pulpitis. Injuries from trauma, such as an avulsed tooth, or fractured tooth. Postoperative complications including alveolar osteitis, bleeding or infection. Restorative Dental Emergencies include Pain management, Infections and soft tissue problems, Crack, fracture and mobility of teeth and dental restorations, Fractured and loose implants, Fractures and swallowing of removable prostheses.

According to the General Dental Council's 'Standards for Dental Professionals', 2009, registered dentists are expected to:

i. Work within your knowledge, professional competence and physical abilities.

ii. Refer patients for a second opinion and for further advice when it is necessary, or if the patient asks.

iii. Refer patients for further treatment when it is necessary to do so. As such, the need for referral may be that the situation lies outside: the knowledge the skill the experience the facilities available to the referring dentist.

2. Dental pain (pulpitis)

Dental pain is the commonest dental emergency and it may occur due to various etiological factors. It is delineated as 'an unpleasant sensory and emotional expertise related to actual or potential tissue damage, or described in terms of such damage. It is one of the most common reasons that why patients seek dental treatment and further to note that various diseases or pathological conditions may be responsible for the initiation of pain. However, pain arising from nondental sources corresponds to myofascial inflammation, cephalalgia headache, maxillary sinusitis, nasal tissues, ears, temporomandibular joints, and neuralgias continually should be thought of and excluded [1].

Odontogenic pain is a pain initiating from the teeth or their supporting structures, the mucosa, gingivae, maxilla, mandible or periodontal membrane.

The major cause of dental pain is inflammation of the dental pulp, most commonly as a result of dental caries (tooth decay), most commonly worldwide, affecting 60–90%

of school children. The second most common infection similar to chronic mycobacterial infections is Periodontal disease (gum disease for example Leprosy, is painless. The periodontal pathogens appear to be singularly and odds-on to cause aggressive periodontal disease. Both *Porphyromonas gingivalis* and *A. actinomycetemcomitans*, along with multiple deep pockets, severe clinical attachment loss is linked with resistance to standard traditional treatments for soft tissues (gingiva). Other risk factors which include smoking and also there is a genetic predisposition responsible to develop this silent painless disease, which may be the leading cause of tooth loss, and is found in almost 5–400% of middle-aged adults.

Initially, dental caries is asymptomatic. Pain does not occur until the decay caused by bacteria reaches near the pulp, and an inflammatory process starts developing. Reversible pulpitis is defined as mild inflammation of the tooth pulp which is caused by caries encroaching on the pulp. Pain is generally triggered by hot, cold, and sweet stimuli which lasts for a few seconds, and resolves spontaneously. If we talk about the treatment then it includes removal of the caries and placement of a dental restoration, or filling. But if the carious lesion persists, it will progress towards irreversible pulpitis, which is a severe inflammation of the pulp. Pain becomes very severe, spontaneous, and persistent in nature, and is poorly localized. The only way to definitively treat irreversible pulpitis is root canal treatment along with appropriate analgesia such as a nonsteroidal anti-inflammatory drug (NSAID).

A severely inflamed pulp will eventually undergo necrosis which may lead to apical periodontitis, which is inflammation around the apex of the tooth. Pain is severe, spontaneous, and persistent, but unlike that of irreversible pulpitis, localizes to the affected tooth. The tenderness to percussion is positive. Management is root canal treatment or extraction. The patient should be referred to a dentist as soon as possible along with prescription of analgesics (**Figure 1**).

Apical abscess is a localized and purulent form of apical periodontitis. Clinically it presents as a fluctuating buccal or palatal swelling, with or without a draining fistula. If pus can drain out from the fistula, the pain is usually not severe in nature. Antibiotics are unnecessary unless concomitant cellulitis is present. Incision and drainage of a fluctuating area should be performed by qualified physician. Definitive treatment is root canal treatment or extraction. Patients should be recalled back to dentist within one or two days and also analgesics should be prescribed.

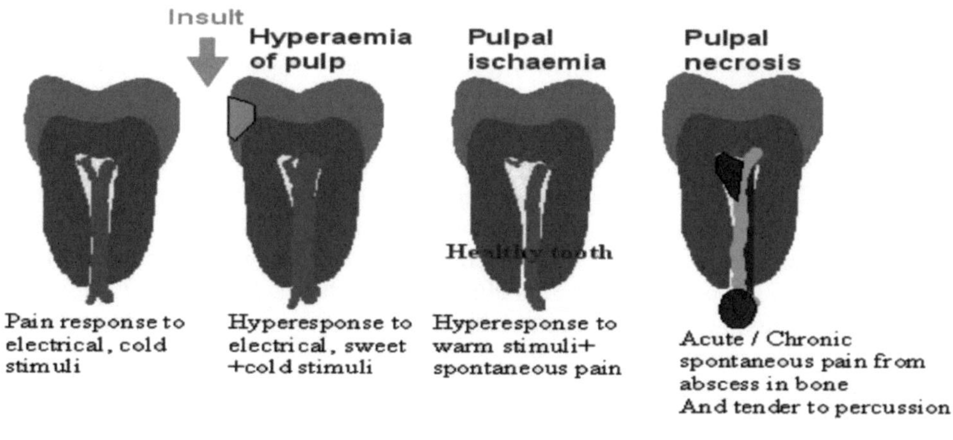

Figure 1.
The stages and characteristics of pulpal pain.

Cellulitis may follow apical periodontitis if the infection spreads to the surrounding tissues and also to the areas of facial space which can lead to facial space infections. Diffuse, tense and painful swelling of the affected tissues may occur. Diagnostic evaluation should focus on determining whether cellulitis remains localized or has spread regionally. Outpatient treatment of patients with localized cellulitis should be treated by the physician with oral antistreptococcal antibiotics, such as oral penicillin 500 mg three times a day in adults or 50 mg/kg/day in children [2].

In case of patient is allergic with penicillin, erythromycin or clindamycin (Cleocin) may be prescribed. In addition, analgesics should be prescribed. Definitive treatment is root canal treatment or extraction, which may be delayed until swelling subsides. Patients should be evaluated by a dentist within one or two days but patient should also advice to return sooner if swelling or pain worsens. If infection spreads into the deep spaces of the head and neck presented with significant swelling, increased risk of life-threatening complications like there is extensive airway involvement. As a general rule, these patients should be hospitalized for a surgical and infectious consultation. Broad-spectrum Intravenous antibiotic therapy should be started immediately and should include coverage for anaerobes.

3. Periodontal origin

Periodontitis can be described as an inflammatory disease of supporting tissues of teeth which is caused by the specific microorganisms or groups of specifics microorganisms which results in progressive destruction of the periodontal ligament and alveolar bone with periodontal pocket formation, gingival recession or both. The main etiological factor is bacterial plaque and calculus. Patients with chronic periodontal disease or patients who have a foreign object impinge in the gingiva may present with an acute periodontal abscess. A gingival abscess is basically a localized, painful and rapidly expanding lesion which involves the marginal gingival or interdental papilla and sometimes in a previously disease-free area. It usually occurs as an acute inflammatory response to foreign substances which has been forced into the gingiva. In its early stage it appears to be a red swelling with a smooth, shiny surface. Within 24 to 48 hours, the lesion is usually fluctuant and pointed, with a surface orifice from which purulent exudates may be seen. If not hindered and allowed to progress, the lesion generally ruptures spontaneously. Acute periodontal abscess presents as a Localized red, ovoid swelling, Periodontal pocket, Mobility, Tooth elevation in socket, Tenderness to percussion or biting, Exudation, Elevated temperature and regional lymphadenopathy.

If it is not treated on time, the abscess may rupture or progress to cellulitis. Oral intervention is incision and drainage within 24 hours of patient referral and debridement of the infected periodontal area. Antibiotics are not prescribed if debridement is successful, because their use remains controversial in these cases.

However, Penicillin is the first drug of choice in the treatment of periodontal abscesses in the UK, being used by 57% of surveyed dentists, followed by amoxicillin (21%) and metronidazole (14%). Amoxicillin, 500 mg (because amoxicillin exhibits an excellent ability to penetrate into both normal and pathologic periodontal tissues and is highly active against many periodontal pathogens) 1.0-g loading dose, then 500 mg three times a day for 3 days. Re-evaluation after 3 days to determine if there is any need for continued or adjusted antibiotic therapy.

4. Pericoronitis

Pericoronitis is inflammation of the soft tissues surrounding the crown of a partially erupted third molar. It occurs when bacterial plaque and food debris accumulate beneath the flap of soft tissue covering the partially erupted third molar. Inflammatory edema, most commonly complicated by trauma from the opposing tooth, which may result in swelling of the flap, pain, tenderness, and a bad taste caused by pus oozing from beneath the flap. Lymphadenopathy is common, and cellulitis and trismus may occur. In severe cases, the oral airway can be compromised. If pericoronitis is well localized, chlorhexidine mouthwashes and irrigation with normal saline and povidone iodine can resolve symptoms in the majority of cases. Localized cases that do not respond to mechanical therapy and more severe untreated cases with spreading cellulitis should be treated with prescribing antibiotic like penicillin and analgesics like NSAIDs prescribed as medication. Patient can be diagnosed in case of symptomatic treatment and refer to the dentists as soon as possible. The intervention of pericoronitis is surgical removal of soft tissue called as operculectomy. If the tooth is impacted, in that case surgical extraction is recommended.

5. Exposed cementum and dentin

Dentinal sensitivity is one of the most common dental emergency conditions. It is characterized by short, sharp pain arising from exposed dentine in response to stimuli, typically thermal, tactile, osmotic or chemical and which cannot be attributed to any other dental defects or pathological conditions. The tooth is having sensitivity from cold fluids or from air which directly affects the pulp of the tooth. The etiological factors are gingival recession, scaling and root planning or wasting disease such as erosion (tooth wear) due to a high acid diet or gastric reflux, the patient may experience generalized dentinal hypersensitivity. The root surface comprised of a thin layer of cementum overlying dentine which may be exposed to oral environment due to aggressive or using wrong tooth brushing technique. Dentine underlying the enamel layer comprised of minute tubules which are fluid filled and connects to the nerve ending in the dental pulp directly. The recent postulate for dental pain includes the osmolality theory, whereby the dentine fluids initiates an action potential within the A delta and C fibers in the pulp when stimulated by mechanical stimulation.

The use of a desensitizing toothpaste and a reduction in acid in the diet will help resolve the symptoms of root sensitivity. Modification and accurate tooth brushing habits along with use of fluoride toothpaste may also reduce the tooth sensitivity symptoms is also recommended. In the case of dental caries, a lost filling or fractured tooth, coverage of the exposed dentine with a temporary restoration will usually relieve the symptoms.

6. Fractured tooth/dental trauma

Dental trauma is most commonly seen in children with a peak age of 12 years old and having a primary tooth. Injury to the teeth and their supporting structure may lead to fractures, lateral or extrusive luxation in which loosening and displacement of the tooth, intrusion where displacement of the tooth vertically into the alveolar bone), and avulsion is a complete displacement of the tooth out of its socket [3]. Tooth fracture may occur on the crown, root or both and in some cases, it may cause exposure to the pulp. Fractures exposing the pulp are often painful, and patients with this condition require timely referral to a dentist. If the crown of a tooth is fractured by trauma and the broken fragment is available, it should be stored in a physiological medium (milk) until a dentist can assess the patient. Definitive treatment may involve root canal therapy or extraction. Coverage of exposed dentine on the fractured crown with a temporary restoration is desirable to protect the underlying pulp tissue [4].

Fracture of the root usually require radiograph and treatment may involve root canal therapy, splinting, or extraction, depending on the exact nature of the root fracture. In case of luxation of tooth if the primary dentition is traumatized and teeth are so loose and are in danger of being aspirated then immediate referral to a dentist for extraction is required [3]. If permanent teeth are involved the dental referral is required for repositioning, splinting, or root canal therapy, along with long term follow-up.

Avulsed teeth are one of the true dental emergency conditions. Primary teeth are never reimplanted [3]. In case of permanent teeth involvement, Immediate on-scene reimplantation is the preferred method of treatment. If the tooth is contaminated, it should be gently rinsed in cold running tap water and then reimplanted. Care should be taken not to touch, rub, or clean the root because it may remove the periodontal ligament fibers and reduce the chance of successful reimplantation. The patient should immediately report to dentist for splinting and antibiotic prophylaxis [5].

7. Placement of temporary restorations

Although it is dubious that general medical practitioners will have temporary filling materials available in their surgeries. Dentine that has been exposed due to caries, a lost filling or tooth fracture can be treated relatively easily by using glass ionomer cement (GIC) or zinc oxide eugenol (ZOE) materials. Mostly GIC materials are available in capsules but a hand-mixed material is also available which consists of a powder, liquid and conditioner. Firstly, the surface of the cavity is painted with the conditioner followed by rinsing and drying and then finally placement of the filling is done. Zinc oxide eugenol materials consist of a powder and liquid (oil of cloves) that are mixed to a putty-like consistency before placement in the tooth.

8. Alveolar osteitis

After extraction, the most common complication is a 'dry socket' in which the clot formation within the socket fails at 3–5 days. It occurs due to the disruption of the clot within the socket. The socket may be filled with food debris along with saliva. Pain usually initiates within 24–72 hours after the extraction of tooth. Pain may vary in frequency and intensity and radiates to the ear and neck which may cause headache, insomnia and dizziness may be present. Redness, swelling, fever or pus formation is uncommon but edema of the surrounding gingiva and regional lymphadenitis is usually present. There is marked halitosis and foul taste. Smoking is a major predisposing environmental factor as it reduces the blood supply. The tissue around the socket appears to be tender and white necrotic bone is exposed in the socket. The incidence of dry socket may vary from 1 to 9%.

Irrigation of the socket using saline or chlorhexidine or powdered sodium perborate and then placement of medicated dressing soaked in bacteriostatic solution (alvogyl paste, bismuth iodoform paraffin paste (BIPP), cotton wool or gauze soaked in iodoform) on ribbon gauze and metronidazole and lidocaine ointment. Analgesics should be prescribed as a short course of non-steroidal anti-inflammatory drug to narcotic based like codeine. Immediate pain relief is usually attained and patients rarely re-present for additional treatment. Patients should be instructed to irrigate the area regularly. If the patient returns with ongoing pain, then osteomyelitis should be excluded and localized bony sequestrate should be excluded.

However, the rate of occurrence is unavoidable. Dry socket condition can only be prevented by copious use of irrigation, antibiotic medicated dressings and maintenance of oral hygiene.

9. Maxillary sinusitis 'mimicking' toothache

Recurrent maxillary sinusitis can result in extensive maxillary tooth pain. When lying down or bending over, the discomfort tends to get worse. On the affected side, there is frequently a sensation of 'fullness.' The discomfort is usually one-sided, dull, throbbing, and constant. Frequently, the patient is sick in general and has a temperature. In temporomandibular disorders (TMD) or neuropathic pain, it might mimic the symptoms of maxillary sinusitis. Unless misdiagnosed, many dental disorders rarely cause chronic discomfort.

Inflammation of the maxillary sinuses is best treated with local and systemic decongestants, and antibiotics may be administered if the condition persists10. Sinus pain is caused by a build-up of pressure in the sinuses. Sinus drainage can be aided by decongestants. In moderate situations, antibiotics are likely to play only a minimal influence. The patient is sent to an otorhinolaryngologist.

Acute necrotizing ulcerative gingivitis is a type of gingival infection that produces ulceration of the interdental gingival papillae. It has the potential to cause widespread devastation. Typically, young to middle-aged adults with low infection resistance are afflicted (diabetes, HIV infection, chemotherapy). Males are more likely to be impacted than females, with predisposing factors including stress, smoking, and poor oral hygiene. Important indications include halitosis, spontaneous gingival bleeding, and a 'punched-out' appearance of the interdental papillae. Patients frequently complain of significant gingival tenderness, which causes pain when eating and brushing their teeth. The ache is dull, profound, and unrelenting. Gums can bleed on their own, and there's an awful taste in the mouth as well as visible halitosis.

Because the infection is anaerobic, treatment is based on surgical principles and comprises superficial debridement, chlorhexidine mouthwashes, and a course of metronidazole pills. A recurrence should be avoided if the causative causes are addressed.

Which tests can assist in diagnosis?

There are several simple tests that may assist in diagnosis of dental pain.

1. **Pulp sensitivity test:** On the cervical third (neck region) of the tooth crown, dry ice on a cotton bud or an ordinary ice stick (made in a plastic or glass tube) is placed. The pulpal tissue is capable of sending nerve impulses and is vital if it responds to the stimuli (pain is the only sensory response from the dental pulp). The absence of a response could imply pulp necrosis.

2. **Percussion test:** A percussion test is performed. The tooth is tapped in the longitudinal axis with an instrument handle. Pain indicates periapical inflammation caused by inflammatory sensitivity of the mechanosensory receptors in the periodontal membrane around the tooth.

3. **Probing:** The health of the gingival tissues can be checked by gently inserting a fine, blunt probe into the gingival sulcus surrounding the tooth. Gum disease caused by inflammation is indicated by bleeding and/or sulcus depths more than 3–4 mm.

4. **Mobility test:** The mobility of a tooth can be tested by holding it firmly between the fingers on the buccal (cheek) and lingual surfaces. Although all teeth have a little amount of mobility (0.5 mm), noticeable movement indicates that the tooth's root has lost bone support.

5. **Palpation:** Tenderness, as well as the type and extent of swelling, may be revealed by careful palpation around the area of concern.

6. **Sinus formation:** Chronic dental abscesses tend to empty the mucosa though buccal aspect causing mucosal sinuses. Rarely lower mandibular teeth with chronic abscesses may drain buccally (below the cheek muscle attachment) or

Diagnosis	Characteristic features	Clinical presentation	complications	Treatment
Reversible pulpitis	Pulpal inflammation	Pain with hot cold and sweet stimuli	Periapical abscess, cellulitis	Restoration
Irreversible pulpitis	Pulpal inflammation	Spontaneous, poorly localized pain	Periapical abscess, cellulitis	RCT, Extraction
Abscess	Localized bacterial infection	Localized pain and swelling	cellulitis	Incision and Drainage, RCT or Extraction
Cellulitis	Diffuse soft tissue bacterial infection	Pain, erythema and swelling	Regional spread	Antibiotics and RCT or Extraction
Pericoronitis	Inflamed gum over partially erupted teeth	Pain, erythema and swelling	Cellulitis	Irrigation, antibiotics if cellulitis is also present
Tooth Fracture	Broken tooth	Clinical examination and Radiography	Pulpitis and sequelae	Restoration with or without RCT, Extraction
Tooth Luxation	Loose tooth	Clinical examination and Radiography	Aspiration, Pulpitis and sequelae	Splinting, with or without RCT, Extraction
Tooth avulsion	Missing tooth	Clinical examination	Ankylosis, Resorption	Reimplantation, splinting

Table 1.
Most common dental emergencies.

inferiorly below the mylohyoid muscle leading to dermal sinuses that are often mistaken for skin lesions remaining immune to routine dermatological remedies

7. **Radiographic examination:** If it's possible to get a screening radiograph, like an orthopantomography, this could help in diagnosis and pinpointing the explanation for the pain. The radiograph shows clearly the apical, periapical and associated structures and tissues. The connection of the maxillary molars and premolars to the ground of the sinus are often examined, and radiographs may reveal recurrent caries or periapical radiolucency's related to a long-time infection (**Table 1**).

10. Conclusion

It has been estimated that one or two life threatening emergencies will occur in the lifetime practice of a general dentist so prompt recognition and efficient management of dental emergencies by a well-prepared dental team can increase the likelihood of a satisfactory outcome. With proper training, thorough preparation, and regular practice, the staff of the dental office will be able to provide appropriate dental care whenever the need arises. To improve access and the quality-of-life care indeed it is essential to identify the need of the use of emergency dental services.

Author details

Navneet Kaur
National Dental College and Hospital, Derabassi, Punjab, India

*Address all correspondence to: kaurparneet1963@gmail.com

IntechOpen

© 2022 The Author(s). Licensee IntechOpen. This chapter is distributed under the terms of the Creative Commons Attribution License (http://creativecommons.org/licenses/by/3.0), which permits unrestricted use, distribution, and reproduction in any medium, provided the original work is properly cited.

References

[1] Okeson JP, Falace DA. Nonodontogenic toothache. Dental Clinical in North America. 1997;**41**:367-383

[2] Goldberg MH, Topazian RG. Odontogenic infections and deep fascial space infections of dental origins. In: Topazian RG, Goldberg MH, Hupp JR, editors. Oral and Maxillofacial Infections. 4th ed. Philadelphia: Saunders; 2002. pp. 158-187

[3] McTigue DJ. Diagnosis and management of dental injuries in children. Pediatrics Clinic in North America. 2000;**47**:1067-1084

[4] Auld DN, Wright GB. The initial management of dento-alveolar trauma in general dental practice. Dental Update. 2010;**37**(5):286-288

[5] Andreasen JO. Traumatic Dental Injuries: A Manual. Copenhagen: Munksgaard; 1999. pp. 34-39

Chapter 2

Perspective Chapter: Early Management of Dental Trauma in the Era of COVID-19

Khairul Bariah Chi Adam, Haszelini Hassan,
Pram Kumar Subramaniam, Izzati Nabilah Ismail,
Nor Adilah Harun and Naziyah Shaban Mustafa

Abstract

Traumatic dental injuries are emergencies that must be treated promptly and properly to reduce the suffering, costs, and time for patients and parents. However, since the coronavirus disease 2019 (COVID-19) outbreak was declared a pandemic on March 11, 2020, most dental care facilities in the affected countries have been completely closed or have been only providing emergency treatment. This can partly be a result of the lack of universal protocol or guidelines regulating the dental care provision during such a pandemic, especially in the management of dental trauma. This lack of guidelines has the potential to both promote the spread of nosocomial COVID-19 through oral health care facilities and deny people in need of immediate treatment. Moreover, ceasing dental care provision during such a period will incense the burden on hospitals' emergency departments that are already struggling with the pandemic. Therefore, this chapter elaborates on the importance of early management of dental trauma by sharing local guidelines and experience with a proposed algorithm for the early management of dental trauma during the emergence of COVID-19.

Keywords: management, dental trauma, COVID-19, guidelines in the management of TDI, algorithm for management of TDI

1. Introduction

Even before the pandemic, dental trauma is one of the world's leading oral health problems that is often neglected [1] leading to a global burden of disease amounting to a US$2—5 million per 1 million inhabitants annually [2]. When the world was hit with a deadly coronavirus in late 2019, the whole world is in a massive total economic and social lockdown to focus on controlling the spread of the infection. The impact it had on the health services is detrimental enough to negatively affect not only the treatment and monitoring of dental trauma patients but also intensify the challenges in new findings and further scientific contributions to dentistry [3, 4].

Before coronavirus disease 2019 (COVID-19), the reported prevalence of dental trauma had varied widely as they depend on various factors such as age, etiology, region, environment, and gender. These injuries may be caused by road traffic accidents, bicycle accidents, assaults, falls, sports, industrial accidents, as well as iatrogenic causes from intraoral procedures. The prevalence of dental trauma in overall groups of patients were ranging from 15% to 30% [2] with an incidence rate of roughly 1—3 per 100 person-years [5, 6]. It was thought that approximately 900 million people had at least one dental trauma in the year 2016 with 1 in 4 adults and one in 6 adolescents having had a history of traumatic dental injuries [1]. The types of dental trauma reported include orofacial soft tissue injuries, maxillomandibular injuries, as well as traumatic dental injuries, in which the majority of the cases were contributed by traumatic dental injuries.

2. Dental trauma and COVID-19: the incidence

The pattern of dental trauma affecting different age groups has been relatively constant for the past many years, with the majority of the cases being contributed by pediatric patients. It was reported that 25% of the dental trauma was affecting the primary dentition, whereas 33% of the dental trauma was found in permanent dentition with the majority of the injuries occurring before the age 1 of 9 [2, 7]. Different age groups were known to have different etiologic factors leading to the presentation of dental trauma. A most common cause of dental trauma in preschool children is due to accidental falls, whereas in school-age children ranging from 7 to 12 years, sports and school fights were the main etiologic factors [2]. Assaults and road traffic accidents are more common etiologic factors among adolescents and adults [6]. This characteristic pattern of etiological factors is significantly affected when the world is hit by the COVID-19 pandemic. Due to the restricted movement order by most government authorities in the world, the changes in the epidemiology of dental trauma were very challenging to acquire for many reasons including the limited oral health emergency services available, as well as the restrictions in the data collection for the epidemiological studies.

Because of the COVID-19 pandemic, school closures, travel restrictions, and cessation of social events have changed the character of dental injuries. It significantly reduced the reported cases of dental trauma during the pandemic period. Few studies done were done in China, India, the UK, and Europe had described a significant reduction in the presentation of dental trauma in the primary and emergency dental services when they compared the dental attendances during a similar period before COVID-19 [8–10]. Some studies in China and the UK even showed that during the pandemic, there was a relatively higher case of dental trauma among preschoolers aged below 6 years, followed by adults [4, 8]. This pattern was different before covid-19 where the majority of the dental trauma cases were contributed by the adults. However, in Europe, it was found that most of the dental trauma was from the adults, with the age group of 20—29 years contributing to more than half of the adult patients [9, 10].

The global lockdown had led to a reduction in road traffic, social violence, group sports, and other school activities. This led to a reduction of dental trauma cases contributed by the mentioned activities. Nonetheless, reports on dental trauma during the pandemic showed that there was a significant increase in accidental falls and bicycle accidents leading to the dental and maxillofacial trauma ranging from 52% to

68% of presentations [8, 9, 11, 12]. This is further followed by interpersonal violence, occupational accidents, and road traffic accidents. A report in the UK also found that assaults from interpersonal and domestic violence had also increased considerably during the pandemic lockdown amounting to approximately 6% compared to a 2.6% prevalence before the pandemic [8]. It is no doubt that the socioeconomic gap that is present in some societies may have contributed to more interpersonal violence when the authority employed the social distancing measure and enforced the "stay-at-home" guidance to flatten the infection curve [13].

Dental trauma can present as an isolated injury or in association with a multisystem traumatic injury. The trend of cases seen in the emergency setting since the COVID-19 emerged has also drastically transformed from a higher number of polytrauma seen in road traffic accidents to a more isolated injury. Soft-tissue facial injuries and traumatic dental injuries caused by the accidental falls were prominent in comparison to maxillomandibular fractures [9, 12]. Since children aged below 6 are those mainly contributing to the number of cases during COVID-19, the diagnosis of traumatic dental injuries was reported to be mainly dentoalveolar injuries which include concussion, luxation, and intrusion injuries to the anterior teeth that may range from 20% to 28% [8, 12]. However, in young adults with permanent dentition, the type of dental trauma presented during the pandemic was reported to be tooth fracture which mainly includes complicated crown fractures ranging from 62% to 75% [8, 9]. Depending on the impact of force from trauma caused by accidental falls or assaults, direct injury mechanisms can contribute to soft tissue injuries usually presenting with a laceration of the lip or chin [14].

The accidental falls with the chin falling first contributed to the indirect forces on the mandibular teeth against the maxillary dentition. The impact of this force often results in complicated crown fractures. The upper central incisors were reported to be most frequently injured [8] regardless of permanent or primary dentition. This trauma is usually accompanied by a condylar and/or mandibular symphysis fracture and intraoral soft tissue and submental laceration. Alveolar fractures were the least number of cases presented during the pandemic phase.

Throughout this unfortunate pandemic phase that had claimed millions of lives, a conclusion can be drawn to the pattern of dental trauma epidemiology which was highly influenced by the social and economic factors. The presentation of dental trauma in the emergency dental services during the COVID-19 pandemic was more likely to be caused by the lower energy injuries caused by falls and assaults that were more likely to be sustained in the home due to the restricted movement and quarantine orders governed by the authorities. Soft-tissue facial injuries accompanied by isolated traumatic dental injuries to the anterior dentition predominated the epidemiology of dental trauma during the COVID-19 pandemic. There is a significant reduction during the pandemic in the more complex dental trauma caused by the high kinetic injuries that would occur outside the homes, such as road traffic accidents and sports injuries.

3. Early management of dental trauma

Initial management when dental trauma occurs on the day of injury has a great influence on healing and the prognosis of the affected teeth. Correct diagnosis and a well-timed treatment will improve outcomes when managing dental trauma, especially in children and adolescents due to growth spurt consideration. Timeliness of treatment provided is a crucial indicator to salvaging the tooth provided an appropriate assessment is conducted and treatment is done according to recommended established guidelines [15–17].

3.1 Dental trauma emergencies

Avulsion, luxation, displaced root fractures, and alveolar fractures require immediate dental treatment. Avulsion of permanent teeth requires timely management, particularly in the first 15 minutes after the traumatic injury [16]. Immediate tooth replantation is strongly advised, however, if this is not possible, the avulsed tooth should be placed in a medium able to preserve the periodontal ligament.

Complicated crown-root fractures (fractures with pulp exposure) should be treated within 24 hours [15]. If tooth fragments are available, they can be reattached once conservative pulp therapy has been completed. However, it is recommended to immerse it in distilled water or saline for 30 minutes before reattachment for rehydration. This process will increase its bonding strength particularly if the fragment is kept dry for long period.

Uncomplicated crown fractures, subluxation, and tooth concussions are not classified as dental emergencies. However, all exposed dentine should be covered promptly within 24 hours, as the patient will experience discomfort due to the sensitivity of exposed dentine. It is crucial to prevent bacterial penetration into the dentinal tubules, thus affecting its long-term prognosis.

Soft tissue injuries also need priority care, and appropriate referral should be made according to the severity of the soft tissue injuries especially in deep through and through lesions and when it involves anatomical aesthetic consideration.

3.2 Assessment checklist

A checklist is recommended to ensure that detailed information regarding the patient and injury is obtained, including [18]:

1. Patient's name, age, gender, address, and contact numbers (including body weight for young patients)

2. Central nervous system symptoms exhibited after the injury e.g., nausea, vomiting, amnesia, double vision, seizures

3. Patient's general health status

4. Details of the injury occurred e.g., when where, and how

5. Treatment the patient received elsewhere

6. History of previous dental injuries

7. Disturbances in the bite

8. Tooth reactions to thermal changes or sensitivity to sweet and sour

9. If the affected teeth are tender to the touch or pain elicited during eating

10. If the patient is experiencing associated pain in the adjacent teeth, jaw, or temporomandibular joint area

The injury must always be thoroughly assessed by both extraoral and intraoral clinical examination and radiographic investigation. The current American Association of Endodontists (AAE) guidelines recommend taking one occlusal and two periapical radiographs with different lateral angulations for all dental injuries, including crown fractures. If cone-beam computed tomography is available, it should be considered for more serious injuries, such as crown/root, root, and alveolar fractures, as well as all luxation injuries.

Additionally, sensitivity tests should be conducted on all teeth involved, including opposing teeth. Cold testing is recommended over electric pulp testing in young patients. Both testing methods should be considered, however, especially when there is no response to one of the two. The pulp might be nonresponsive for several weeks after a traumatic injury, so a pulp test should be done at every follow-up appointment until a normal response is obtained.

3.3 Clinical management

Dental trauma can be categorized into two groups: fractures and luxation injuries. Fractures are further divided by type: crown, crown-root, and root fractures. Any dental tissue injuries that lead to pulp exposure, is considered a complicated fracture. However, if the pulp is not exposed to the oral environment, it is an uncomplicated fracture.

Tetanus prophylaxis administration should be considered for contaminated wounds even though the patient may have had previous immunization history. Broad-spectrum antibiotics against gram-positive organisms such as penicillin, and cephalosporin, are the drugs of choice for soft tissue injuries with oral cavity communication.

4. Barriers to early management of dental trauma during COVID-19

Traumatic dental injury (TDI) can occur even via a low-kinetic trauma which can happen anywhere relating to falls, sports, and collisions with objects and people. Hence, it is the most common type of dental-related trauma to occur. TDI is also a condition that requires urgent attention, being more so since its management can be more daunting if the case involves young patients with primary dentition or mixed dentition stage [19]. This form of trauma despite not being life-threatening in most cases can cause significant distress to the patient as well as their parents as there are substantial physical, aesthetical, and psychological consequences. In the urgent setting, dental trauma care revolves around the tenet that it is intended to stop the pain, and restore oral function and esthetics whilst reducing dental anxiety [20]. In the long-term setting, the treatment should avoid infection propagation and smooth progression of growth to permanent dentition if the situation involves young children group.

The proper steps of management are essential to mitigate the undesired short- and long-term consequences [21]. Even in cases of properly reviewed young patients with a history of severe dental trauma during the deciduous or mixed dentition stage may present with consequences years later leading to issues with permanent dentition succession problems [22, 23]. Despite clear guidelines being spelled out for the management of TDI; COVID-19 concern takes precedence which indicates that the usual standard of care may not be the feasible option. In a situation, with the COVID-19 pandemic still being rampant amongst the population, many barricades impact the ideal provision or acquisition of care for dental trauma. These barriers are represented at many points including dental healthcare regulation policy, patients' concerns, dental service providers' concerns, dental amenities issues as well as other limitations.

Some studies have reported that patients are more than hesitant to obtain dental care due to fear of COVID-19 transmission [9, 24]. This concern is very much allayed by the fact that most dental treatment revolves around the implementation of aerosol-generating procedures (AGP). Hence the risk of transmission is increased [25, 26]. During dental AGP several thousand droplets are aerosolized where larger droplets gravitate quickly to surfaces whilst smaller droplets tend to evaporate allowing dry microscopic pathogens to remain air-borne and freely circulating via air convection [26]. The basic understanding of COVID-19 in terms of its novel and rapid transmission instills this dread even more amongst the public [4]. A study done in Nigeria by Ajayi and Arigbede [27] implies that patients choose to defer from seeking treatment for dental-related emergencies as it is their perception that such ailments are not life-threatening, hence it would simply resolve them on their own. Ahmad et al. [28] also communicated that patients' refusal for seeking urgent dental treatment includes dental fear, perception of need, sterilization concerns, lack of awareness, and discomfort at the long wait in the emergency or dental outpatient clinic. This is due to the notion that the emergency waiting area could be harboring active COVID-19 patients. Hence, this cavalier approach of wait and see by the patient towards dental trauma is not just limited to the population with limited access to health care provisions.

Additionally, many do believe in the notion that if there are no symptoms or if the symptoms resolve, no further treatment is necessary after the dental trauma. In some other situations, it is the patient's concern about the high treatment cost incurred upon seeking dental trauma treatment, especially since COVID-19 has diminished livelihood and devastated job opportunities. Another report suggests that the reluctance of patients even in developed nations to seek treatment for trauma or non-trauma-based dental condition is due to the loss of the employer-sponsored dental insurance coverage caused by the pandemic [29]. Even in the post-lockdown phase, the impact of COVID-19 has far-reaching consequences as there is an opinion considering younger patients are not able to comply with the period of preoperative and postoperative isolation that might be required in tandem with dental trauma management due to their commitments towards their employment, children at school or care for elderly family members [30]. Dental trauma care for elderly patients is also another concern as they are at greater risk of developing severe reactions and morbidities related to the COVID-19. This opinion is supported by a recently cited United Kingdom study have noted a reduction of TDI cases in patients aged range of 50 years of age [9].

The next loci impeding the management of dental trauma revolves around the dental service provider force as well as the amenities that are involved in the treatment. One concern is the limitation of available dental care providers as many dental staffs may have redeployed to the frontline for COVID-19 testing or triaging roles as well as being furloughed thus limiting access to dental care [29]. A web-based survey done in Brazil divulged that many dentists who attended emergency or dental trauma patients proceeded so without auxiliary dental staff support to minimize infection spread and due to manpower restrictions [31]. From another viewpoint, limiting the number of dental personnel during AGP is essential to minimize the propagation of

COVID-19 though this is likely to draw the procedure time even longer than the usual. In the private sector, dental practitioners are burdened by financial issues resulting from reduced working hours and limited dental procedures that could be performed. On the other hand, public health workers including dental practitioners have experienced stress and depression during the pandemic period caused by increased workload, constant changes in the infection control protocols, social distancing, self-isolation, and caring for deteriorating patients [32]. These conditions could impede their standard of care during the management of dental trauma as well. In addition, older dental practitioners and staffs are more cautious when dealing with dental trauma cases since they are in the more susceptible age group in terms of COVID-19 severe reaction [33]. Younger dental practitioners reported lower anxiety in the same manner whilst the older dental practitioners face greater family and job concerns as well as financial considerations [33].

Next, the adjoining dental amenities can also be a barrier in the treatment of dental trauma as will be expounded here. The use of an intraoral radiograph to assess dental trauma for conditions like an intrusion, lateral luxation or crown-root fracture is ideal during the initial treatment phase for such conditions. It is one of the most common forms of radiographic technique in dental imaging. However, the use of intraoral radiographs involves placement of the radiograph film inside the mouth leading to stimulation of salivary secretion and activation of gag reflex leading to etching and coughing [3, 29]. This is undoubtedly not suitable as the dispersion of droplets and bioaerosols will be increased. This situation is made worse by the fact that most dental procedures are the aerosol-generating type as the tools used as air-driven handpieces, ultrasonic scalers, piezotomes, cautery units as well air-water syringes [25]. Dental avulsion, intrusion, and luxation injuries routinely require the placement of splint using composite resin requires the use of air-drying syringe while removing the splints requires bur cutting and suctioning. Hence the issue of minimizing the use of such tools during the management of dental trauma would be a barrier to providing sound treatment.

Based on the UK Office for National Statistics, dental practitioners and auxiliary staff deal with their patients in proximity inferring the possibility of increased exposure to general disease and COVID-19 [34] due to splashback of saliva or bioaerosols. Efforts to minimize and reduce the salivary viral load are another concern that could hinder the treatment of dental trauma in patients with a high risk of COVID-19 especially the routine mouthwash such as chlorhexidine may not be effective against COVID-19 [35, 36]. Disinfection of tools and surfaces of the dental clinical surfaces for COVID-19 includes a waiting period to allow the aerosols generated in the previous session to dissipate. This means an increase in waiting time and further delays in the provision of treatment, especially in healthcare facilities with high trauma case flow [29]. Additionally, the use of fumigation is not considered a practical option in dental surgery as it will further increase the waiting time for starting the procedure [3]. Additionally, methods to minimize follow-up for dental trauma management are also a hindrance as a treatment for such condition usually requires frequent follow-up to ensure no morbidities ensues.

Next, the limitation in healthcare facilities and policies are identified as potential blockades in the provision of dental trauma emergency care during the COVID-19 pandemic. It is not unusual to observe that during budget deductions in hospital or emergency services; dental benefits or dental treatment budgets are among the first service to receive cuts [29]. This is likely to hamper further the effort in providing sound dental care for trauma cases. Additionally, most dental healthcare facilities can be under great strain to provide personal protective equipment (PPE) for their staff and to stay ahead of the curve in the evolving infection control policies regarding COVID-19 [9]. The next challenge includes the availability of a negative pressure room for dental trauma procedures which will be very ideal; however, most if not all dental facilities still lack such options as most dental operatories are clustered in open spaces without physical barriers. Other limitation includes the availability of teledentistry in most dental healthcare centers as well as emergency centers. Teledentistry is a viable tool for triaging and follow-up assessment by dental practitioners without direct contact with patients [37]. Some challenges may still ensue in the implementation of teledentistry in all dental healthcare facilities as there is the need for dental personnel to acclimatize to this new technology, whilst managing, sharing, and disseminating personal-medical information on their patients.

Overall, the hindrance or limitations mentioned above must be addressed expediently to minimize the delay of comprehensive dental trauma treatment secondary to COVID-19 limitations as it will inevitably create a backlog of cases. Health issues in the oral cavity will most likely occur in such cases especially if regular follow-ups and care are not available. In addition, the consequence of substandard dental trauma treatment will flare up, especially in cases involving children with deciduous or mixed dentition as it could affect permanent dentition and thus increase the need for further dental care in the future. Finally, the current implementation of biosafety in clinical dental practices may compromise the cost of dental consultation and reduce the consultation time.

5. Guidelines in the management of dental trauma during COVID-19

5.1 Available guidelines and proposed algorithm in the management of traumatic dental injuries

In the era of the early COVID 19 pandemic, most dental practices were forcibly closed and it was uncertain whether dental services in the hospitals would be able to cope with patients suffering from dental trauma. However, research also has revealed that patients are hesitant to go to a hospital out of worry for the potential risk of contracting COVID-19 [9]. Therefore, it is important to weigh the benefit of managing traumatic dental injuries to the primary dentition and minimizing the risk of transmission of COVID-19 to patients and staff. In published interim guidance for the provision of essential oral health services during the COVID-19 pandemic, it was advised that routine non-essential oral health care to be delayed until there has been sufficient evidence of control in COVID-19 transmission rates at the national, sub-national, or local level [38–42]. This is mainly due to the prolonged duration and the proximity of dental healthcare workers to the patient's facial region. The dental procedures involve close contact and exposure to saliva, blood, and handling sharp instruments; stratifying the dental healthcare workers as high risk of being infected with COVID-19 or passing the infection to patients.

Multiple guidelines were written in conjunction with this cause on resuming general dental services and principles for acute care during the pandemic such as the new 2020 IADT trauma guidelines [20, 38–42]. The focus of the updated guideline was mainly on general information in certain sections, and a table of complications with the recommendation of longer follow-up (yearly till 5 years and beyond). In intrusive injuries, for example, the current recommendation is only to observe and review as opposed to extraction of the primary teeth. More emphasis is placed on conservative treatment rather than pulpotomy or extraction in injuries such as crown fractures and luxation [20].

While the new IADT guideline advocates conservative treatment options following traumatic injuries to the primary dentition during the COVID-19 pandemic, the British Society of Paediatric Dentistry (BSPD) and Dental Trauma UK suggest treatment options should focus on either observation or extraction [43]. This approach minimizes the number of face-to-face contacts and reduces aerosol-generating procedures. The BSPD has published consensus guidelines on the management of dental trauma concerning the COVID-19 pandemic, including acute management of traumatic injuries and follow-up care. Remote consults are recommended during follow-up to assess oral hygiene, healing, and complications. If deemed necessary, the patient is seen in the clinic for detailed assessment and treatment. All follow-ups could be made through remote consults for root fractures 1 week, 4 weeks, and 1-year intervals after the injury. For enamel-dentine fractures, the follow-up could also be remote, and the recommended time is 8 weeks.

In supporting tissue injuries, for example in lateral luxation and intrusion, which have higher risks of sequels and require more frequent follow-ups, the guideline recommends that remote consult be performed. Remote consult for review at 1-week for all supporting tissue trauma and, depending on the type of trauma, at 8 weeks, 6 months, and 1 year of follow-up are required. Post-injury advice should include care not to further traumatize the injured teeth while eating and encouraging the patients to return to normal function as soon as possible; oral hygiene instructions that include cleaning the affected area with a soft brush or cotton swab combined with an alcohol-free chlorhexidine gluconate mouth rinse.

In the meantime, the Scottish Dental Clinical Effectiveness Programme published a guide on the management of acute dental problems during the COVID-19 pandemic [44]. In the cases of dental injuries that don't require urgent medical attention, patients are advised to clean the affected area with mild antiseptic and to apply ice packs and pressure on the injured soft tissue to stop bleeding. Urgent care is recommended for avulsed, luxated, or fractured teeth. In the case of the avulsed primary tooth, they should not be re-implanted, instead, it is recommended for self-help and consultation that include appropriate analgesia followed by advice on a soft diet.

In tandem with guidelines by the BSPD and Dental Trauma UK as well as the Scottish Dental Clinical Effectiveness Programme, the King's College Hospital has published new standard operating procedures specifically for the COVID-19 pandemic, published by Ilyas et al. [45] in June 2020. This guideline is also recommended on telephone advice only or a dental visit to perform extraction as management of primary tooth trauma during the pandemic. Telephone advise only is given for all cases of dental trauma that does not interfere with occlusion/airway risk. Only enamel-dentine fractures and pathological mobility, causing occlusal interference/airway risk are recommended to be seen urgently for treatment.

The Royal College of Surgeons of England also published the recommendations for pediatric dentistry during the COVID-19 pandemic of COVID-19 [46]. These guidelines recommended that no routine dentistry should be provided for children during this pandemic and treatment should be deferred to minimize the risk of transmission of the disease to patients, staff, and the public. They also recommended that urgent management is only indicated in pulp exposure or severe luxation that carries a potential airway risk or is severely interfering with occlusion for primary teeth. To reduce the need for AGP, extraction may be the preferred treatment option for children with pulpal symptoms.

The aim of trauma management should be to minimize the number of visits required and the number of AGPs provided. Outcomes should be optimized by giving evidence-based initial management with a low risk of complications requiring further intervention.

In Malaysia, a guideline or standard operating procedures were published urgently in view of the pandemic in early 2020. During the early phase of COVID-19, all dental clinics in Malaysia were to suspend their services except for emergency dental treatment including dental trauma. Therefore, all dental trauma cases were channeled to hospitals for urgent management. Following that, more revised protocols focusing on PPE and patient screening were published to allow the opening of dental services again with restrictions. The ministry of health published the guideline on "Management of COVID-19 screening in dental clinics" and circulated

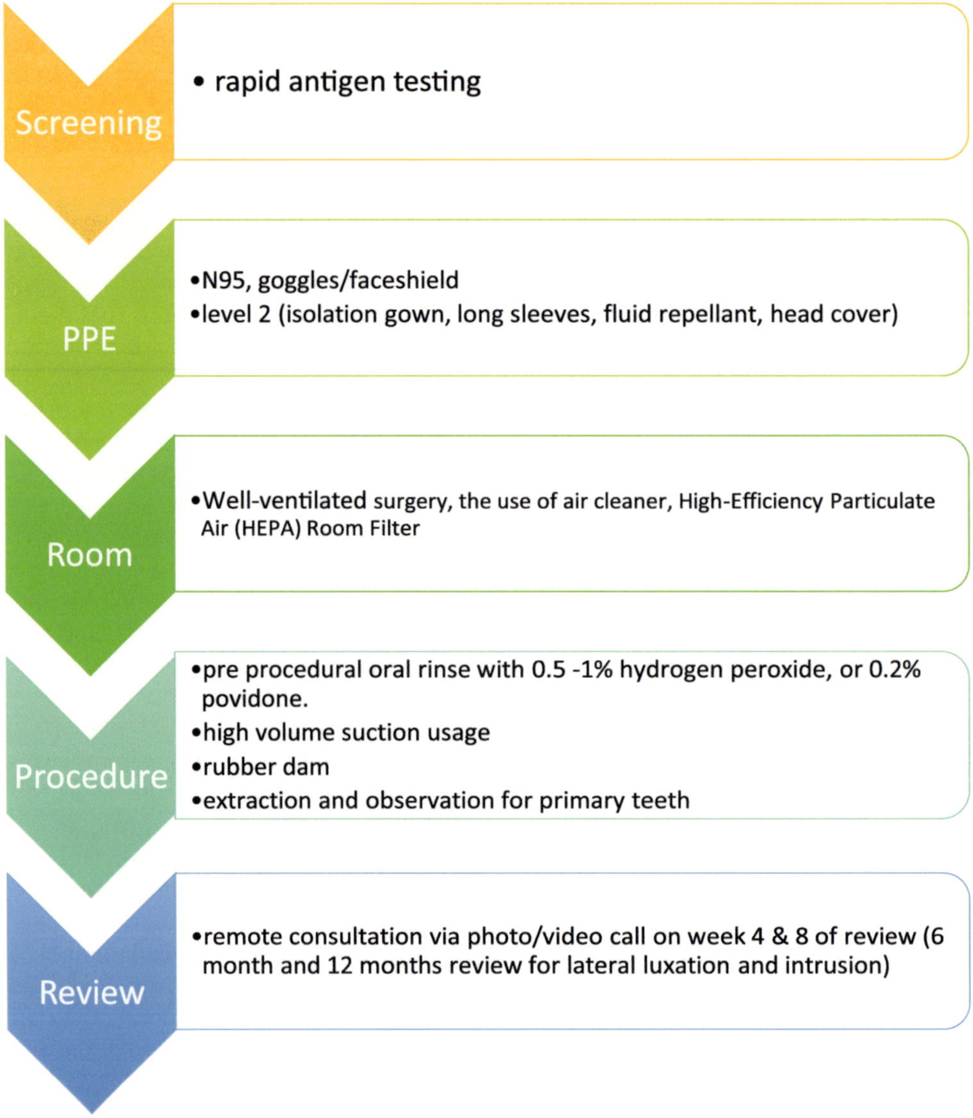

Figure 1.
Proposed algorithm for management of TDI during COVID-19.

it in January 2020 concerning the Interim Guidelines Novel Coronavirus (nCov) in Malaysia. This document mainly addressed the concerns on the identification and handling of positive COVID-19 patients or Person Under Investigation (PUI) at the point of screening/triage prior to dental treatment. Several amendments had been made to the protocols to ensure it is updated and kept abreast with other international guidelines given their rapid change of management.

In summary, there are some similarities observed in published guidelines during the pandemic. Regarding treatment options for example, although some guidelines recommended conservative treatments (i.e., pulpotomy, composite build-ups, root canal treatment, and repositioning and splinting) during the COVID-19 pandemic, BSPD Dental Trauma UK, The Royal College of Surgeons of England as well as King's College Hospital protocol, however, suggest treatment options should focus on either observation or extraction. These guidelines recommended that a more definitive treatment, such as tooth extraction, may avoid recurring visits to the dental office and thus reducing the risk of exposure to COVID-19. Following an acute injury, most of the guidelines are encouraged remote consultation (e.g., telephone, photographs, or video conferencing) that can help clinical teams to clarify a provisional diagnosis and treatment. An effective remote consultation may also reduce the face-to-face time in the clinic, thereby maximizing the potential use of the clinic and minimizing PPE usage. Only selected cases may require an initial face-to-face consultation to ensure an accurate diagnosis where remote consultation is not possible, or diagnosis is uncertain. Follow-up appointments are necessary to assess healing, oral hygiene, and complications in the intervals of 1 week up to 5 years of the review were recommended with the intervals of remote and face-to-face consultation. Beginning a road to recovery will require "new normal" management. As part of the recovery, clinicians are recommended to completely re-evaluate how services are prioritized and delivered. Relieving children of pain must take priority over routine dental care services [47]. These guidelines are likely to evolve as dental services return to normal, at which point this guide will be withdrawn in preference for the new 2020 IADT trauma guidelines.

Below is the summary of the proposed management algorithm for dental trauma during the pandemic following various guidelines worldwide (**Figure 1**).

6. Conclusions

Traumatic dental injuries are among the dental emergencies that must be addressed as early as possible to ensure the survival of the tooth with good treatment outcomes and a better prognosis. In a long run, this reduces the number of visits, number of treatments, and cost as well as the time of treatment needed in the future. During the COVID-19 pandemic, the etiology of the injury has also shifted to accidental falls, and interpersonal and domestic violence since most countries implemented the movement restriction orders, school closure, and travel restrictions—all accounting for to stay home policy. The incidence of TDI across many countries has shown a change in age predilection and the characteristics of dental injury.

Special management protocols for immediate dental trauma management have been forwarded by many guidelines and various modified measures have been suggested to reduce and regulate droplet and aerosol contamination in the emergency dental setting has been discussed. This includes the screening of the patients before procedures, reduction or avoidance of droplet/aerosol generation in emergency dental situations, the disinfection of the treatment field, application of a rubber dam, and pre-procedural antiseptic mouth rinse, and the dilution and efficient removal of contaminated air utilizing the air filter. Some cases are even consulted via teledentistry to reduce the face-to-face contact between the dental healthcare worker and patients during pandemics.

With the available guidelines for treating dental diseases during the COVID-19 pandemic time, some dental practices can safely return and restart operations, other practices may choose to remain closed or limit services to only those critical or emergency procedures that cannot be delayed due to expected risks and existing safeguards.

Acknowledgements

This work was supported by International Islamic University Malaysia.

Conflict of interest

All named authors have no conflict of interest, financial or otherwise.

Notes/thanks/other declarations

We declare no conflicts of interest in any of the related issues.

Author details

Khairul Bariah Chi Adam*, Haszelini Hassan, Pram Kumar Subramaniam, Izzati Nabilah Ismail, Nor Adilah Harun and Naziyah Shaban Mustafa
Department of Oral Maxillofacial Surgery and Oral Diagnosis, Kulliyyah of Dentistry, International Islamic University Malaysia, Kuantan, Malaysia

*Address all correspondence to: bariah@iium.edu.my

IntechOpen

© 2022 The Author(s). Licensee IntechOpen. This chapter is distributed under the terms of the Creative Commons Attribution License (http://creativecommons.org/licenses/by/3.0), which permits unrestricted use, distribution, and reproduction in any medium, provided the original work is properly cited. (cc) BY

References

[1] Petti S, Glendor U, Andersson L. World traumatic dental injury prevalence and incidence, meta-analysis-one billion living people have had traumatic dental injuries. Dental Traumatology. 2018;**34**(2):71-86. DOI: 10.1111/edt.12389

[2] Andersson L. Epidemiology of traumatic dental injuries. Journal of Endodontics. 2013;**39**(3):S2-S5

[3] Bhanushali P, Katge F, Deshpande S, Chimata VK, Shetty S, Pradhan D. COVID-19: changing trends and its impact on future of dentistry. International Journal of Dentistry. 2020;**2020**:1-6

[4] Guo H, Zhou Y, Liu X, Tan J. The impact of the COVID-19 epidemic on the utilization of emergency dental services. Journal of Dental Sciences. 2020;**15**(4):564-567

[5] Andreasen JO, Andreasen FM, Andersson L. Textbook and Color Atlas of Traumatic Injuries to the Teeth. Hoboken, New Jersey: Wiley-Blackwell 2007; 2007

[6] Glendor U, Andersson L. Public Health Aspects of Oral Diseases and Disorders: Dental Trauma. London; Chicago: Quintessence Pub ©2007; 2007

[7] Renapurkar SK, Abubaker O. Diagnosis and management of dentoalveolar injuries. In: Fonseca RJ, editor. Oral and Maxillofacial Surgery. 3rd ed. St Louis, MO: Elsevier; 2018

[8] Yang Y, Zhang W, Xie L, Li Z, Li Z. Characteristic changes of traumatic dental injuries in a teaching hospital of Wuhan under transmission control measures during the COVID-19 epidemic. Dental Traumatology. 2020;**36**(6):584-589. DOI: 10.1111/edt.12589

[9] Woolley J, Djemal S. Traumatic dental injuries during the COVID-19 pandemic. Primary Dental Journal. 2021;**10**(1):28-32. DOI: 10.1177/2050168420980994

[10] Luzzi V, Ierardo G, Bossù M, Polimeni A. Paediatric oral health during and after the COVID-19 pandemic. International Journal of Paediatric Dentistry. 2021;**31**(1):20-26. DOI: 10.1111/ipd.12737

[11] Surendra G, Perera I, Ranasinghe A, Kumarapeli V, Tham R, Wickramaratne P. Pattern and causes of oral and maxillofacial injuries presented to a tertiary care public dental hospital in strictly imposed COVID-19 lockdown scenario. Oral. 2020;**1**(1):3-14

[12] Puglia FA, Hills A, Dawoud B, Magennis P, Chiu GA, Adams A, et al. Management of oral and maxillofacial trauma during the first wave of the COVID-19 pandemic in the United Kingdom. British Journal of Oral and Maxillofacial Surgery. 2021;**59**(8):867-874

[13] Home Affairs Committee. Home Office Preparedness for Covid-19 (Coronavirus): Domestic Abuse and Risks of Harm Within the Home. Available from: https://publications.parliament.uk/pa/cm5801/cmselect/cmhaff/321/32105.htm#footnote-112 [Last accessed: 13 April 2021]

[14] Levin L, Day PF, Hicks L, O'Connell A, Fouad AF, Bourguignon C, et al. International Association of Dental Traumatology guidelines for the management of traumatic dental injuries: general introduction. Dental

Traumatology. 2020;**36**(4):309-313. DOI: 10.1111/edt.12574

[15] DiAngelis AJ, Andreasen JO, Ebeleseder KA, Kenny DJ, Trope M, Sigurdsson A, et al. International Association of Dental Traumatology guidelines for the management of traumatic dental injuries: 1. Fractures and luxations of permanent teeth. Dental Traumatology. 2012;**28**(1):2-12. DOI: 10.1111/j.1600-9657.2011.01103.x

[16] Andersson L, Andreasen JO, Day P, Heithersay G, Trope M, DiAngelis AJ, et al. International Association of Dental Traumatology guidelines for the management of traumatic dental injuries: 2. Avulsion of permanent teeth. Dental Traumatology. 2012;**28**(2):88-96. DOI: 10.1111/j.1600-9657.2012.01125.x

[17] Malmgren B, Andreasen JO, Flores MT, Robertson A, DiAngelis AJ, Andersson L, et al. International Association of Dental Traumatology guidelines for the management of traumatic dental injuries: 3. Injuries in the primary dentition. Dental Traumatology. 2012;**28**(3): 174-182. DOI: 10.1111/j.1600-9657.2012. 01146.x

[18] Sigurdsson A. Treating dental trauma. The Journal of Multidisciplinary Care: The Decision in Dentistry. September 2019;**5**(8):32-34, 37. [Internet]. 2017. Available from: https:// decisionsindentistry.com/

[19] Needleman HL. The art and science of managing traumatic injuries to primary teeth. Dental Traumatology. 2011;**27**(4):295-299. DOI: 10.1111/j. 1600-9657.2011.01005.x

[20] Day PF, Flores MT, O'Connell AC, Abbott PV, Tsilingaridis G, Fouad AF, et al. International Association of Dental Traumatology guidelines for the management of traumatic dental injuries: 3. Injuries in the primary dentition. Dental Traumatology. 2020;**36**(4):343-359. DOI: 10.1111/edt.12576

[21] Goswami M, Rahman B, Singh S. Outcomes of luxation injuries to primary teeth-a systematic review. Journal of Oral Biology and Craniofacial Research. 2020;**10**(2):227-232

[22] Qassem A, da Martins NM, VPP d C, Torriani DD, Pappen FG. Long-term clinical and radiographic follow-up of subluxated and intruded maxillary primary anterior teeth. Dental Traumatology. 2015;**31**(1):57-61. DOI: 10.1111/edt.12135

[23] Ranka M, Dhaliwal H, Albadri S, Brown C. Trauma to the primary dentition and its sequelae. Dental Update. 2013;**40**(7):534-542. DOI: 10.12968/denu.2013.40.7.534

[24] Vanka S, Jan AS, Alhazmi STF, Alsubhi BM, Allehyani RS, Wali O, et al. Barriers of dental services utilization during COVID-19 pandemic. International Journal of Medical Dentistry. 2020;**24**:523-530

[25] Harrel SK, Molinari J. Aerosols and splatter in dentistry. The Journal of the American Dental Association. 2004;**135**(4):429-437

[26] James R, Mani AK. Dental aerosols: A silent hazard in dentistry. International Journal of Science and Research. 2016;**5**(11):1761-1763

[27] Ajayi D, Arigbede A. Barriers to oral health care utilization in Ibadan, southwest Nigeria. African Health Sciences. 2013;**12**(4)

[28] Ahmad W, Farhat Bukhari S, Aslam M, Irfan F, Fatima R, Ali M. Barriers in access and utilization of dental care: assessment and

recommendations using Delphi technique. Journal of the Pakistan Dental Association. 2019;**28**(01):13-17. Available from: http://www.jpda.com.pk/barriers-in-access-and-utilization-of-dental-care-assessment-and-recommendations-using-delphi-technique/

[29] Kalenderian E, Xiao Y, Spallek H, Franklin A, Olsen G, Walji MF. COVID-19 and dentistry: challenges and opportunities for providing safe care. Patient Safety Network. 2022. Available from: https://psnet.ahrq.gov/primer/covid-19-and-dentistry-challenges-and-opportunities-providing-safe-care

[30] Mackay ND, Wilding CP, Langley CR, Young J. The impact of COVID-19 on trauma and orthopedic patients requiring surgery during the peak of the pandemic. Bone & Joint Open. 2020;**1**(9):520-529. DOI: 10.1302/2633-1462.19.BJO-2020-0108.R1

[31] Faccini M, Ferruzzi F, Mori AA, Santin GC, Oliveira RC, RCG d O, et al. Dental care during COVID-19 outbreak: a web-based survey. European Journal of Dentistry. 2020;**14**(S 01):S14-S19. DOI: 10.1055/s-0040-1715990

[32] Fauziah YA, Rulianto M, Binarsa DB. Challenges of dentistry in coronavirus pandemic. Malaysian Journal of Medicine and Health Sciences. 2021:162-164

[33] Jungmann SM, Witthöft M. Health anxiety, cyberchondria, and coping in the current COVID-19 pandemic: which factors are related to coronavirus anxiety? Journal of Anxiety Disorders. 2020;**73**:102239

[34] Office for National Statistics. Which Occupations have the Highest Potential Exposure to the Coronavirus (COVID-19)?. Available from: https://www.ons.gov.uk/employmentandlabourmarket/peopleinwork/employmentandemployeetypes/articles/whichoccupationshavethehighestpotentialexposuretothecoronaviruscovid19/2020-05-11

[35] Kawana R, Kitamura T, Nakagomi O, Matsumoto I, Arita M, Yoshihara N, et al. Inactivation of human viruses by povidone-iodine in comparison with other antiseptics. Dermatology. 1997;**195**(2):29-35

[36] Farzan A, Firoozi P. WhichMouthwashe is Appropriate for Eliminating Coronaviruses? A mini literature review. Journal of "Regeneration, Reconstruction & Restoration." 2020;**5**(e2)

[37] Talla PK, Levin L, Glogauer M, Cable C, Allison PJ. Delivering dental care as we emerge from the initial phase of the COVID-19 pandemic: teledentistry and face-to-face consultations in a new clinical world. Quintessence International. 2020;**51**(8):672-677

[38] Blackhall KK, Downie IP, Ramchandani P, Kusanale A, Walsh S, Srinivasan B, et al. Provision of emergency maxillofacial service during the COVID-19 pandemic: a Collaborative Five Centre UK Study. British Journal of Oral and Maxillofacial Surgery. 2020;**58**(6):698-703

[39] Ayub K, Alani A. Acute endodontic and dental trauma provision during the COVID-19 crisis. British Dental Journal. 2020;**229**(3):169-175

[40] Jamal M, Shah M, Almarzooqi SH, Aber H, Khawaja S, el Abed R, et al. Overview of transnational recommendations for COVID-19 transmission control in dental care settings. Oral Diseases. 2021;**27**(S3): 655-664. DOI: 10.1111/odi.13431

[41] American Dental Association Official Website. What Constitutes a

Dental Emergency?. 2020. Available from: https://success.ada.org/~%7B%7D/media/CPS/Files/Open Files/ADA_COVID19_Dental_ Emergency_DDS.pdf

[42] American Dental Association ADA. Interim Guidance for Management of Emergency and Urgent Dental Care. Updated 4 January 2020. 2020. Available from: https://www.ada.org/~%7B%7D/media/CPS/Files/COVID/ADA_Int_Guidance_Mgmt_Emerg-Urg_Dental_COVID19?utm_source=adaorg&utm_medium=VanityURL& utm_content=interimguidance-flowcharts&utm_campaign=covid-19

[43] Day P, Djemal S, Albadri S. BSPD. Permanent dentition acute management of traumatic injuries and follow-up care during the COVID-19 pandemic. Available from: http://www.bspd.co.uk/Portals/0/Guidelines/Permanent%20Dentition%20Trauma%20Guideline%20COVID-19_NEW%20150620.pdf [Accessed 20 November 2020]

[44] SDCEP. Management of Acute Dental Problems during COVID-19 Pandemic. 2020. Available from: https://www.sdcep.org.uk/wp-content/uploads/2020/03/SDCEP-MADP-COVID-19-guide-300320.pdf

[45] Ilyas N, Agel M, Mitchell J, Sood S. COVID-19 pandemic: the first wave - an audit and guidance for pediatric dentistry. British Dental Journal. 2020;**228**(12):927-931

[46] Royal College of Surgeons Recommendations for Paediatric Dentistry during the Recovery Phase of the COVID-19 Pandemic. 2021. Available from: https://www.rcseng.ac.uk/dental-faculties/fds/coronavirus

[47] Malini SK, Innes NP, Raggio DP, Araujo MP, Robertson MD, Jayaraman J. Coronavirus disease (COVID-19): characteristics in children and considerations for dentists providing their care. International Journal of Paediatric Dentistry. 2020;**30**(3):245-250. DOI: 10.1111/ipd.12653

Chapter 3

Perspective Chapter: Update and Making-Decisions in Dental Traumatology

Blanca del Carmen Migueláñez Medrán, Nuria Delgado Castro, Elena Riad Deglow and Álvaro Zubizarreta Macho

Abstract

Dental traumatology is highlighted as an unexpected emergency event which can occur at any moment, age, sex, and gender. Crown fractures account for most traumatic injuries occurring in the permanent dentition. A complete radiographic examination is considered essential in order to assess the state of the pulp, the degree of root development, and the existence of any pathologies affecting the supporting tissues. These examinations also provide a useful tool for subsequent comparisons with those conducted after treatment, ensuring adequate clinical follow-up. Additionally, avulsion of permanent teeth has been highlighted as one of the most relevant dental injuries; therefore, the prognosis of this traumatic event has been directly related to the treatment decision-making process and the time passed since the accident. In addition, dental trauma is also one of the most frequent emergency situations seen in Pediatric Dentistry; moreover, the dental injury of the temporary teeth could also affect to the permanent teeth; hence, it is necessary to perform an exhaustive clinical and radio diagnostic exam to allow a correct diagnosis and a predictable treatment plan. Therefore, the creation of action protocols makes it possible to simplify and facilitate decision-making under stressful situations for patients and clinicians.

Keywords: dental fracture, dental traumatology, permanent dentition, primary dentition, tooth avulsion

1. Introduction

Avulsion of permanent teeth has been highlighted as one of the most relevant dental injuries; it has been reported to make up between 0.5 and 16% of all dental injuries [1, 2]. Additionally, the prognosis of this dental injury is directly related to the treatment decision-making process and the time passed since the accident [3–6]; it is therefore essential to inform society and keep professionals updated so that the decision-making chain is as optimal as possible and leads to a predictable prognosis [7, 8]. Currently, dental replantation is the treatment of choice; however, certain scenarios prevent it from being carried out immediately, including extensive caries, periodontal disease, uncooperative patients, immunosuppression, or heart disease, which require individualized treatment procedure. Additionally, the final decision must be made with the consent of the parents. Therefore, the creation of action protocols makes it possible to simplify and facilitate decision-making under stressful situations for patients and clinicians. For this reason, guides developed by scientific societies are published in the most popular media, so that they might reach the majority of society and clinicians. 2. Treatment guidelines and decision-making for dental fractures.

1.1 Crown fractures

Crown fractures account for most traumatic injuries occurring in the permanent dentition. The most common etiology of this type of injury is accidental falls, contact sports, traffic accidents, or accidents at work.

A complete radiographic examination is considered essential in order to assess the state of the pulp, the degree of root development and the existence of any pathologies affecting the supporting tissues. These examinations also provide a useful tool for subsequent comparisons with those conducted after treatment, ensuring adequate clinical follow-up [9].

1.1.1 Enamel fissures (enamel infraction)

These types of fractures are located on the vestibular surface of the anterior teeth and may go unnoticed because there is no loss of tooth structure. Clinically, they appear as fissures that do not cross the amelo-dentinal junction [10, 11], and they are usually revealed when light is targeted perpendicular to the major axis of the tooth (transillumination).

Vitality tests are usually positive3, although they may be temporarily negative after any impact [9].

The presence of crack lines in the enamel should alert the clinician to the possibility of injury to the surrounding supporting structures (e.g. luxation). In such cases, there may visible changes in dental color.

Fissures limited to enamel generally do not require treatment. In selected cases, to avoid potential staining by external agents, the enamel surface can be sealed [9, 11].

The long-term prognosis of this type of lesion is very good, with tooth survival approaching rates of 100%.

1.1.2 Fracture without pulp exposure (uncomplicated crown fracture)

Fortunately, this type of fracture occurs more frequently than those with pulp involvement.

On initial examination, thermal tests may be negative for a certain period of time (primarily if the lesion coexists with a luxation), but with this type of fracture there is usually sensitivity to thermal changes due to dentine exposure (more prevalent in younger teeth due to the larger diameter of the dentin tubules and the proximity of the fracture to the pulp), pressure changes, and dehydration [9, 11].

Just like with enamel fissures, the surrounding tissues should be routinely examined to exclude other pathologies that might affect the supporting tissues.

The primary goal of treatment is to achieve adequate esthetics and function. Nowadays, with composite resins [12] and the use of adequate bezels to mask the fracture line, it is possible to attain very satisfactory results [13].

Another therapeutic option involves the fixation of the detached crown segment with a total acid etching technique and the application of composite resins at the fracture line. This type of fixation is more predictable the larger the fragment is, and if it is a single fragment (smaller and multiple fragments have a worse prognosis) [9]. Before being bonded to the remaining tooth structure, the fragment must be rehydrated [11].

According to different authors, failures in this type of restorations can be attributed to:

1. Failure of the bonding system.

2. Cohesive fractures of the composite resin.

3. Color instability.

4. Recurrent caries.

5. Horizontal tensile forces exerted either on the restoration or on the bonded fragment [9].

1.1.3 Crown fracture with pulp exposure (complicated crown fracture)

In this case, visible loss of tooth structure is evident, and a slight hemorrhage can be observed at the site of pulp exposure. In cases in which there is a delay in treatment, and particularly in young teeth, a pulp polyp may be observed.

Due to this pulp exposure, the teeth are often sensitive to thermal and pressure changes.

Radiographs are very useful for diagnosis, mainly to assess the extent of the lesion and to determine the degree of root development, in order to choose the most appropriate treatment option for each individual case.

The primary objective of treatment is the preservation of pulp vitality without inflammation, to achieve the formation of a hard tissue barrier [9, 13].

The prognosis of treatment will depend on:

1. State (maturity or immaturity) of the apex: This is perhaps the most important factor. Pulp conservation is desirable in teeth with immature apexes, whereas in teeth with closed apexes, pulp tissue can be removed.

2. Time elapsed between the lesion and treatment.

3. Extent of pulp exposure: The smaller the size of the exposure, the greater the likelihood of dentin bridging.

4. Existence of other surrounding hard tissue injuries, e.g. luxation, as it compromises the neurovascular supply to the pulp, compromising pulp vitality.

5. Existence of prior trauma: Healing capacity is considerably decreased in teeth that have already suffered a previous trauma [9].

Treatment of teeth with an open/immature apex should be as conservative as possible, trying to maintain pulp vitality. The therapeutic options that can be considered are as follows:

- *Direct pulp capping*: This is used in small pulp exposures in which treatment can be carried out in less than 24 h and the bleeding stops when pressure is applied with cotton wool.

  Pulp capping, which may consist of applying glass ionomer cement (GIC) or mineral trioxide aggregate (MTA) before placing the restoration to prevent bacterial invasion [14].

- *Partial pulpotomy* (*Cvek pulpotomy*): The treatment of choice if the trauma occurred more than 24 h before. It consists of removal of the damaged tissue until clinically healthy pulp is available [15].

  Depending on the size of the pulp exposure, it may be performed partially or coronally. This treatment be used in both mature and immature teeth.

  After removal of the affected pulp and controlling the bleeding, Calcium Hydroxide (CaH) or MTA is placed. Zinc oxide eugenol or another cement can be placed on top. After 3 months, if appropriate sensitivity has been preserved and a dentin barrier can be observed via radiographic examination, definitive reconstruction can be carried out.

- *Coronal pulpotomy*: Consists of removing the entire coronal pulp while keeping the root pulp intact. For this procedure, the root pulp must be healthy [16]. It is performed in immature permanent teeth if the inflammation is larger than 2 mm in order to achieve complete root development1, or currently even on teeth with a closed apex. An optimal treatment result would include the formation of a dentine bridge under the CaH or MTA veneer used [17].

- *Deep pulpotomy*: In this case, coronal pulp and the coronal third of the root portion are removed.

  As in the previous cases, bleeding must be controllable (hemostatic agents can be used). The material of choice is CaH [9], although calcium silicate–based cement is also used [18].

  Despite advances in both technique and materials used, it is particularly difficult to assess the state of the pulp in root canals, so the prognosis of this therapeutic option remains controversial.

- *Non-vital teeth*: Teeth with complete root formation can be treated with standard endodontic procedures, producing a predictable outcome.

  Teeth without complete root formation have a poorer prognosis, as cessation of the neurovascular supply leads to incomplete apex closure, thinner root walls, and, in some cases, even an unfavorable crown-root ratio [19].

  The apexification procedure allows for complete root development by forming an apical hard tissue barrier [20].

  This was traditionally carried out using CaH, which induced apex closure until complete apical closure was achieved, enabling conventional endodontic treatment. Nowadays, MTA is used to achieve apical closure in a single step [19], and even platelet-rich plasma is used in combination with MTA [21].

If CaH is used, endodontic reopening of the tooth is performed when the clinician observes the desired apical closure radiographically, and the existence of the apical barrier is checked with a file.

If MTA is used, after proper opening and cleaning of the canal, the MTA is loaded into a dental plate holder and placed at the apex with the aid of a thick paper tip 1–2 mm shorter than the estimated working length and a thick stripper until a 4–5 mm thick plug is formed. When the plug is deemed to be adequate, a radiographic check of the plug is necessary, and once the MTA has set, the root canal can be filled [9].

1.2 Intra-alveolar root fractures

These represent a much lower percentage than coronal fractures. Furthermore, they are much less common in the primary dentition and in teeth with immature apexes (these tend to dislocate rather than fracture). These types of fractures can be located horizontally or vertically with respect to the major axis of the tooth and involve enamel, dentine, and cementum [9, 13]. Vertical fractures usually have a worse prognosis, the tooth is not usually restorable, and often the only option is to extract the tooth.

Horizontal fractures, depending on their location, can affect the coronal, middle, or apical third.

Clinically, the affected teeth will appear as if they were extruded. As the trauma usually comes from the vestibular side, we will often also find the tooth is slightly lingually inclined, in addition to exhibiting mobility, bleeding from the gingival sulcus, and positive percussion. In terms of vitality, both fragments may be necrotic, or the coronal fragment may be endodontically treated and the apical fragment may still be vital.

The diagnosis of an intra-alveolar fracture is sometimes complicated by the small separation of fragments at the time of impact. This separation usually increases over the following days, which often makes diagnosis easier as the fracture line can be seen on the radiographic scan if the beam is directed at approximately the same angle as the fracture line. This is usually easier when the fracture is more horizontal rather than oblique. Therefore, in a patient with a possible intra-alveolar fracture, several radiographs should be taken, changing the degree of angulation [9]. If the radiographic projections do not give us the information we need, it is advisable to perform a CBCT (Cone Beam Computed Tomography) to determine the location, extension, and trajectory of the fracture [12].

The different types of scarring between fragments were first classified by Andreasen and Hjorting-Hansen [22] into four different categories (**Table 1**).

Calcifying fusion of fragments	There is radiographic evidence of fracture but no radiolucent lesion between the two fragments
Band of connective tissue between fragments	There is a narrow radiolucent image between the fragments
Bone formation between fragments	Bone deposition can be observed in the diastasis area
Granulation tissue between fragments	The space between the two fragments is wider and radiolucent

Table 1.
Types of scarring observed in fragments [22].

Internal resorption	This is not a frequent finding in intra-alveolar fractures. It is a pulp reaction to a chronic inflammatory process in the form of lacunae or spaces that appear within the root canal 14
External resorption	Occurs in the form of resorption in those areas close to the fracture, beginning on the external or lateral surface of the tooth root 15
Pulp survival with canal obliteration	Calcification of the canal lumen, although the vitality of the tooth is sometimes preserved
Loss of the osseous crest	More frequent when the fracture affects the coronal third and extends into the gingival sulcus. Very poor prognosis

Table 2.
Sequelae of intra-alveolar fractures [9].

In addition, intra-alveolar fractures present four types of sequelae, which are summarized in **Table 2**.

The treatment and prognosis of the tooth will depend largely on the location of the root fracture: whenever possible, it is advisable to reduce the fracture by repositioning the coronal fragment in an appropriate position. If it is very mobile, it should be splinted passively and flexibly (semi-rigid) [23].

If the fracture affects both the crown and the root but there is no pulp exposure, the fractured fragment should be reconstructed [12].

In the case of an intra-alveolar fracture, it should be noted that vitality tests may initially be negative. If the diagnosis of loss of vitality is confirmed, or if it is confirmed that the root of an immature tooth is not continuing to develop, endodontic treatment should be carried out. Depending on the case, treatment of both fragments can be carried out in several ways:

- Endodontic treatment of the coronal fragment.
- Endodontic treatment of the coronal fragment and extraction of the apical fragment.
- Treatment of both fragments (coronal and apical).
- Treatment of the apical fragment and extraction of the coronal fragment [9].

2. Introduction of the treatment guidelines and decision-making for avulsed permanent teeth

2.1 Patient recommendations

Traumatic events occur suddenly and unexpectedly, and first aid responses for an avulsed permanent tooth is usually performed by a guardian, teacher, or parents, who call the dental clinic asking for instructions on how to respond to the traumatic event. Afterwards, it is necessary to confirm that it is a permanent tooth that has been avulsed, as a primary tooth should not be replanted. Subsequently, clinicians should provide the following recommendations [24]:

1. Keep the patient and the guardian, teacher, and/or parents calm.

2. Encourage them to find the avulsed permanent tooth and pick it up by the crown, trying to avoid damaging the root and therefore the periodontal ligament cells.

3. Rinse the avulsed permanent tooth gently with a saline solution or milk to remove dirt, taking care not to apply heavy pressure to avoid damaging the periodontal ligament [25].

4. Encourage the guardian, teacher, and/or parents to immediately replant the avulsed permanent tooth on the alveolus, preferably before blood clot formation, which could complicate replantation of the avulsed permanent tooth. It must be taken into consideration that the guardian, teacher, and/or parents are not specialists and that bleeding and stress can make replantation difficult.

5. Some situations preclude immediate replantation of avulsed permanent teeth, for example if the patient is uncontrolled or non-cooperative, unconscious, or presenting with vital injuries requiring urgent attention. In such cases, it is recommended to store and transport the avulsed permanent tooth in a wet medium such as milk, Hank's Balanced Salt solution (HBSS), saliva, or saline solution to avoid dehydration of the periodontal ligament tissue which is responsible for the fixation of the root to the alveolus [24, 25]. Finally, it is recommended to emphasize that time may affect the prognosis of the avulsed permanent teeth, since most of the periodontal ligament cells do not survive after 30 minutes of extra-alveolar dry time [26, 27].

6. Go immediately to a dental clinic to be attended by a clinician, both to follow the preceding guidelines/treatments and to perform the autotransplantation of the permanent tooth.

In addition, the International Association of Dental Traumatology (IADT) has developed the free app "ToothSOS", which provides useful information for patients affected by dental injury.

2.2 Management and decision-making for avulsed permanent teeth

Once the patient arrives to the dental clinic, the clinician should ask whether or not it was possible to replant the avulsed permanent tooth. If the tooth was replanted on the alveolus, the clinician should verify that the tooth has been replanted correctly by comparing the angulation and incisal border with respect to the adjacent teeth, as well as by using a periapical radiograph. However, if the tooth could not be successfully replanted on the alveolus, the clinician should first analyze the condition of the periodontal ligament fibers according to the classification of the IADT in order to obtain useful information regarding the prognosis of the avulsed permanent tooth [28]:

Most of the periodontal ligament fibers are viable, since the tooth was replanted immediately or within the first 15 min after the accident.

The periodontal ligament fibers are damaged, as the extra-oral dry time did not exceed 60 min, despite being stored in a wet medium.

Most of the periodontal ligament fibers are non-viable, as the extra-oral dry time exceeded 60 min.

Regardless of treatment prognosis, replantation should be the treatment of choice; that being said, the stage of development of the avulsed permanent tooth is an important factor.

2.2.1 Management of avulsed permanent teeth with closed apex

Three different scenarios can occur, depending on the replantation site and length of extra-oral dry time:

2.2.1.1 Mature permanent tooth replanted immediately at the accident site

If the avulsed permanent tooth with closed apex has been replanted at the injury site, the clinician should follow the following recommendations:

1. Administer local anesthesia, preferably without a vasoconstrictor.
2. Clean the damaged area, removing any traces of dirt and blood with a saline serum or chlorhexidine.
3. Verify that the tooth has been replanted correctly by comparing the angulation and incisal border position with respect to the adjacent teeth, in addition to with a periapical radiograph. If the tooth was not correctly replanted, try to gently reposition it.
4. Splint the avulsed tooth using a 0.016″/0.4-mm diameter wire attached to the tooth and adjacent teeth for 2 weeks, avoiding invading the gingival margin [29]. However, the splint should be more rigid and left for 4 weeks if there is an associated alveolar or jawbone fracture.
5. Perform the root canal treatment after 15 days.
6. Prescribe systemic antibiotics.
7. Check tetanus vaccine status.
8. Monitor outcome with a follow-up appointment.

2.2.1.2 Avulsed permanent tooth stored in wet medium for less than 60 min

The medium used to store depends on the accident location; however, tissue culture media such as milk or HBSS are recommended to preserve the viability of periodontal ligament cells.

1. Gently rinse the avulsed permanent tooth with saline solution or milk to remove any dirt, taking care not to apply heavy pressure to avoid damaging the periodontal ligament.
2. Leave the tooth hydrated in a moist environment while you examine the patient and take their medical history.

3. Administer local anesthesia, preferably without a vasoconstrictor.

4. Gently irrigate the socket with saline, removing the coagulum for easier replantation of the avulsed tooth.

5. Examine the alveolus to rule out any fractures in the alveolar walls. If there is a fracture of the alveolar walls, replace the fragment.

6. Gently replant the avulsed tooth, picking it up by the dental crown (**Figure 1**).

7. Verify that the tooth has been replanted correctly by comparing the angulation and incisal border position with regard to the adjacent teeth, as well as with a periapical radiograph. If the tooth was not correctly replanted, try to gently reposition it.

8. Splint the avulsed tooth using a 0.016″/0.4-mm diameter wire attached to the tooth and adjacent teeth for 2 weeks.

9. Suture any cuts or lacerations.

10. Perform the root canal treatment after 15 days.

11. Prescribe systemic antibiotics.

12. Check tetanus vaccine status.

13. Monitor outcome with a follow-up appointment.

2.2.1.3 Extra-oral dry time longer than 60 min

1. Gently rinse the avulsed permanent tooth with a saline solution or milk to remove any dirt, taking care not to apply heavy pressure to avoid damaging the periodontal ligament.

2. Leave the tooth hydrated in a moist environment while you examine the patient and take their medical history.

3. Administer local anesthesia, preferably without a vasoconstrictor.

4. Gently irrigate the socket with saline, removing the coagulum for easier replantation of the avulsed tooth.

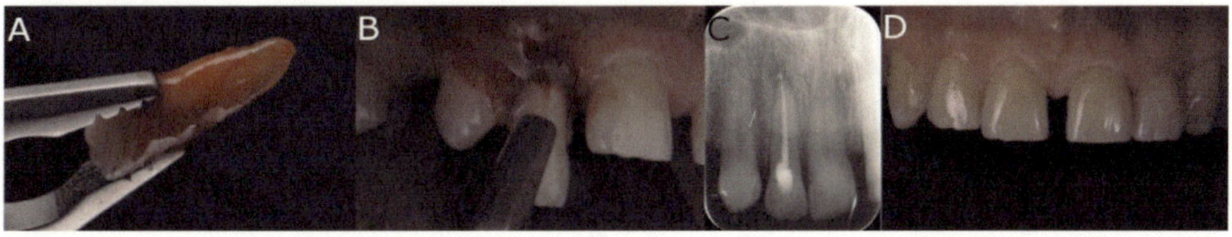

Figure 1.
(A) Avulsed permanent tooth held by the dental crown, (B) replantation procedure, (C) root canal treatment after 15 days, and (D) 6 months follow-up after replantation.

5. Examine the alveolus to rule out any fractures in the alveolar walls. If there is a fracture of the alveolar walls, replace the fragment.

6. Gently replant the avulsed tooth, picking it up by the dental crown (**Figure 1**).

7. Verify that the tooth has been replanted correctly by comparing the angulation and incisal border position with regard to the adjacent teeth, as well as with a periapical radiograph. If the tooth was not correctly replanted, try to gently reposition it.

8. Splint the avulsed tooth using a 0.016″/0.4-mm diameter wire attached to the tooth and adjacent teeth for 2 weeks.

9. Suture any cuts or lacerations.

10. Perform the root canal treatment after 15 days.

11. Prescribe systemic antibiotics.

12. Check tetanus vaccine status.

13. Monitor outcome with a follow-up appointment.

2.2.2 Management of avulsed permanent teeth with open apex

Three different scenarios can also occur here, depending on the replantation site and length of extra-oral dry time:

2.2.2.1 Immature permanent tooth replanted immediately at the accident site

If the avulsed permanent tooth with closed apex has been replanted at the injury site, the clinician should follow the following recommendations:

1. Administer local anesthesia, preferably without a vasoconstrictor.

2. Clean the damaged area with a saline solution or chlorhexidine, removing any traces of dirt or blood.

3. Verify that the tooth has been replanted correctly by comparing the angulation and incisal border position with regard to the adjacent teeth, as well as with a periapical radiograph. If the tooth was not correctly replanted, try to gently reposition it.

4. Splint the avulsed tooth using a 0.016″/0.4-mm diameter wire attached to the tooth and adjacent teeth for 2 weeks, avoiding invading the gingival margin [29]. However, the splint should be more rigid and left for 4 weeks if there is an associated alveolar or jawbone fracture.

5. Pulp revascularization must be the first treatment choice, as it enables the development of the root process; however, clinicians should be aware of inflammatory root resorption. Should pulp revascularization fail, apexogenesis or apexification procedures must be initiated.

6. Prescribe systemic antibiotics.

7. Check tetanus vaccine status.

8. Monitor outcome with a follow-up appointment.

2.2.2.2 Avulsed immature permanent tooth stored in wet medium for under 60 min

The medium used to store depends on the accident location; however, tissue culture media such as milk or HBSS are recommended to preserve the viability of periodontal ligament cells.

1. Gently rinse the avulsed permanent tooth with a saline solution or milk to remove any dirt, taking care not to apply heavy pressure to avoid damaging periodontal ligament [30, 31].

2. Leave the tooth hydrated in a moist environment while you examine the patient and take their medical history.

3. Administer local anesthesia, preferably without a vasoconstrictor.

4. Gently irrigate the socket with saline, removing the coagulum for easier replantation of the avulsed tooth.

5. Examine the alveolus, ruling out any fractures in the alveolar walls. If there is a fracture of the alveolar walls, replace the fragment.

6. Gently replant the avulsed tooth, picking it up by the dental crown (**Figure 1**).

7. Verify that the tooth has been replanted correctly by comparing the angulation and incisal border position with regard to the adjacent teeth, as well as with a periapical radiograph. If the tooth was not correctly replanted, try to gently reposition it.

8. Splint the avulsed tooth using a 0.016″/0.4-mm diameter wire attached to the tooth and adjacent teeth for 2 weeks.

9. Suture any cuts or lacerations.

10. Pulp revascularization must be the first treatment choice, as it enables the development of the root process; however, clinicians should be aware of inflammatory root resorption. Should pulp revascularization fail, apexogenesis or apexification procedures must be initiated.

11. Prescribe systemic antibiotics.

12. Check tetanus vaccine status.

13. Monitor outcome with a follow-up appointment.

2.2.2.3 Extra-oral dry time longer than 60 min

1. Gently rinse the avulsed permanent tooth with a saline solution or milk to remove any dirt, taking care not to apply heavy pressure to avoid damaging periodontal ligament.

2. Leave the tooth hydrated in a moist environment while you examine the patient and take their medical history.

3. Administer local anesthesia, preferably without a vasoconstrictor.

4. Gently irrigate the socket with saline, removing the coagulum for easier replantation of the avulsed tooth.

5. Examine the alveolus, ruling out any fractures in the alveolar walls. If there is a fracture of the alveolar walls, replace the fragment.

6. Gently replant the avulsed tooth, picking it up by the dental crown (**Figure 1**).

7. Verify that the tooth has been replanted correctly by comparing the angulation and incisal border position with regard to the adjacent teeth, as well as with a periapical radiograph. If the tooth was not correctly replanted, try to gently reposition it.

8. Splint the avulsed tooth using a 0.016″/0.4-mm diameter wire attached to the tooth and adjacent teeth for 2 weeks.

9. Suture any cuts or lacerations.

10. Pulp revascularization must be the first treatment choice, as it enables the development of the root process; however, clinicians should be aware of inflammatory root resorption. Should pulp revascularization fail, apexogenesis or apexification procedures must be initiated.

11. Prescribe systemic antibiotics.

12. Check tetanus vaccine status.

13. Monitor outcome with a follow-up appointment [28].

3. Introduction of the treatment guidelines and decision-making for traumatic dental injuries (TDI) in temporary teeth

Dental trauma is one of the most frequent emergency situations seen in Pediatric Dentistry, especially in notable hospitals or dental clinics, or those linked to schools or sports centers. Dental trauma often happens in the schoolyard or in sports facilities where children practice some sport without the presence of the parents, who are notified by the institution, go to pick up their child, and come to us bewildered, nervous, and scared regardless of the severity of the blow.

The situation is one of tension, anguish, and chaos, further exacerbated by the presence of blood, crying, having to dental fragments or missing teeth... Therefore, when these situations reach us, we must prioritize their attention and transmit our sense of calm to the patient and their family members. In addition, in cases of multiple traumas, time is essential for the best possible prognosis and evolution of the case.

Once the anamnesis and medical history have been taken, we collect data on the accident, how it happened, where, how long ago, whether it is the first time the area has been hit, whether there is pain, bleeding, dental dyschromia, changes in bite, or if you have had any neurological symptoms that force us to prioritize another type of medical assessment by professionals from another specialty.

Then, once in the clinical area, we must wash the patient's face and thoroughly clean the injured areas with saline solution and gauze pads, using 5-ml syringes for areas that are difficult to access, such as the back of the vestibule. Often once this cleaning has been carried out, the diagnosis is nothing more than the most banal of injuries, despite the initial appearance of the blow (**Figure 2**) [32–40].

It is important to highlight that when a tooth suffers a trauma, no matter how slight, the neurovascular bundle that innervates it and supplies it with nutrients through the apical foramen is always involved. This can undergo compression or stretching that may well evolve without any complications, or it may evolve to necrosis that requires treatment. For this reason, it is essential that we monitor the evolution of the pulp over time and that we follow up on the signs and symptoms that may appear, sometimes several months after the trauma [41].

With regard to this evolution of the pulpal state of a tooth that has suffered a trauma, any change in color or darkening of the tooth become especially important. Many traumas give rise to a more or less immediate darkening of the color of the tooth due to internal bleeding that enters through the dentinal tubules, resulting in dyschromia. This tone lightens in the days after the trauma, although it does not usually disappear completely, but it does not indicate any pulpal degenerative processes at all. It is important that we note the color of the tooth during the initial exploration of the trauma, assessing whether there has been a change in shade or not; if the darkening of the tooth occurs gradually, becoming increasingly darker over time, this would be a sign of pulpal degeneration and necrosis (**Figure 3**) [42–45].

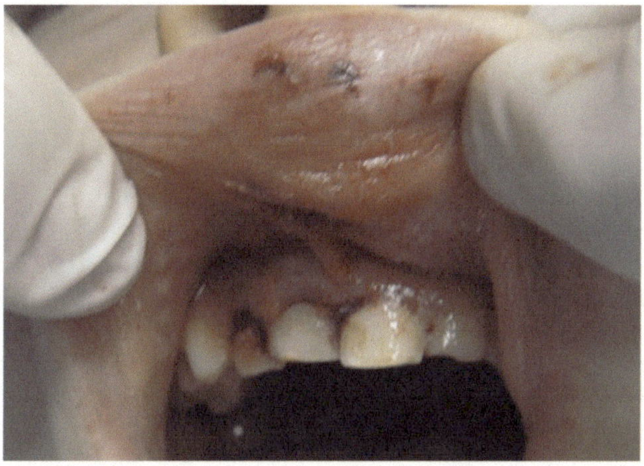

Figure 2.
Trauma in temporary teeth prior to thorough cleaning of the area.

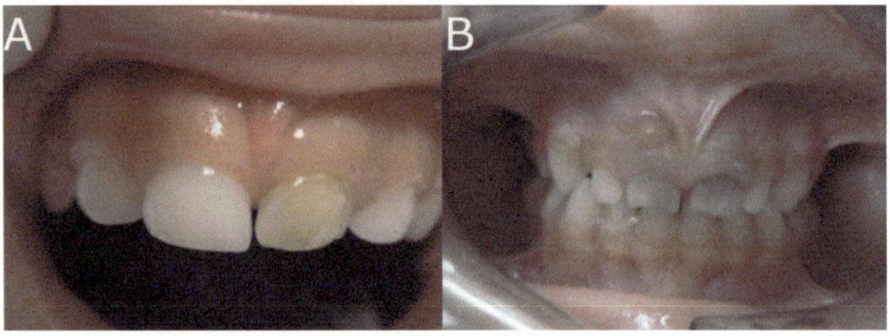

Figure 3.
(A) Dyschromia of 61 caused by internal bleeding at the time of injury and (B) dyschromia of 51 and 61 caused by pulp necrosis.

Essentially, when assessing our case, we must classify injuries according to the tissues affected: soft tissues, periodontal ligament, dentin-pulp complex, and bone tissue, doing our best to explain to the parents that each tissue has a unique healing capacity and rhythm requiring different types of care and/or treatment. As a general rule, soft tissues heal in 3–4 days when following the specific guidelines for their care, the periodontal ligament in 7–10 days, depending on the degree of severity, and the pulp can suffer direct effects that require immediate treatment to avoid potential long-term complications, a condition that we will diagnose later if observed during the follow-up appointments that we schedule after the trauma.

Dental trauma can affect both primary and permanent dentition, and many times traumas that occur in temporary dentition can even affect permanent dentition regardless of the age at which they occur, given the intimate contact between the roots of temporary incisors and the germs of permanent incisors. In fact, the younger the patient is when a primary tooth suffers trauma, the more severe the consequences may be for the future permanent tooth, given the immaturity of its formation at the time of the trauma. These possible consequences of injuries must be kept in mind when writing the accident damage report, as it is often the insurance companies that bear the cost of immediate treatment, follow-up appointments to assess their evolution, and treatment of any complications or sequelae should they occur [46–49].

3.1 Dental tissue injuries involving pulp

3.1.1 Crown infraction

This is an incomplete fracture of the enamel without any loss of dental substance. They are small fissures that can be vertical, horizontal, or diagonal, generally diagnosed because the hemorrhage itself deriving from the soft tissues stains the surface of the dental crown, making crown infractions evident. It can also be diagnosed using transillumination, aiming the light beam from the palatal position to be able to visualize the fracture lines on the buccal surface of the crown. Treatment for this type of injury depends on the case, ranging from a simple supply of fluoride to remineralize the area to polishing of the fissure and application of fluoride, or even sealing of the fissure if so required.

However, the most important thing that we must not overlook is that at the moment of the blow, the neurovascular bundle suffers, and the evolution of the pulp must be monitored after 1, 3, and 6 months to monitor the evolution of the pulp.

Given that vitality tests in children are uncertain, we will base our pulp monitoring on assessing the absence of clinical signs over time, such as darkening of tooth color, appearance of fistulae or swelling of the attached gingiva at the level of the dental apex, and/or mobility. Radiographically, we must also ensure that the root development of the tooth continues to advance over time, narrowing the lumen of the canal and thickening the dentin of its walls, as well as ensuring the absence of atypical root resorption or apical focus.

3.1.2 Uncomplicated fracture of the crown

This is a fracture limited to enamel or enamel and dentin in which there is already loss of substance. Treatment depends on the affected tissues and can range from application of fluoride, if it is only a small loss of enamel, to rounding and polishing of sharp edges and application of fluoride if the loss of enamel is greater or damages the tongue or lip of the patient. If there is exposed dentin, it is always necessary to reconstruct, either with composite materials or by replacing the fragment, although in temporary dentition this latter option is not very frequent (**Figure 4**).

Again, the most important thing that we must not forget is the neurovascular bundle. It is necessary to monitor evolution at 1, 3, and 6 months to monitor the evolution of the pulp. Assess pulp vitality at these appointments, controlling for the absence of clinical signs over time, such as darkening of tooth color, appearance of fistulae or swelling of the attached gingiva at the level of the dental apex, and/or mobility. Radiographically, we must also ensure that the root development of the tooth continues to advance over time, narrowing the lumen of the canal and thickening the dentin of its walls, as well as ensuring the absence of atypical root resorption or apical focus. It is not uncommon for these injuries to lead to pulpal necrosis in the long term, requiring a pulpectomy of the tooth to be carried out later (**Figure 5**).

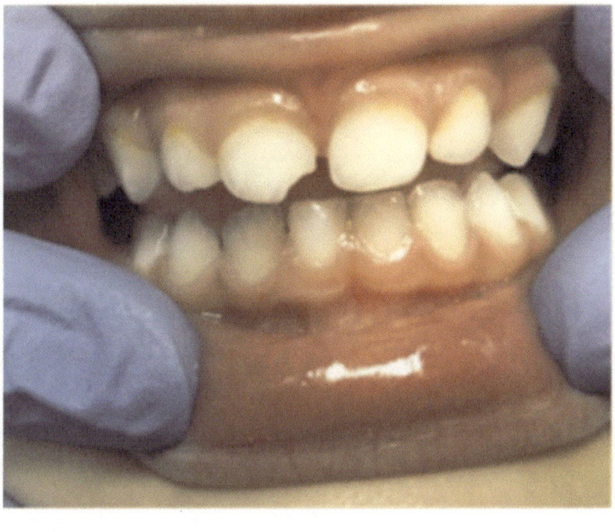

Figure 4.
Enamel and dentin fracture of a 51 without pulp exposure.

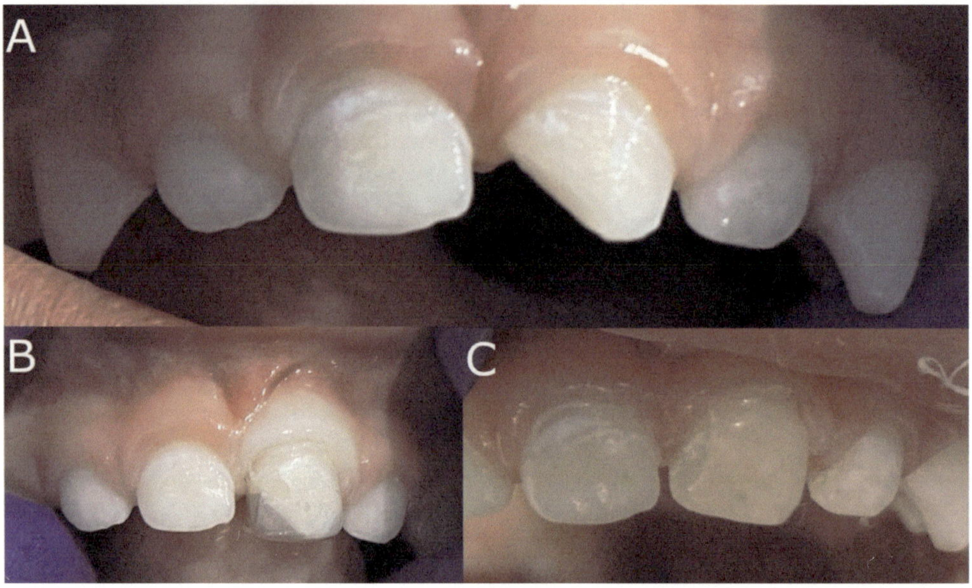

Figure 5.
Uncomplicated fracture of tooth 61 in a 3-year-old patient. Reconstruction with preformed crown and composite resin.

3.1.3 Complicated crown fracture

This is a fracture of enamel and dentin with pulp exposure. In these cases, if the tooth is restorable and the physiological resorption is still slight, pulp treatment can be carried out, generally a pulpectomy and restoration with composite materials. If pulp exposure was minimal (<1 mm) and recent (<1 h), direct pulp capping (DPR) could be carried out with bioactive materials such as MTA or Biodentine™ before restoration with composite materials. If the tooth is not restorable or the physiological resorption is already very advanced, extraction would be the treatment of choice (**Figures 6** and 7).

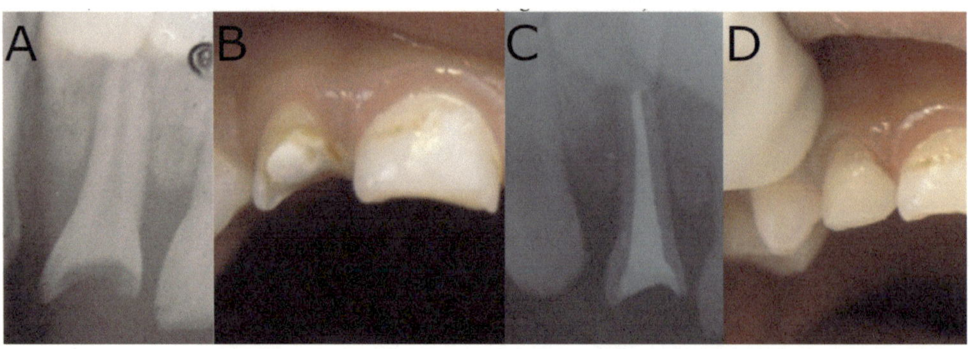

Figure 6.
Complicated crown fracture of tooth 52. Pulpectomy with iodoform paste and reconstruction with composite resin in tooth 52.

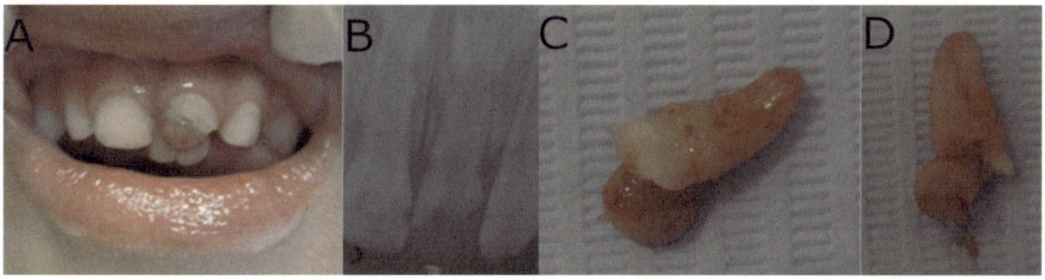

Figure 7.
Complicated fracture of tooth 61 with presence of pulp polyp in a 2-year-old patient. X-ray of teeth 51–61. Tooth extraction of tooth 61.

3.1.4 Uncomplicated crown and root fracture

This is a fracture of enamel, dentin, and cement without pulp exposure. These fractures are difficult to diagnose; pain may appear when chewing. To tailor the treatment, it will be necessary to remove the coronal fragment under local anesthesia and assess whether it is possible to restore it or not. If restoration is not possible, extraction will have to be carried out.

3.1.5 Complicated crown-root fracture

This is a fracture of enamel, dentin, and cementum with pulp exposure. In primary dentition, they often follow the longitudinal axis of the tooth. In this case, and when the fracture covers more than a third of the clinical root, the treatment of choice is extraction. When the fracture covers less than a third of the clinical crown, after extracting the coronal fragment under local anesthesia, the possibility of restoration is assessed. If it is restorable, a pulpectomy and reconstruction with composite materials is carried out (**Figure 8**).

It is very common to find this type of fracture in maxillary primary first molars as a result of the violent closure of the mandible against the maxilla after a contraction injury caused by trauma to the chin. For this reason, with this type of trauma it is very important to examine the crowns of the upper molars, always trying to separate their cusps with the probe in order to diagnose them. If we do not take this precaution, the most common outcome is that the fracture goes unnoticed and the patient arrives at the consultation weeks after the trauma presenting with pain and inflammation in one

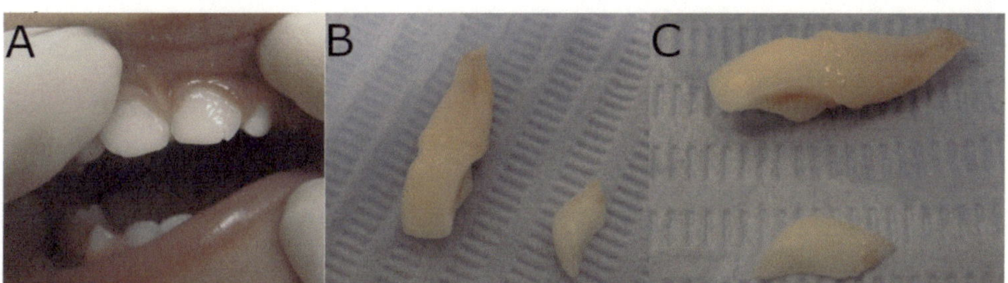

Figure 8.
Complicated crown-root fracture and extraction of tooth 61.

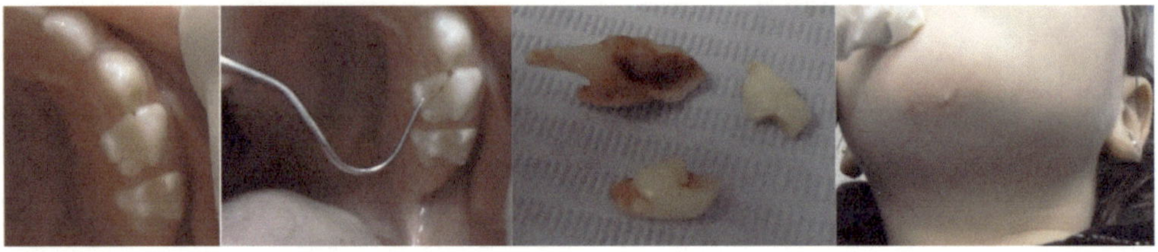

Figure 9.
Complicated crown-root fracture of tooth 64. Using the probe to separate the cusps. Extraction of tooth 64. Healed injury on the chin.

side of the face and an almost healed lesion on the chin. By exploring the upper molars, we can identify the fracture (**Figure 9**).

3.1.6 Root fracture

This is a dentin and cement fracture with pulp involvement that can affect the apical third, middle third, or coronal third. Clinical experience tells us that most root fractures are diagnosed as incidental findings over time; this is because only 20–44% of root fractures result in pulpal necrosis. For this reason, we must take a preventative approach, monitoring the evolution of the case with a follow-up appointment at 1, 3, and every 6 months to assess the pulpal response. In most cases, obliteration of the duct occurs as a reparative response, without any associated clinical symptoms. If necrosis occurs, the treatment would involve the extraction of the coronal fragment; the apical fragment must be left so as not to damage the germ of the permanent tooth. A vital apical fragment is usually resorbed without problem. There are times when the root fracture is very apical and we can perform a pulpectomy up to the fracture line and restore with composite materials, subsequently monitoring the evolution of the case (**Figure 10**) [50–66].

3.2 Periodontal tissue injuries

3.2.1 Concussion

This is an incomplete rupture of the periodontal fibers, with hemorrhage and edema of the same but without mobility or displacement of the tooth. There may be percussion tenderness but no radiological signs.

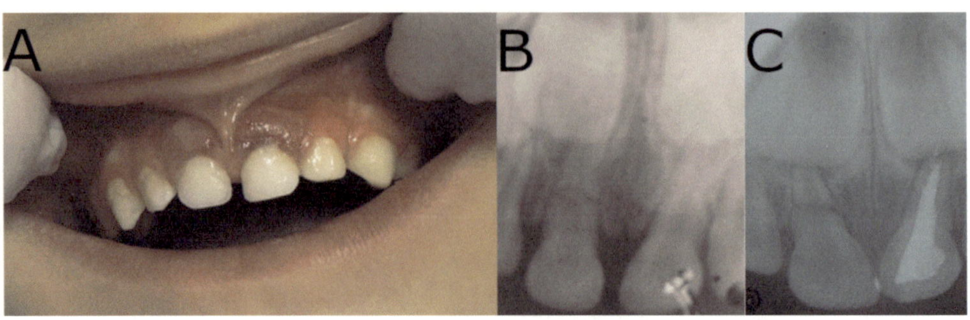

Figure 10.
Root fracture of 51. Clinical appearance. Root fracture of tooth 51. X-ray. 1-year follow-up.

3.2.2 Subluxation

This is damage to the supporting tissue, which results in mobility but not displacement of the tooth. Sensitivity to percussion and occlusal forces is increased, and upon radiographic examination, an increase in the space of the periodontal ligament can be seen.

The treatment for both concussion and subluxation is to recommend resting the area to allow the damaged periodontal fibers to heal. Depending on the child's age, emphasis must be placed on reducing the use of bottles and pacifiers, limiting the use of teethers, following a bland diet, following extreme hygiene measures, and once again, scheduling a follow-up appointment at 1, 3, and 6 months to monitor pulpal evolution as any trauma, no matter how slight, can damage the neurovascular bundle and lead to long-term pulpal complications. During these follow-up appointments, the color of the tooth becomes important, because while darkening of the clinical crown is a very noticeable sign for parents and can alert us to pulpal necrosis, it is common in this type of trauma; at the time of the blow, a small internal hemorrhage occurs, resulting in immediate dental darkening. It is important not to confuse this dyschromia with that caused by pulpal necrosis, and for this reason, care must be taken to note the color of the tooth in the first assessment or to ask the parents about the color change. When it comes to staining due to hemorrhage immediately after trauma, the color tends to lighten over time, unlike in cases of necrosis, in which the color darkens over time (**Figure 11**) [41].

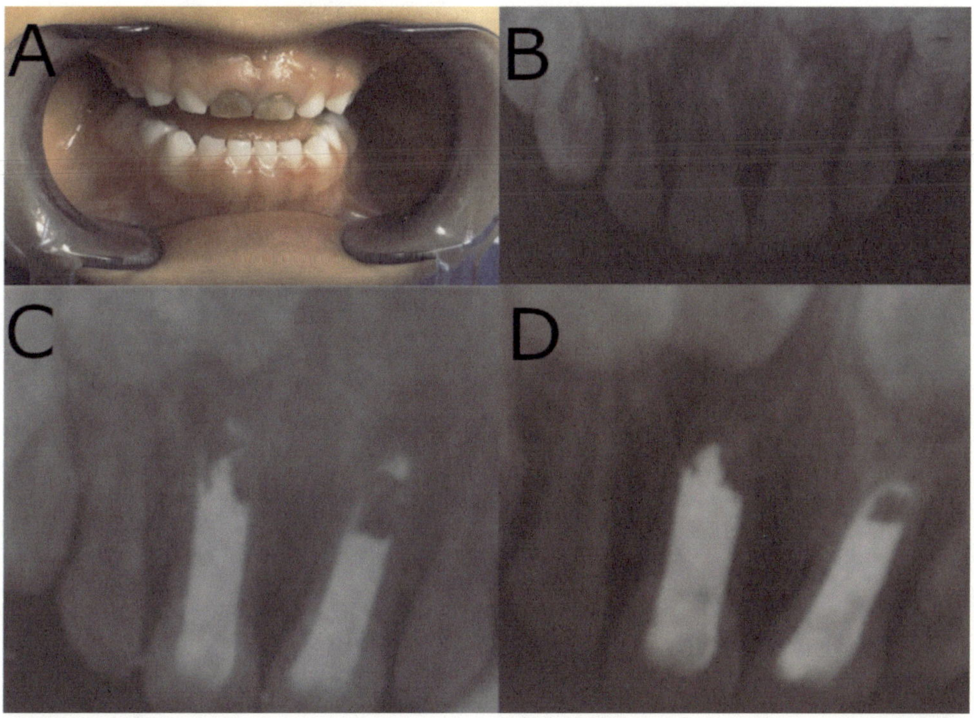

Figure 11.
Injuries 2 years ago to teeth 51–61 in a 4-year-old patient with no prior dental assistance. X-ray of teeth 51–61, apical focus with pulp necrosis. Pulpectomy of teeth 51–61 at a very early stage of root development. Evolution 1 year after treatment.

3.2.3 Intrusive luxation

This is the movement of the tooth into the socket. It is associated with a comminuted fracture of the alveolar bone. Sometimes we see part of the tooth in the intraoral examination and it is easy to diagnose, and other times the tooth completely disappears inside the socket and an X-ray is needed to diagnose it because the parents believe that it has been lost and they simply have not found it at the site of trauma. In temporary dentition, the treatment will be to monitor the evolution over time, as it is common for the tooth to re-erupt to its position in the arch. Clinical and radiographic controls must be performed at 1, 3, and 6 months. During these follow-up evaluations, it is most common to see that the tooth is advancing on the path towards re-eruption, being closer to the occlusal plane, and it is usually almost complete at 6 months. In addition to monitoring the eruption, as in the previous cases, pulp vitality must also be monitored. If after 6 months of follow-up, the tooth has not undergone any progress or has been the origin of an infectious process while still in the place of inclusion, we must schedule the extraction of the piece (**Figures 12–14**) [50, 67].

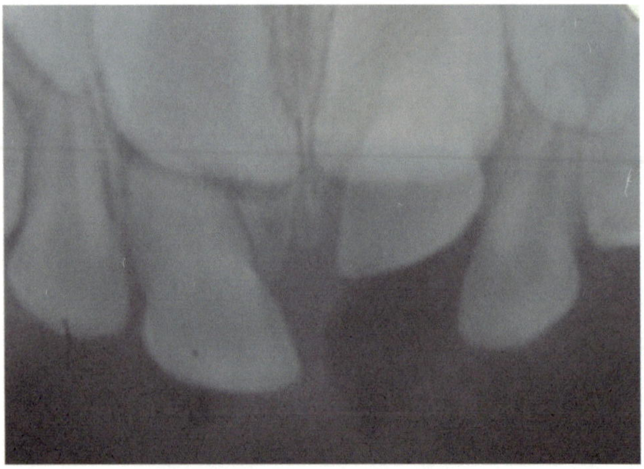

Figure 12.
X-ray. Intrusion of tooth 61.

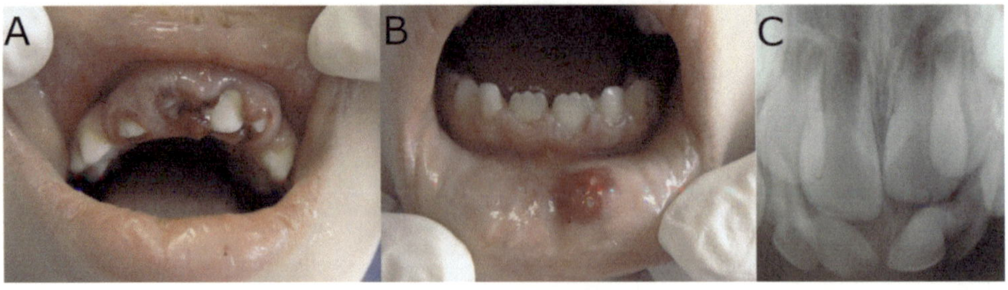

Figure 13.
Intrusion of teeth 52–51–61–62. Clinical photos and radiography.

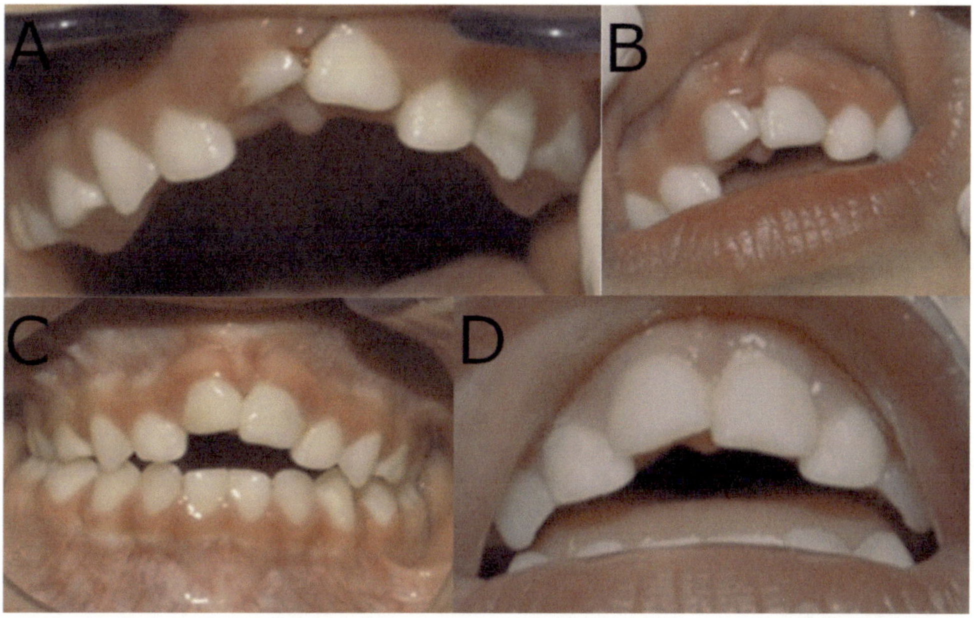

Figure 14.
Intrusion of 51–61. 1-, 3-, and 6-month follow-up.

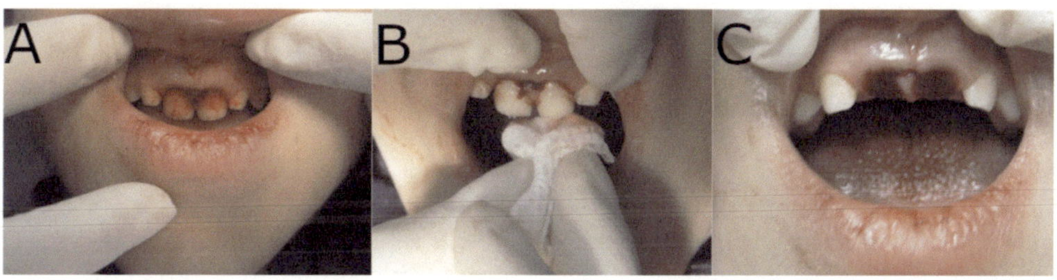

Figure 15.
Extrusive luxation of tooth 51–61. Tooth extraction.

3.2.4 Extrusive luxation

Movement of the tooth out of the alveolus as a result of a sharp blow. Radiographic examination always shows the increase in the periodontal space. The neurovascular bundle may be completely ruptured. In temporary dentition, we should not reposition the tooth in the alveolus due to the risk of damaging the germ of the permanent tooth in formation, so the treatment of choice is extraction (**Figure 15**).

3.2.5 Lateral luxation

This is a lesion to the supporting tissue of the tooth with its deviation in an axial direction. The most frequent cause is a horizontal impact that forces the crown towards the palatal wall and the apex towards the vestibular wall, resulting in occlusal interference and bleeding through the groove. It is always accompanied by a fracture of the alveolar process, so there is no mobility since the tooth is impacted on the cortical bone. Upon radiographic examination, the widening of the periodontal space

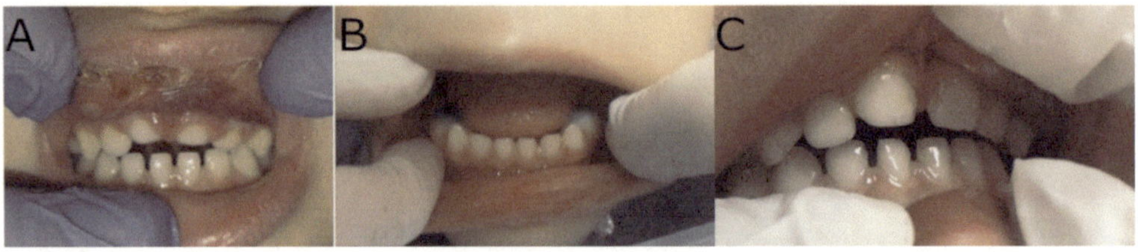

Figure 16.
Intrusion of tooth 51–61 and palatine luxation of tooth 62 with occlusal interference. Bite lifts on tooth 74–84 to physiologically correct the luxation of tooth 62. Follow-up at 1 week.

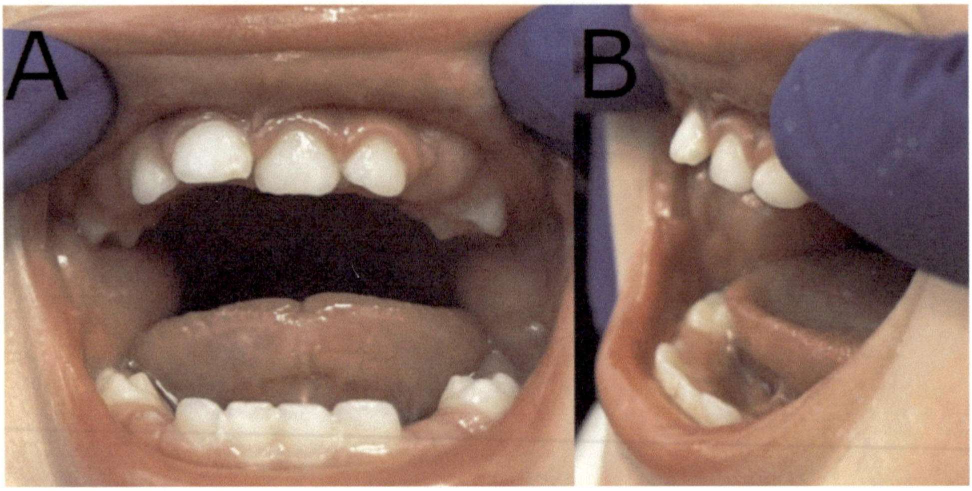

Figure 17.
Palatine luxation of tooth 61 in an 18-month-old baby.

is visible. In temporary dentition, we should never reposition the tooth in its original position due to the danger of damaging the germ of the permanent tooth in formation, but if the displacement is small, we can keep the tooth in the mouth and relieve the occlusion by placing bite lifts to gently reposition it spontaneously with the help of the tongue. If the displacement of the tooth is larger, tooth extraction is recommended (**Figures 16** and **17**) [50–66].

3.2.6 Avulsion

This is the complete expulsion of the tooth from the alveolus. In temporary dentition, we should never replant an avulsed tooth due to the danger of damaging the permanent tooth in formation. There are different fixed or removable therapeutic procedures to replace lost pieces early in the deciduous dentition (**Figure 18**) [49].

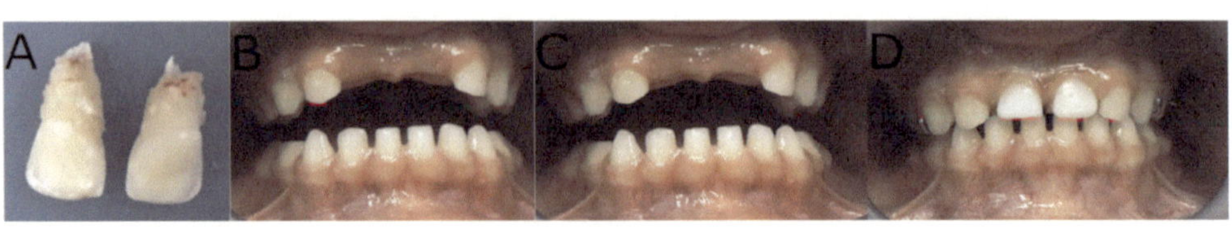

Figure 18.
Avulsion of teeth 51–61 in a 4-year-old patient. Replacement with removable acrylic plate.

4. Bone tissue injuries

4.1 Comminuted fracture of alveolar bone

Internal breakage of the alveolar bone that usually occurs as a result of an intrusion or lateral dislocation.

4.2 Fracture of the alveolar wall

This can be a fracture of the facial or lingual wall (**Figure 19**).

4.3 Alveolar process fracture

A fracture of the alveolar process may also include the alveolus.

In this type of bone fractures, we need to splint for consolidation, often with 0.12–0.14 braided wire anchored to the teeth with composite. On many occasions, the teeth that we use to anchor the splint have to be extracted, but first we use them as anchors. We let them consolidate and heal the bone fracture, and after that is when we plan the corresponding dental extractions. In conclusion, we must prioritize bone healing and never extract a tooth when there is a fracture of the wall or alveolar process until it has consolidated (**Figures 20–22**).

5. Gum or oral mucosa injuries

5.1 Laceration of gum or oral mucosa

Superficial or deep injury to the epithelium that is usually produced by a sharp instrument. For treatment, the wound must be irrigated with saline. If the edges can be approximated, we suture and close by first intention; if they cannot be approximated, we will control the bleeding with compression and close by second intention. We must always give recommendations to the patient and their parents for exhaustive

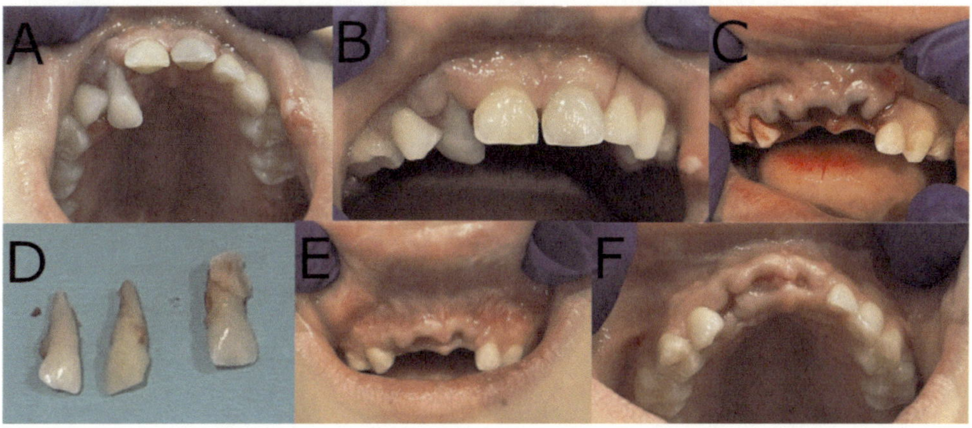

Figure 19.
Superior maxillary vestibular alveolar wall fracture between tooth 61 and 62 and palatine luxation of 52. 1-day follow-up.

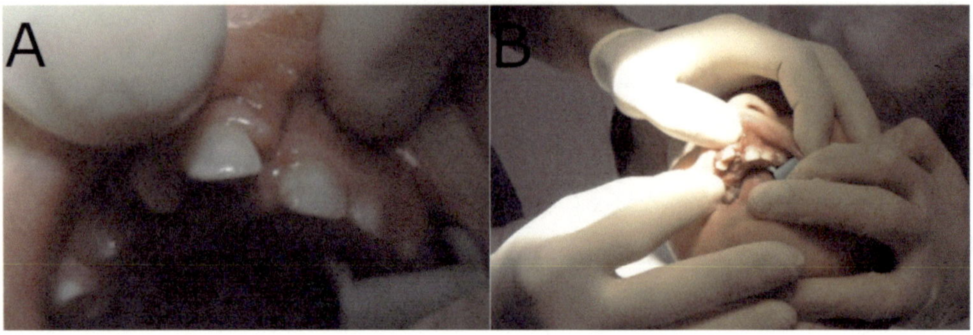

Figure 20.
Fracture of the superior alveolar process in an 18-month-old patient.

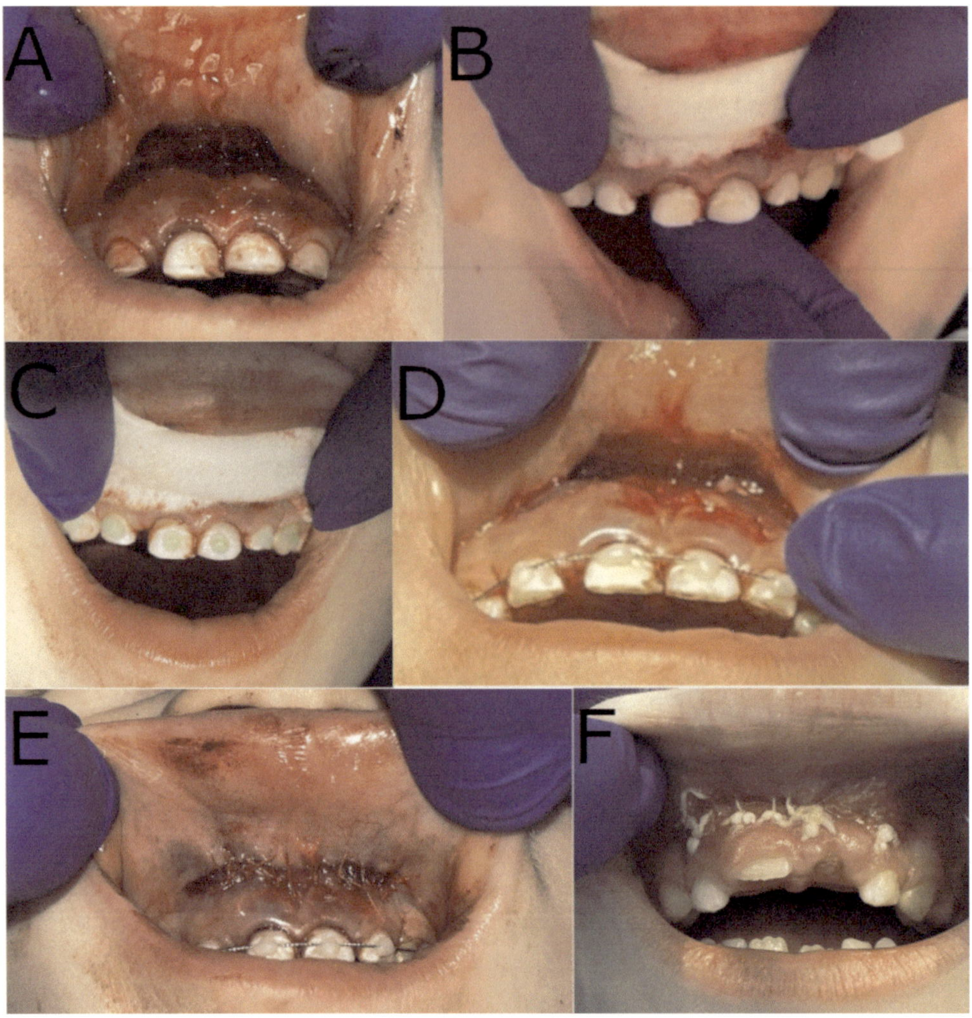

Figure 21.
Alveolar process fracture in a 5-year-old patient. Splinting and suture. 1-month follow-up.

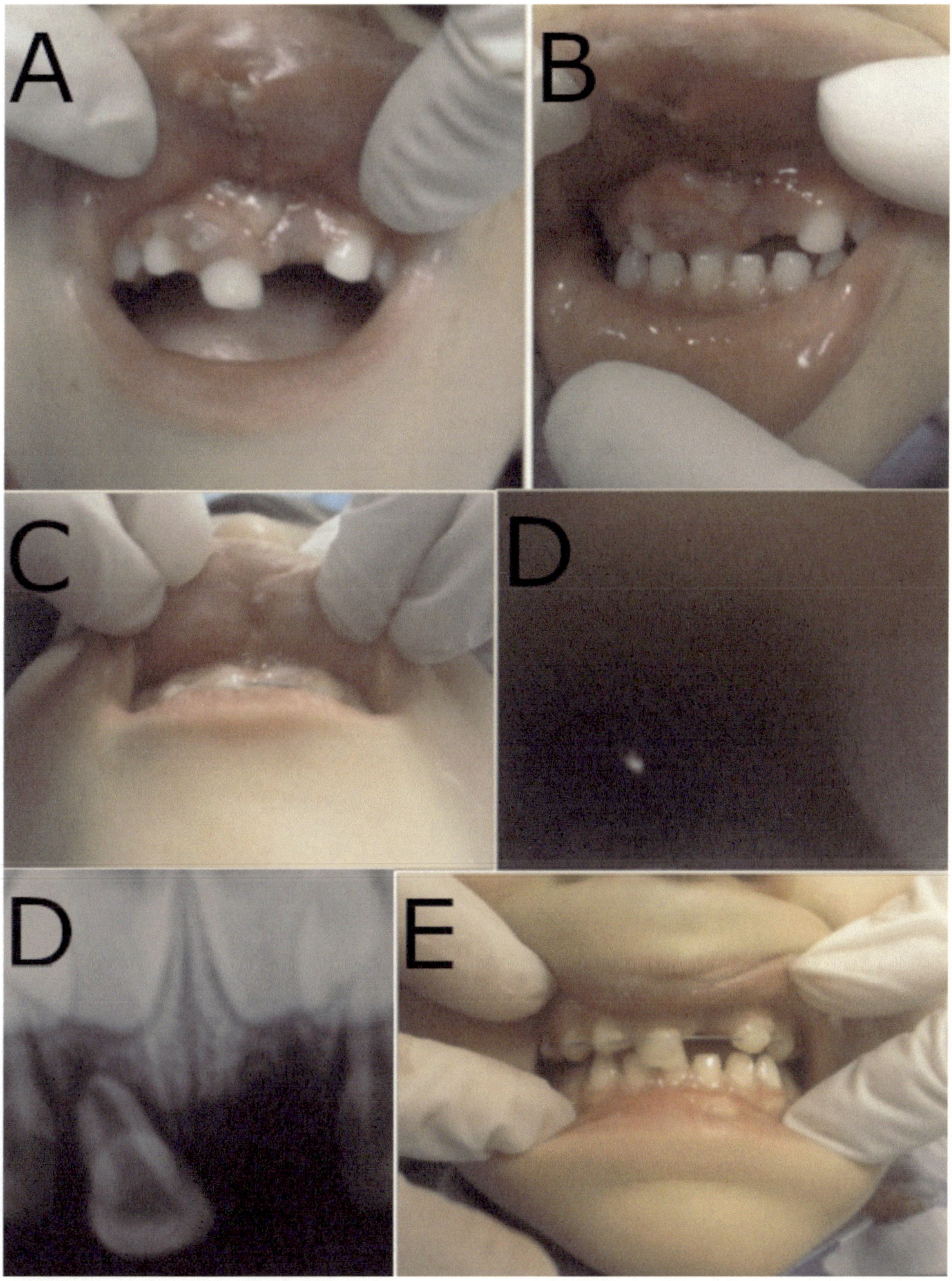

Figure 22.
Avulsion of tooth 61, luxation of tooth 51, superior alveolar process fracture with occlusal interference and foreign body in upper lip of a 5-year-old patient. Radiographic control. Soft tissue and periapical radiography. Splinting and bite lifts on teeth 74–84.

cleaning of the area, application of chlorhexidine gel, analgesic and anti-inflammatory treatment, and antibiotic therapy if necessary, depending on whether the injury occurred in a dirty environment or depending on the condition of the instrument that caused the injury (**Figure 23**).

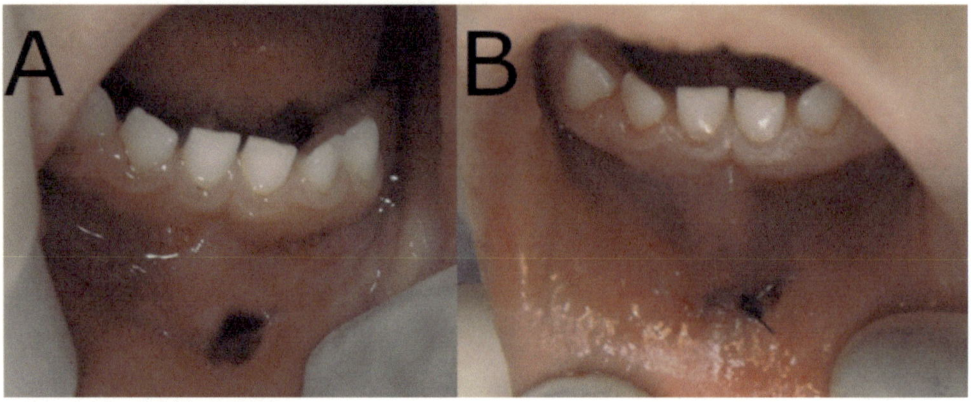

Figure 23.
Laceration on the internal side of the lip in a 5-year-old patient. 10-day follow-up.

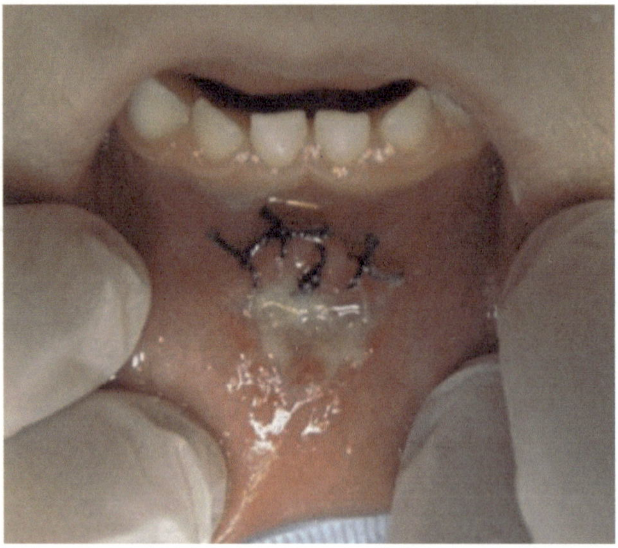

Figure 24.
Four days post-injury with fibrin at the edge of the lesion as a result of lip traction and new tearing.

If we suture the inner area of the lips, we must remember that they should not be revealed to visualize the wound because it is very likely that the margins of the injury will tear again and end up healing by secondary intention (**Figures 24–27**).

5.2 Contusion of gum or oral mucosa

This is an injury caused by blunt force trauma with blunt surfaces. It causes edema and hematoma of the subcutaneous tissue, while the skin and mucosa remain intact. Generally, this type of injury only requires analgesic anti-inflammatory treatment, and we recommend the application of a cold compress. We must remember that it is important that when we see an injury of this type on the chin, the crowns of the upper molars must be examined very thoroughly, as it is very common for fractures to occur

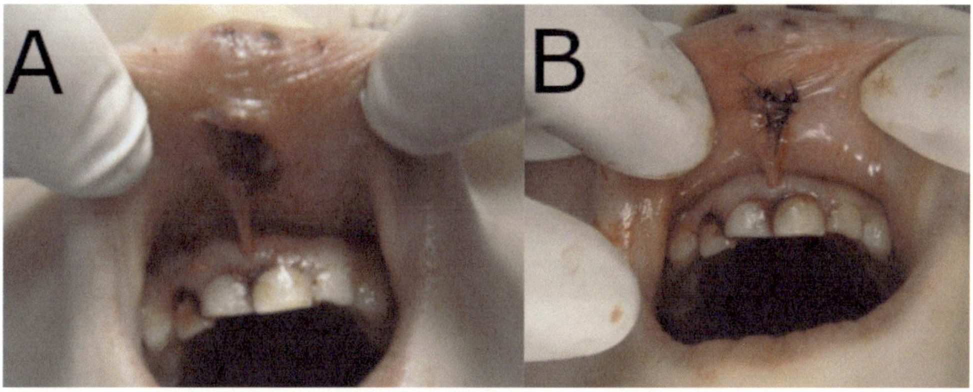

Figure 25.
Upper lip laceration in a 4-year-old patient. Suture.

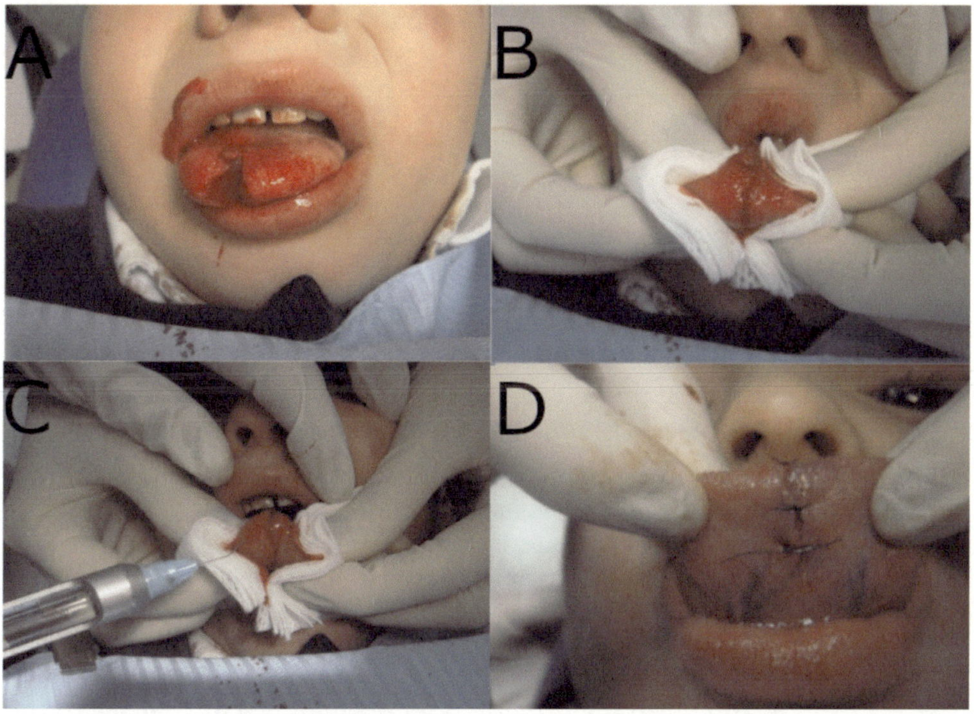

Figure 26.
Tongue laceration in a 4-year-old patient. Suture.

due to the counterblow, and we do not inspect carefully, we will not be able to diagnose these until the appearance of later complications (**Figure 28**).

5.3 Abrasion of the gum and oral mucosa

This occurs due to friction trauma. It removes the reticular and papillary layer of the epidermis, exposing the bleeding reticular layer of the dermis. There is continuity of the tissue and it is painful given the nerve endings of the dermis. A thorough

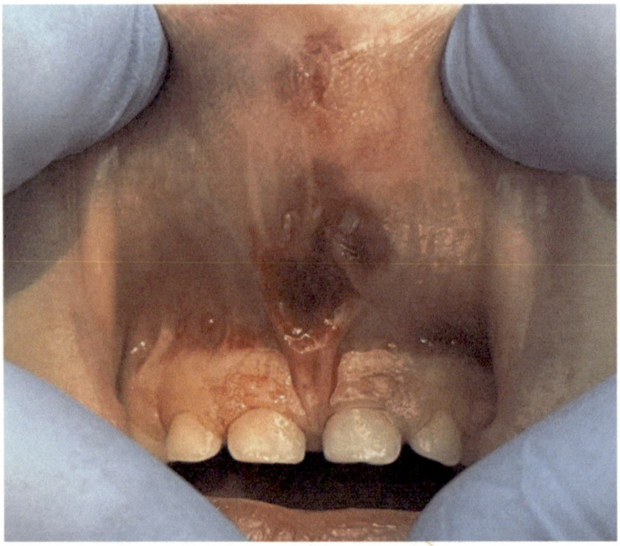

Figure 27.
Laceration of upper lip brace in a 4-year-old patient.

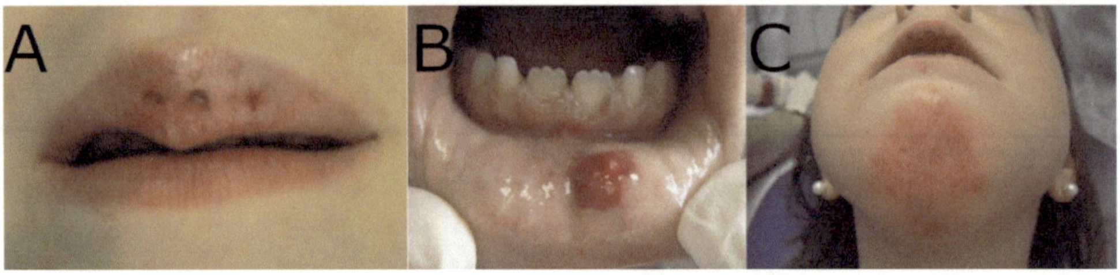

Figure 28.
Contusions on the skin and mucosa of the lip and chin.

cleaning of the area must be carried out to avoid the retention of dirty particles that can lead to infections or permanent discoloration. It scars by secondary intention, and as treatment recommendations we must insist on cleaning the area, application of chlorhexidine gel, analgesic anti-inflammatory treatment, and antibiotic and anti-tetanus prophylaxis (**Figures 29–31**) [50–66].

6. Affectation of the permanent teeth as a consequence of injuries to the temporary dentition

As we discussed previously, trauma to the primary dentition may have consequences for the permanent dentition. These consequences may be due to:

- Direct impact of the root of the temporary tooth on the germ of the permanent tooth. This can result in:

    a. Displacement of the tooth inside the bone, altering its eruption trajectory in the future. The permanent tooth may erupt out of place, have delayed eruption, or even fail to erupt.

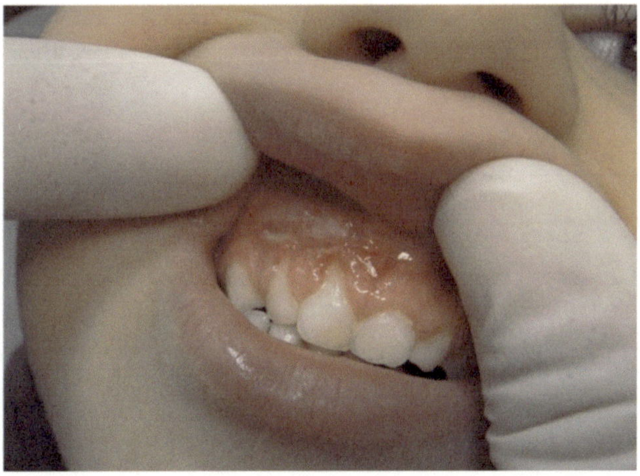

Figure 29.
Gum abrasion on teeth 51–52 in a 4-year-old patient.

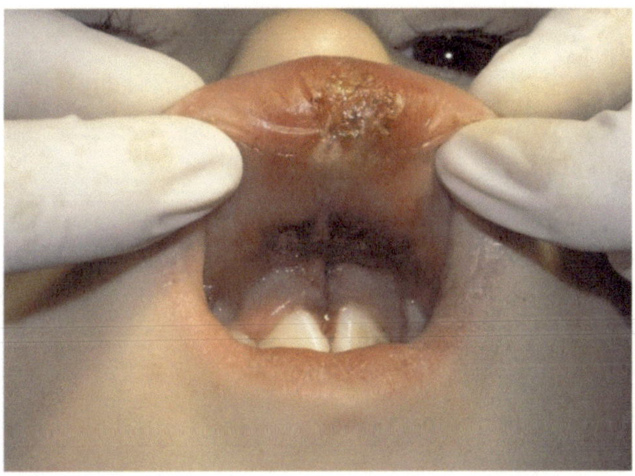

Figure 30.
Upper lip abrasion in a 7-year-old patient.

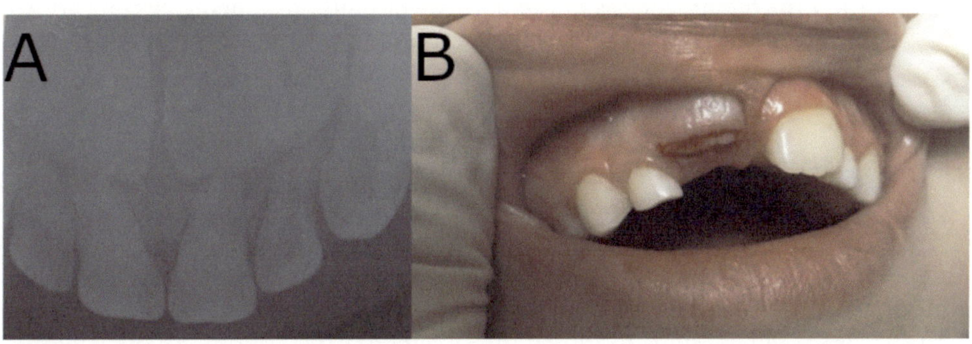

Figure 31.
Extraction of teeth 51 and 61 involved in a trauma with abrasion of the gum. Periapical radiography.

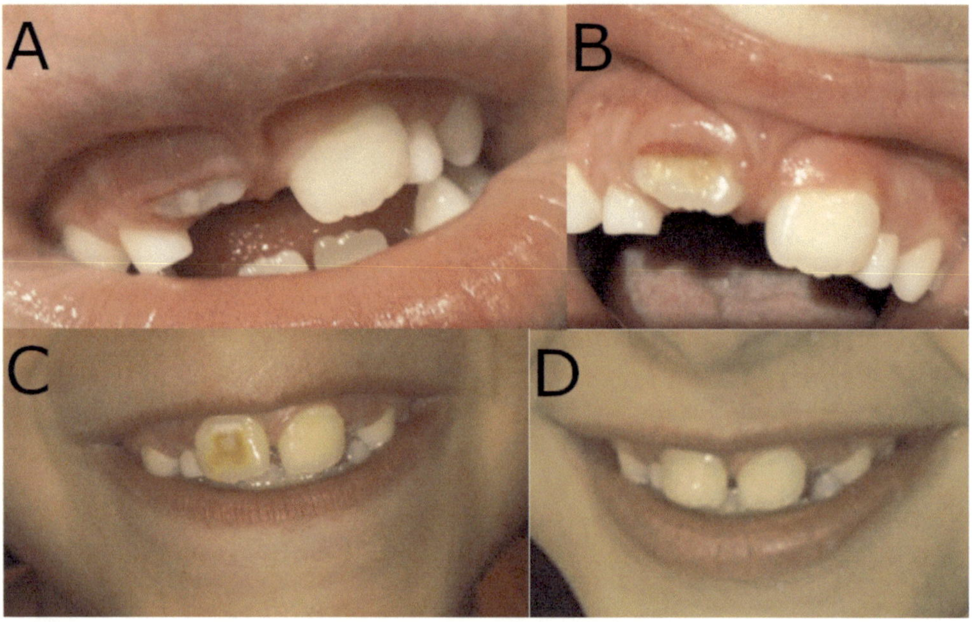

Figure 32.
Ulectomy. Eruptive delay of 11 by intrusion of 51 after 2 years. 48-hour and 7-day follow-up. Alteration in the structure and dyschromia due to impaction of the apex of tooth 51. Esthetic restoration of tooth 11, 6 years after the causing trauma.

b. If there is an impaction of the apex of the temporary tooth in the structures in formation of the permanent tooth, after eruption we may observe areas of hypoplasia, hypomineralization, dilacerations, or other alterations in the structure or tooth shape.

- Injuries resulting from an infection present over a period of time. Silent, long-term necrosis of the neurovascular bundle of the primary tooth may:

  a. Accelerate resorption of the primary tooth root and alter the timing of tooth replacement.

  b. Alter the odontogenesis of the permanent tooth, producing circumscribed chromatic lesions or structural alterations on the buccal surface of the crown of the permanent incisors (**Figure 32**) [35, 46–49].

7. Discussion

Crown fractures, regardless of the degree of involvement of the tooth, are the most common fractures in the permanent dentition. They are usually caused by contact sports or accidental falls.

In all cases, a radiographic examination should be carried out to provide an idea of the best therapeutic option in each case and to evaluate the surrounding tissues for any associated soft tissue lesions [9].

Treatment in cases of fissures limited to enamel usually consists of simply observing and monitoring the tooth or some authors even suggest sealing the enamel surface [9].

If the lesion affects enamel and dentine but there is no pulp involvement, there are several therapeutic options: if the fragment is available, it can be bonded to the tooth surface with the help of composite resins [9, 12] or the fractured segment can be directly restored with reconstructions made of composite resins [13, 14].

Finally, in the most complicated cases in which pulp tissue exposure occurs, it is necessary to evaluate whether the camera pulp or healthy root pulp can be maintained in those cases in which complete root development has not finalized [9, 14]. For this purpose, there are available different therapeutic options, depending on the pulp involvement, which are as follows:

- Direct pulp capping [15].
- Partial pulpotomy (Cvek pulpotomy) [16].
- Coronal pulpotomy [17].
- Deep pulpotomy [9, 18].

In those clinical situations in which the pulp is necrotic, the degree of root development will also be assessed, so that in teeth with an open apex, apexification with CaH or MTA [18–20] will be chosen, and in teeth with a closed apex, the relevant endodontic treatment will be carried out.

Intra-alveolar root fractures occur much less frequently than coronary fractures and even less frequently in the primary dentition or teeth with immature apex. They can be horizontal (better prognosis) or vertical (worse prognosis).

As with coronal fractures, it is essential to carry out a correct radiographic examination, modifying the degree of angulation of the fracture in multiple shots [9, 13]. Currently, CBCT (Cone Beam Computed Tomography) is also used for a correct diagnosis by image, which helps us to locate the fracture and even the direction and extent [12].

The treatment of intra-alveolar fractures depends mostly on the location of the fracture, but in any case, when possible, semi-rigid splinting of the fragments should be attempted [23]. Since vitality tests can be confusing at first, the treatment options available for intra-alveolar fractures are as follows:

- Endodontic treatment of the coronal fragment.
- Endodontic treatment of the coronal fragment and extraction of the apical fragment.
- Treatment of both fragments (coronal and apical).
- Treatment of the apical fragment and extraction of the coronal fragment [9].

The most relevant factors related to the prognosis of the avulsed teeth are the storage medium and the extra-oral dry time; therefore, previous studies have been conducted in order to assess the management procedures and behavior that are most recommendable in this scenario [63]. Zeissler-Lajtman et al. reported that cling film possibly could be used as an alternative transport medium for a storage period of up to 6 h [64]. However, De Brier et al. reported that although milk was shown to extend the periodontal ligament cell viability before replantation compared with saline or tap water, Hank's balanced salt solution, propolis, oral rehydration salts, rice water, and cling film media have also demonstrated efficacy at preserving the cell viability [65]. Additionally, Adnan et al. concluded that milk is the most recommended storage medium individually, based not only on PDL cell viability, but also practical considerations [66].

Moreover, the management procedures and making decisions after the accident comprising dental avulsion are also relevant for the long-term prognosis of these teeth. Therefore, some approaches have been performed in order to improve the attachment of the periodontal cells. Parthasarathy et al. performed an interdisciplinary approach to regenerate the osseous defect including the placement of PRF membrane around the root surface [68]. However, Schjøtt et al. analyzed the efficacy of Emdogain to promote regeneration of the periodontal tissues of avulsed teeth and reported that the teeth were all extracted, the ankylosis sites removed and the root and socket treated with Emdogain. After 6 months all teeth showed recurrence of ankylosis and concluded that Emdogain was not able to prevent or cure ankylosis [69]. Recently, Aksel et al. analyzed cell- or stem cell-based regenerative medicine and concluded that this approach has a promising future for the regeneration of periodontal regeneration of avulsed teeth [67].

Currently, studies agree that the highest prevalence of trauma in primary dentition is subluxation, followed by lateral dislocation and avulsion. This is due to the fact that, in children, the resistance capacity of the bone and the periodontal ligament is high given their elasticity and absorbs most of the energy of the impact, in addition, anatomically, the primary teeth have small crowns and short roots, trait that may favor dislocations over fractures.

It is important to know and establish an appropriate follow-up and/or treatment guideline in each case according to the complexity of the trauma. In fact, most of the sequelae derived from trauma are the consequence of inadequate treatment, lack of follow-up or not having acted within the necessary period of time.

Many times, this delay in the time of action is a consequence of the patient not coming to our consultations until a few weeks after the trauma. We must make parents and caregivers aware that in the event of any dental trauma, professional attention should be sought, since early diagnosis and treatment is essential, as well as monitoring the evolution of the case over time, to avoid unfavorable prognoses.

The international guidelines for dental traumatology agree that the early diagnosis and treatment of traumatisms will frequently determine the medium and long-term prognosis of the teeth involved in the trauma. For this reason, it is essential to have a clear action protocol that facilitates the dentist's decision-making to achieve an adequate immediate or deferred treatment based on the evidence, as well as a follow-up that allows early detection of an unfavorable evolution of the case, establishing a change in the mode of action. This will be the basis for the success of the treatment.

It should not be forgotten that even the slightest trauma to the primary dentition can have direct or indirect consequences on the permanent dentition given the close relationship between the apex of the root of the primary teeth and the permanent tooth in formation, and that these consequences they will be even more severe the younger the patient is at the time of impact due to the degree of immaturity in the formation of the permanent tooth germ. It is another of the key points that parents, caregivers and other health professionals must be made aware of so as not to downplay dental trauma in young patients [70].

8. Conclusions

In both types of fractures, a complete radiographic examination is essential for a proper diagnosis and treatment of the lesion. The surrounding tissues should always be evaluated regardless of the type of injury. In addition, one of the most decisive characteristics in terms of treatment is the degree of root development of the tooth and whether or not there is pulp exposure, characteristics which in most cases are what will indicate which treatment option will be more accurate.

It is recommended to maintain the avulsed teeth in a wet storage medium; preferably milk, Hank's Balanced Salt solution (HBSS), saliva, or saline solution and visit a dentist under 60 min after injury.

Dental trauma is the result of the interaction of many factors, so the success of treatment is unpredictable. Most professionals follow the general guidelines of the IADT to perform treatments on traumatized teeth, although clinical experience, good behavior management and continuous updating on the knowledge of trauma are essential for the dentist when it comes to treat and monitor these injuries.

Prevention and information on how to act at the scene of the accident by people close to the child is essential to carry out a favorable treatment, as well as instilling in the population the importance of going to a qualified professional whenever a fall or a blow is involved the oral cavity.

In this chapter we have tried to capture in a simple way the recommendations, most frequent situations and the most effective way of proceeding when dealing with trauma in primary dentition, as a result of the clinical experience of professionals in a reference center for diagnosis and treatment. of dental trauma emergencies and supported by the most current bibliography.

Conflict of interest

The authors declare no conflict of interest.

Author details

Blanca del Carmen Migueláñez Medrán[1], Nuria Delgado Castro[2], Elena Riad Deglow[3] and Álvaro Zubizarreta Macho[3,4]*

1 Faculty of Health Sciences, Alfonso X el Sabio University, Madrid, Spain

2 Department of Pediatric Dentistry, San Rafael Hospital, Madrid, Spain

3 Faculty of Health Sciences, Department of Implant Surgery, Alfonso X el Sabio University, Madrid, Spain

4 Faculty of Medicine, University of Salamanca, Department of Surgery, Spain

*Address all correspondence to: alvaro.zubizarreta@usal.es

IntechOpen

© 2022 The Author(s). Licensee IntechOpen. This chapter is distributed under the terms of the Creative Commons Attribution License (http://creativecommons.org/licenses/by/3.0), which permits unrestricted use, distribution, and reproduction in any medium, provided the original work is properly cited.

References

[1] Glendor U, Halling A, Andersson L, Eilert-Petersson E. Incidence of traumatic tooth injuries in children and adolescents in the county of Västmanland, Sweden. Swedish Dental Journal. 1996;**20**(1–2):15-28

[2] Andreasen JO, Andreasen FM, Tsilingaridis G. Avulsions. In: Andreasen JO, Andreasen FM, Andersson L, editors. Textbook and Color Atlas of Traumatic Injuries to the Teeth. Oxford: Wiley Blackwell; 2019. pp. 486-520

[3] Andersson L, Bodin I, Sörensen S. Progression of root resorption following replantation of human teeth after extended extraoral storage. Endodontics & Dental Traumatology. 1989;**5**(1): 38-47. DOI: 10.1111/j.1600-9657.1989.tb00335.x

[4] Andersson L, Bodin I. Avulsed human teeth replanted within 15 minutes—A long-term clinical follow-up study. Endodontics & Dental Traumatology. 1990;**6**(1):37-42. DOI: 10.1111/j.1600-9657.1990.tb00385.x

[5] Barrett EJ, Kenny DJ. Survival of avulsed permanent maxillary incisors in children following delayed replantation. Endodontics & Dental Traumatology. 1997;**13**(6):269-275. DOI: 10.1111/j.1600-9657.1997.tb00054.x

[6] Andreasen JO, Andreasen FM, Skeie A, Hjørting-Hansen E, Schwartz O. Effect of treatment delay upon pulp and periodontal healing of traumatic dental injuries—A review article. Dental Traumatology. 2002;**18**(3): 116-128. DOI: 10.1034/j.1600-9657.2002.00079.x

[7] Kargul B, Welbury R. An audit of the time to initial treatment in avulsion injuries. Dental Traumatology. 2009; **25**(1):123-125. DOI: 10.1111/j.1600-9657.2008.00732.x

[8] Bastos JV, de Souza I, Côrtes M, Andrade Goulart EM, Colosimo EA, Gomez RS, et al. Age and timing of pulp extirpation as major factors associated with inflammatory root resorption in replanted permanent teeth. Journal of Endodontia. 2014;**40**(3):366-371. DOI: 10.1016/j.joen.2013.10.009

[9] Berman LH, Blanco L, Cohen S. Manual clínico de traumatología dental. 1st ed. Madrid, España: Elsevier; 2008

[10] IDCDA. Application of the International Classification of Diseases to Dentistry and Stomatology IDCDA. 3rd ed. Geneva: WHO; 1995

[11] Bourguignon C, Cohenca N, Lauridsen E, Flores MT, O'Connell AC, Day PF, et al. International association of dental traumatology guidelines for the management of traumatic dental injuries: 1. Fractures and luxations. Dental Traumatology. 2020;**36**:314-330

[12] Andreasen FM, Andreasen JO. Crown fractures. In: Andreasen JO, Andreasen FM, Andersson L, editors. Textbook and Color Atlas of Traumatic Injuries to the Teeth. 4th ed. Oxford, UK: Blackwell; 2007. pp. 280-305

[13] Andreasen JO, Bakland LK, Flores MT, Andreasen FM, Andersson L. Traumatic Dental Injuries: A Manual. 3rd ed. Wiley-Blackwell: Chichester, UK; 2011

[14] Hilton TJ, Ferracane JL, Mancl L. Northwest practice-based research collaborative in evidence-based dentistry (NWP). Comparison of CaOH with

MTA for direct pulp capping: A PBRN randomized clinical trial. Journal of Dental Research. 2013;**92**(7 suppl):16-22

[15] Cvek M. Partial pulpotomy in crown-fractures incisors—Results 3 to 15 years after treatment. Acta Stomatologica Croatica. 1993;**27**:167-173

[16] Alqaderi H, Lee CT, Borzangy S, Pagonis TC. Coronal pulpotomy for cariously exposed permanent posterior teeth with closed apices: A systematic review and meta-analysis. Journal of Dentistry. 2016;**44**:1-7

[17] Jepsen K, Dommisch E, Jepsen S, Dommisch H. Vital root resection in severely furcation-involved maxillary molars: Outcomes after up to 7 years. Journal of Clinical Periodontology. 2020; **47**(8):970-979

[18] Guerrero F, Mendoza A, Ribas D, Aspiazu K. Apexification: A systematic review. Journal of Conservative Dentistry: JCD. 2018;**21**(5):462-465

[19] Nicoloso GF, Pötter IG, Rocha RO, Montagner F, Casagrande L. A comparative evaluation of endodontic treatments for immature necrotic permanent teeth based on clinical and radiographic outcomes: A systematic review and meta-analysis. International Journal of Paediatric Dentistry. 2017;**27**: 217-227

[20] Yadav P, Pruthi PJ, Naval RR, Talwar S, Verma M. Novel use of platelet-rich fibrin matrix and MTA as an apical barrier in the management of a failed revascularization case. Dental Traumatology. 2015;**31**:328-331

[21] Andreasen JO, Hjorting-Hansen E. Intra-alveolar root fractures: radiographic and histologic study of 50 cases. Journal of Oral Surgery. 1967;**25**: 414-426

[22] Fernandes M, De Ataide I, Wagle R. Tooth resorption part I – pathogenesis and case series of internal resorption. Journal of Conservative Dentistry: JCD. 2013;**16**(1):4-8

[23] Fernandes M, De Ataide I, Wagle R. Tooth resorption part II – external resorption: Case series. Journal of Conservative Dentistry: JCD. 2013;**16**(2): 180-185

[24] Flores MT, Al Sane M, Andersson L. Information to the public, patients and emergency services on traumatic dental injuries. In: Andreasen JO, Andreasen FM, Andersson L, editors. Textbook and Color Atlas of Traumatic Injuries to the Teeth. Oxford, UK: Wiley Blackwell; 2019. pp. 992-1008

[25] Adnan S, Lone MM, Khan FR, Hussain SM, Nagi SE. Which is the most recommended medium for the storage and transport of avulsed teeth? A systematic review. Dent Traumatol. 2018;**34**(2):59-70. DOI: 10.1111/edt.12382

[26] Andreasen JO. Effect of extra-alveolar period and storage media upon periodontal and pulpal healing after replantation of mature permanent incisors in monkeys. International Journal of Oral Surgery. 1981;**10**(1): 43-53. DOI: 10.1016/s0300-9785(81)80007-5

[27] Barbizam JV, Massarwa R, da Silva LA, da Silva RA, Nelson-Filho P, Consolaro A, et al. Histopathological evaluation of the effects of variable extraoral dry times and enamel matrix proteins (enamel matrix derivatives) application on replanted dogs' teeth. Dental Traumatology. 2015;**31**(1):29-34. DOI: 10.1111/edt.12131

[28] Fouad AF, Abbott PV, Tsilingaridis G, Cohenca N, Lauridsen E,

Bourguignon C, et al. International association of dental traumatology guidelines for the management of traumatic dental injuries: 2 Avulsion of permanent teeth. Dent Traumatol. 2020; **36**(4):331-342. DOI: 10.1111/edt.12573

[29] Kwan SC, Johnson JD, Cohenca N. The effect of splint material and thickness on tooth mobility after extraction and replantation using a human cadaveric model. Dental Traumatology. 2012;**28**(4):277-281. DOI: 10.1111/j.1600-9657.2011.01086.x

[30] Zeissler-Lajtman A, Connert T, Kühl S, Filippi A. Cling film as storage medium for avulsed teeth. An in vitro pilot study. Swiss Dent J. 2017;**127**(11): 954-959 Corrected and republished in: Swiss Dental Journal;**127**(11):960–963

[31] De Brier N, Dorien O, Borra V, Singletary EM, Zideman DA, De Buck E, et al. Storage of an avulsed tooth prior to replantation: A systematic review and meta-analysis. Dental Traumatology. 2020;**36**(5):453-476. DOI: 10.1111/edt.12564

[32] Parthasarathy R, Srinivasan S, Vikram C, Thanikachalam Y, Ramachandran A. An interdisciplinary management of avulsed maxillary incisors: A case report. Cureus. 2022; **14**(4):e23891. DOI: 10.7759/cureus.23891

[33] Schjøtt M, Andreasen JO. Emdogain does not prevent progressive root resorption after replantation of avulsed teeth: A clinical study. Dental Traumatology. 2005;**21**(1):46-50. DOI: 10.1111/j.1600-9657.2004.00295.x

[34] Aksel H, Zhu X, Gauthier P, Zhang W, Azim AA, Huang GT. A new direction in managing avulsed teeth: Stem cell-based de novo PDL regeneration. Stem Cell Research & Therapy. 2022;**13**(1):34. DOI: 10.1186/s13287-022-02700-x

[35] Boj JR, Catalá M, García Ballesta C, Mendoza A, Planells P. Odontopediatría. La evolución del niño al adulto joven. Vol. 28. Ripano and Ergón; 2011. pp. 361-363

[36] Barbería E. Atlas de odontología infantil para pediatras y odontólogos. Vol. 6. Ripano and Ergón; 2005. pp. 89-103

[37] Lam R. Epidemiology and outcomes of traumatic dental injuries: A review of the literature. Australian Dental Journal. 2016;**61**:4-20

[38] Pinkham JR, Casamassimo PS, McTigue DJ, Fields HW, Nowak AJ. Pediatric Dentistry. Infancy Through Adolescence. 4th ed. St Louis, Missouri: Elsevier Inc.; 2005. pp. 236-256

[39] Andreasen JO, Andreasen FM. Dental Traumatology: Quo-Vadis. Endodontics & Dental Traumatology. 1990;**6**:78

[40] Zaleckiene V, Peciuliene V, Brukiene V, Drukteinis S. Traumatic dental injuries: Etiology, prevalence and possible outcomes. Stomatologija. 2014; **16**(1):7-14

[41] Fried I, Erickson P, Schwartz S, Keenan K. Subluxation injuries of maxillary primary anterior teeth: Epidemiology and prognosis of 207 traumatized teeth. Pediatric Dentistry. 1996;**18**:145-151

[42] Holan G, Fuks AB. The diagnostic value of coronal dark gray discoloration in primary teeth following traumatic injuries. Pediatric Dentistry. 1996;**18**: 224-227

[43] Holan G. Development of clinical and radiographic signs associated with

dark discolored primary incisors following traumatic injuries: A prospective controlled study. Dental Traumatology. 2004;**20**:276-287

[44] Cardoso M, de Carvalho Rocha MJ. Association of crown discoloration and pulp status in traumatized primary teeth. Dental Traumatology. 2010;**26**: 413-416

[45] Holan G. Long-term effect of different treatment modalities for traumatized primary incisors presenting dark coronal discoloration with no other signs of injury. Dental Traumatology. 2006;**22**:14-17

[46] Borum MK, Andreasen JO. Sequelae of trauma to primary maxillary incisors. I. Complications in the primary dentition. Endodontics & Dental Traumatology. 1998;**14**:31-44

[47] Jácomo DRDES, Campos V. Prevalence of sequelae in the permanent anterior teeth after trauma in their predecessors: A longitudinal study of 8 years. Dental Traumatology. 2009;**25**: 300-304

[48] Ravn JJ. Developmental disturbances in permanent teeth after intrusion of their primary predecessors. Scandinavian Journal of Dental Research. 1976;**84**:137-141

[49] Christophersen P, Freund M, Harild L. Avulsion of primary teeth and sequelae on the permanent successors. Dental Traumatology. 2005;**21**:320-323

[50] García C, Mendoza A. Traumatología Oral en Odontopediatría. Diagnóstico y tratamiento integral. Ripano and Ergón; 2003. pp. 271-296

[51] Day P, Flores MT, O'Connell A, et al. International Association of Dental Traumatology guidelines for the management of traumatic dental injures: 3. Injuries in the primary dentition. Dental Traumatology. 2020;**36**:343-359

[52] Verdugo Lugo LR, Hachity Ortega JA, de Celis R, Quintan GN. Diagrama de flujo para trauamatismos en niños y adolescentes. Odontologia Pediatrica. 2021;**29**(1):11-22

[53] Flores MT. Traumatic injuries in the primary dentition. Dental Traumatology. 2002;**18**(6):287-298

[54] Moule A, Cohenca N. Emergency assessment and treatment planning for traumatic dental injuries. Australian Dental Journal. 2016;**61**:21-38

[55] Flores MT, Malmgren B, Andersson L, Andreasen JO, et al. International Association of Dental Traumatology. Guidelines for the management of traumatic dental injuries. III. Primary teeth. Dental Traumatology. 2007;**23**:196-202

[56] Nicolau B, Castonguay G, Madathil S, Vuong T, Almeida TDD. Periodontal diseases and traumatic dental injuries in the pediatric population. Pediatric Clinics of North America. 2018;**65**(5):1051-1061

[57] Azami-Aghdash S, Ebadifard Azar F, Pournaghi Azar F, et al. Prevalence, etiology, and types of dental trauma in children and adolescents: Systematic review and meta-analysis. Medical Journal of the Islamic Republic of Iran. 2015;**29**(4):234

[58] Flores MT, Holan G, Borum M, Andresen JO. Injuries to the primary dentition. In: Andreasen JO, Andreasen FM, Andersson L, editors. Textbook and Color Atlas of Traumatic Injuries to the Teeth. 4th ed. Oxford, UK: Blackwell Munksgaard; 2007. pp. 516-541

[59] Malmgren B, Andreasen JO, Flores MT, et al. International Association of Dental Traumatology. Guidelines for the management of traumatic dental injuries. Injuries in the primary dentition. Dental Traumatology. 2012;**28**(3):174-182

[60] Cohenca N, Silberman A. Contemporary imaging for the diagnosis and treatment of traumatic dental injuries: A review. Dental Traumatology. 2017;**33**:321-328

[61] Needleman HL. The art and science of managing traumatic injuries to primary teeth. Dental Traumatology. 2011;**27**:295-299

[62] Rocha MJ, Cardoso M. Survival analysis of endodontically treated traumatized primary teeth. Dental Traumatology. 2007;**23**:340-347

[63] Avsar A, Topaloglu B. Traumatic tooth injuries to primary teeth of children aged 0–3 years. Dental Traumatology. 2009;**25**:323-327

[64] Cunha RF, Pugliesi DM, Percinoto C. Treatment of traumatized primary teeth: A conservative approach. Dental Traumatology. 2007;**23**:360-363

[65] Kupietzky A, Holan G. Treatment of crown fractures with pulp exposure in primary incisors. Pediatric Dentistry. 2003;**25**:241-247

[66] Rocha MJ, Cardoso M. Federal University of Santa Catarina endodontic treatment of traumatized primary teeth—Part 2. Dental Traumatology. 2004;**20**:314-326

[67] Colak I, Markovic D, Petrovic B, Peric T, Milenkovic A. A retrospective study of intrusive injuries in primary dentition. Dental Traumatology. 2009; **25**:605-610

[68] Andreasen JO, Bakland LK, Flores MT, Andreasen FM, Andersson L. Traumatic Dental Injuries: A Manual. 3rd ed. Chichester, UK: Wiley-Blackwell; 2011. pp. 54-57

[69] Altun C, Cehreli ZC, Güven G, Acikel C. Traumatic intrusion of primary teeth and its effects on the permanent successors a clinical follow-up study. Oral Surgery, Oral Medicine, Oral Pathology, Oral Radiology, and Endodontics. 2009;**107**:493-498

[70] Spinas E, Melis A, Savasta A. Therapeutic approach to intrusive luxation injuries in primary dentition. A clinical follow-up study. European Journal of Paediatric Dentistry. 2006;7: 179-186

Chapter 4

Perspective Chapter: Teeth Avulsion

Manal Abdalla Eltahir, Randa Fath Elrahman Ibrahim and Hanan Alharbi

Abstract

Tooth avulsion refers to total displacement of the tooth out of its alveolar socket. This chapter discusses the causes of avulsion for both primary and permanent dentition in addition to the prevalence of avulsion comparing it between before and during COVID-19 era. Successful outcomes depend on procedure conduction with immediate replantation of the avulsed tooth and good handling of the tooth keeping the tooth in suitable available storage media till a professional service is obtainable. Management of this type of dental trauma necessitates awareness and collaboration between the lay personal at the site of injury in addition to the important role of different dental professional. After replantation of the avulsed tooth, it should be kept immobile with preservation of the functional (physiological) mobility by application of suitable splint. There are adjunctive therapies including antibiotics, analgesics, mouth washes, and tetanus vaccines. Endodontic therapy should be initiated within 7–10 days from the time of avulsion, where the outcomes generally might be favorable or unfavorable. Newly emergent teledentistry played important role in the treatment of tooth avulsion, especially during COVID-19 period.

Keywords: avulsion, replantation, storage media, antibiotic, splinting, open apex, closed apex, trauma, dental emergency, teledentistry, tooth replantation

1. Introduction

Tooth avulsion is a very serious traumatic dental injury (TDI) as tooth loss may remarkably compromise the patient in both functional and psychological aspects [1, 2].

Among all dental traumas, avulsion of the permanent tooth accounts for up to 16% of all dental injuries and constitutes the most serious one. It is considered as one of the few emergency situations in dentistry [3]. By definition, tooth avulsion refers to the total displacement of the tooth out of its alveolar socket (**Figure 1**) [4]. Presence of the tooth outside the socket leads to deterioration of the pulp and periodontal ligaments (PDLs) due to the lack of blood and nerve supply to their cells in addition to the unfavorable external environment such as dryness and possible contamination [5]. This may end up with periodontal attachment damage, pulp necrosis, and eventually tooth loss [6]. The maxillary central incisors are the most frequently involved teeth; boys and the age group of 7–11 years old are more susceptible to this type of trauma [7].

IntechOpen

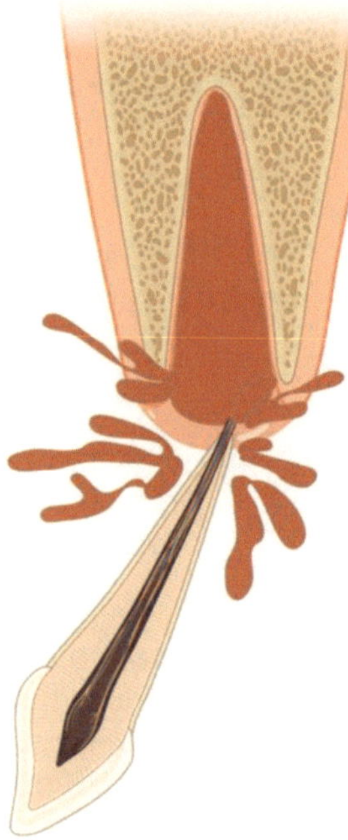

Figure 1.
Tooth avulsion refers to the total displacement of the tooth out of its alveolar socket.

1.1 Epidemiology of avulsed teeth before and during COVID-19 pandemic

The prevalence and incidence of reported traumatic dental injuries (TDIs) have significantly been affected during COVID-19 pandemic. In a retrospective analysis conducted at King's College Hospital Dental Institute in London, UK, there was around 46% reduction in presented cases with TDIs during the COVID-19 compared to the year before for the same period of time [8]. With respect to avulsion injuries, the study revealed a remarkable decline in cases by around 93%. It also showed an increase in the mean delay in presentation following TDIs from 2.4 days the year before to 5.3 days during COVID-19 [8]. The reasons behind these changes were mostly related to the lockdown and forcible closure of dental practices during the pandemic. Although the urgent dental cares services in hospitals were mostly available worldwide, patients were hesitant to reach out to such centers due to the perceived fear of acquiring viral infections. Other studies also showed the same steep reduction in reported TDIs and traumatic injuries generally during COVID-19 [8–10].

According to previous studies, demographic data of reported cases has not differed between COVID-19 and years before except having less admitted cases in group age older than 70-year-old [8].

1.2 Causes

The etiology of tooth avulsion varies according to the type of dentition. Avulsion in primary dentition is typically a result of hard objects hitting the teeth, whereas avulsion in permanent dentition is generally a result of falls, fights, sport injuries, automobile or bicycle accidents, and domestic abuse. In permanent and primary dentition, avulsion generally occurs in the maxilla, and the most affected teeth are the maxillary central incisors (**Figure 2**). Increased overjet and incompetent lips were identified as potential etiological factors in such avulsion cases [11–13]. In rare cases, iatrogenic teeth avulsion during other procedures might happen and were reported in the literature [14–17].

2. Management of the avulsed tooth

Several factors should be considered [18], when treating a patient with an avulsed permenant tooth (**Figure 3**):

1. Patient's age

2. Medical status

3. Root development

4. Development of the dentition and of the face

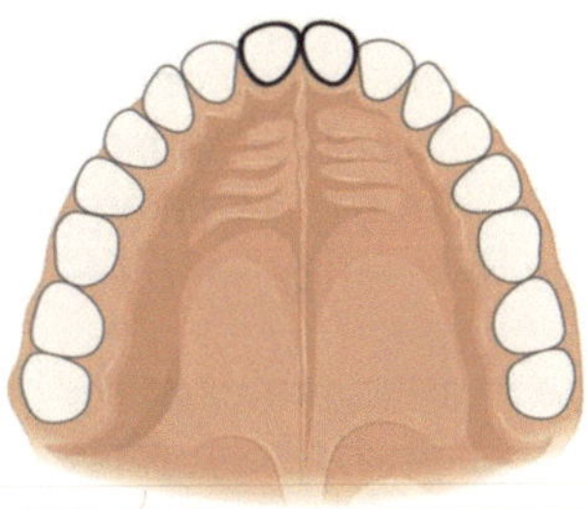

Figure 2.
Maxillary central incisors are the most frequently involved teeth in avulsions.

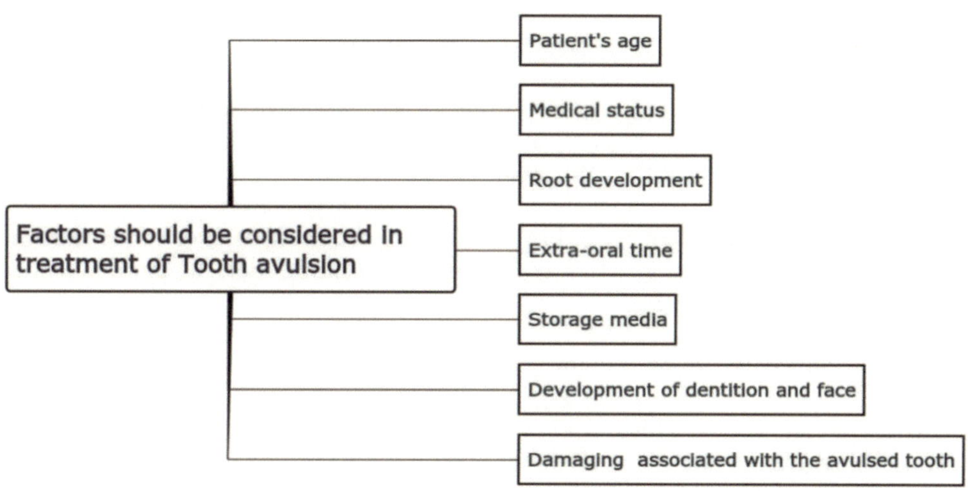

Figure 3.
Factors should be considered in the treatment of tooth avulsion.

5. Extra-oral time

6. Storage medium

7. Damage associated with the avulsed tooth

2.1 Emergency treatment/management (at the site/and at the clinic)

Multidisciplinary approach in avulsion injuries is essential and considered a cornerstone during the management process. Though the management of avulsions is highly dependent on the early actions taken following the trauma and the time spent till reaching out healthcare services, this is furthermore affected during COVID-19 pandemic due to international lockdowns and restricted accessibility to hospitals. Such times clearly signify the importance of public awareness of first-aid measures in TDIs, especially avulsion.

International guidelines have been proposed to address TDIs and avulsions injuries. According to the International Association of Dental Traumatology (IADT) guidelines [19–21] and the European Society of Endodontology position statement [22], certain systematic approach has to be adopted to treat teeth avulsions. Obviously, tooth avulsion leads to necrosis of disrupted pulp which requires endodontic treatment.

We will be talking about the management for teeth avulsion and treatment choices during COVID-19. Best approach to treat an avulsed permanent tooth is immediate replantation. Whether the case is admitted to emergency clinic or people at trauma site are instructed on phone, the following steps are to be considered:

- Take self-precautions while treating others at the emergency cite including wearing masks and personal protective equipment (PPE) if possible, to avoid viral infections. However, gold standard treatment always should be provided, even if dental aerosol-generating procedures (AGPs) are likely to be involved [23].

- Calm the patient down.

- Always aim for immediate replantation. If replantation cannot be done at the trauma site by surrounding peoples/parents/others, the tooth has to be stored as soon as possible in a storage media; milk, Hanks' Balanced Salt Solution (HBSS), saliva, saline, or water. This is to avoid root surface dehydration. Then tooth can be replanted immediately at the emergency clinic.

- Before replantation, tooth could be rinsed under running milk or saline to clean any dirt. It must be hold by the crown without touching root. Replanting primary teeth is contraindicated.

- After tooth replantation, patient is asked to bite on gauze.

History: Review patient history in case of any other injury (potentially more serious) is involved, simultaneously. If any vomiting, headache, unconsciousness, or drowsiness are reported, this should be further investigated at the hospital, and also, if there is a previous injury to the teeth or the alveolar bone or if the occlusion has further changed.

How, when, and where the trauma/accident happened are all questions that should be answered. This will further help in evaluating the trauma for legal and insurance purposes. Any suspected abuse should be reported to local authority.

Anesthesia: administering local anesthesia is always recommended, preferably without vasoconstrictor [20].

Recent guidelines have detailed the plan on replanting tooth according to two main factors:

1. Extra-oral dry time: being less or more than 60 min.

2. Root maturation: closed or open apex.

For extra-oral dry time, it is used to assess periodontal ligament (PDL) cells' viability. The soonest the tooth is replanted, within 15 min, the most likely PDL cells are viable. When the extra-oral dry time exceeds 60 min, it is more likely that PDL cells are nonviable. In all situations, it is recommended to replant the tooth acknowledging that prognosis is best when replantation is within 15 min and poorest when it is after 60 min [20]. Ankylosis-related (replacement) root resorption is an expected outcome in cases of late tooth replantation [18, 20, 24].

2.2 Factors might influence the success of replantation

These factors are the patient's general health, the maturity of the root, the time the tooth is out of its socket, storage medium [11, 25–27], extra-alveolar permanence period, means of preservation, contamination, manipulation, and conditions of the avulsed tooth [28], and also relevant factors such as type of splint used and time of permanence (**Figures 4** and 5).

2.3 Storage media

Successful healing after replantation may occur only if the damage to the PDL cells was minimal. Immediate replantation of the avulsed tooth into the socket at the site of the trauma has been suggested to prevent further damage to the PDL cells left on the root surface from desiccation. As this is not always attainable since the lay person at the trauma site may lack the skill and the willingness to try this procedure. In such situations, it is recommended to put the avulsed tooth temporarily in a storage medium capable of preserving PDL cells viability. Thus, the extra-alveolar dry time and the type of storage medium are the most critical factors. Prolonging the duration of dry storage causes necrosis of the PDL cells after 30–60 min and decreases greatly the chances of healing after replantation [29].

2.3.1 Characteristics of the ideal storage medium [29]

- No or minimal microbial contamination.

- Readily available or accessible.

- Physiologically compatible pH and osmolality to maintaining PDL cell viability.

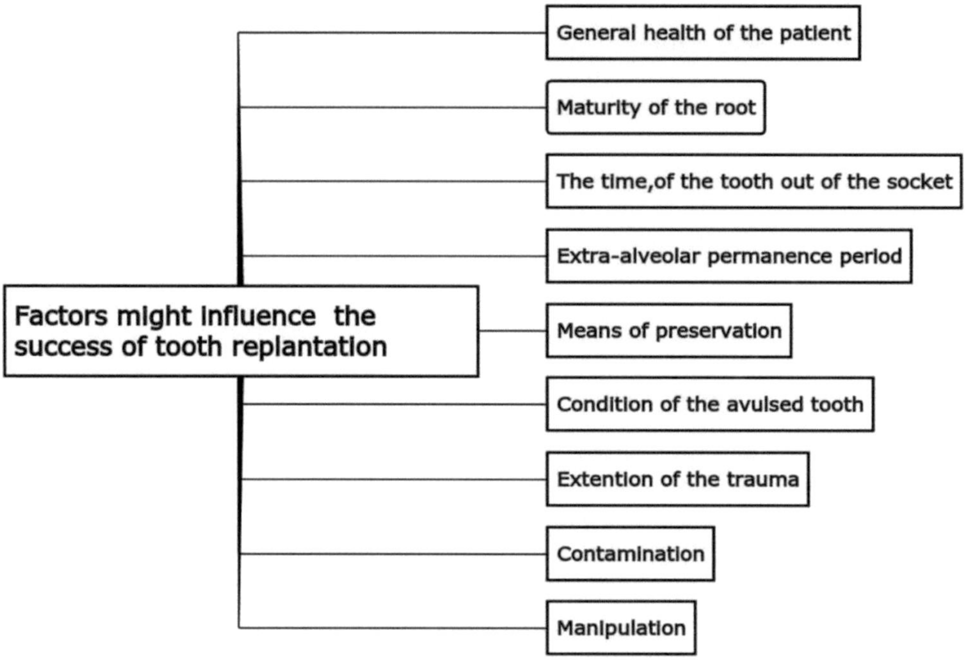

Figure 4.
Factors might influence the success of tooth replantation.

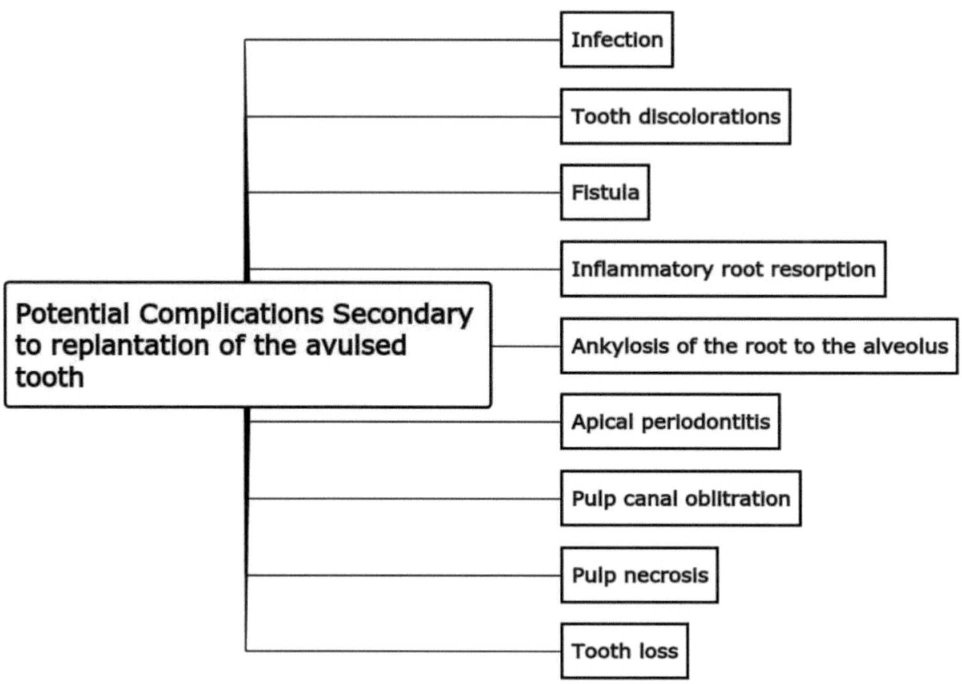

Figure 5.
Potential complications following tooth replantation.

- The pH of the environment should be around 6.6–7.8 to maintain cell growth.
- Optimal osmolality is 230–400 mOsmol/kg.21 as it affects water absorption of the cells.

2.3.2 Types of storage media

In their quest for an ideal storage media, a wide variety of materials have been tested by a lot of researchers for their role as potential storage media. The recent guidelines of IADT recommend in descending order of preference, milk, HBSS (Hanks' Balanced Salt Solution), saliva, or saline as suitable and convenient storage mediums. Water is considered a poor medium but is better than dry storage. Other materials, some with promising results, include ViaSpan, propolis, and egg white [20, 30].

2.3.2.1 Milk

Many authorities recognized milk as the most recommended storage medium for avulsed teeth. The ease of obtaining it at accident sites makes it a practical choice. The physiological properties of milk are significantly better than other solutions, and pH (6.5–7.2) and osmolality (270 mOsm/kg) are compatible with PDL cells. Milk contains a combination of nutritional substances such as amino acids, carbohydrates, and vitamins capable of maintaining PDL cell viability. In addition, the presence of epithelial growth factor stimulates the proliferation and regeneration of epithelial cell rests of Malassez and activates the alveolar bone resorption. Hence, the bone tissue may be isolated from the tooth and decreases the chances of ankylosis [30, 31]. However, it should be noted that few reports argued that replanted teeth stored in milk were subject to ankylosis [32–34].

2.3.2.2 HBSS (Hanks' Balanced Salt Solution)

The HBSS is a sterile, isotonic, and physiologically balanced standard saline solution which is used in biomedical research to support the growth of many cell types. It is a nontoxic solution, biocompatible with PDL cells; its pH (7.2) and osmolality (320 mOsm/kg) are balanced and considered almost ideal. It is composed of glucose, sodium, calcium, potassium, and magnesium ions.

HBSS is highly recommended for its ability to provide long-term preservation of PDL cells viability and proliferation capacity. Its ingredients may further help to reconstitute the depleted cellular components of the PDL. HBSS is commercially available as "Save-A-Tooth." However, it is not found at most of the accident sites; this makes it an impractical storage medium [20, 29, 31, 32, 34].

2.3.2.3 Saliva

The only advantage of saliva as a storage media is its ease of availability immediately on almost all accident sites. However, it presents a possible source of bacterial contamination for PDL cells. Its osmolality (60–70 mOsm/kg) is considerably lower than the physiological osmolality; thus, cells stored in saliva show swelling and membrane damage. Saliva is better than tap water or dry storage, but it can be used only for very short storage time [29–31].

2.3.2.4 Saline

Normal saline, a 0.90% NaCl solution, has a physiological osmolality of 280 mOsm/kg which is compatible with the PDL cells. However, it is deficient in the essential nutrients, such as glucose, magnesium, and calcium which are needed to the normal metabolic functions of the cells of the PDL. Moreover, the hypotonic properties of saline induce rapid cellular lysis. Therefore, saline is not a good storage media unless for short periods only [29, 31].

2.3.2.5 Viaspan

Viaspan is a cell culture media widely used for storing and transporting organs to be transplanted. It has 320 mOsm/kg osmolality and 7.4 pH which favors cell growth and viability of the PDL cells. It is nearly an ideal material for storage of avulsed teeth for long periods. However, its high cost, short vitality expiration, and the limited access to it especially at the accident sites make it difficult to find and use this storage medium [31, 35].

2.3.2.6 Egg white

Egg white is considered a good storage media because of its high protein content, vitamins, and water. It is easily accessible and lacks microbial contamination with a pH of 8.6–9.3 and osmolality of 258 mOsmol/kg. Thus, it favors PDL cells viability and healing and presents a suitable choice for extended storage time [29, 31].

2.3.2.7 Tap water

Tap water has an approximate osmolality of 30 mOsm/kg and a pH of 7.4–7.79. It is not considered a suitable storage medium for avulsed teeth. It has bacterial contamination; its hypotonicity and nonphysiologically pH and osmolality favor the PDL cell lysis. Cells stored in water did not maintain their viability. However, it is better than dry storage and should be used only when there are no other alternatives (**Table 1** and **Figure 6**) [29, 31].

Storage media	Osmolality (mOsmo/kg)	pH	Efficacy	Accessibility
Milk	270	6.5–7.2	✓	✓
HBSS	270–290	7.2–7.3	✓	
Saliva	60–70	6.3		✓
Saline	280	7		✓
Viaspan	320	7.4	✓	
Egg white	258	8.6–9.3	✓	✓
Tap water	30	7.4 7.79		✓

Table 1.
Characteristics of storage media.

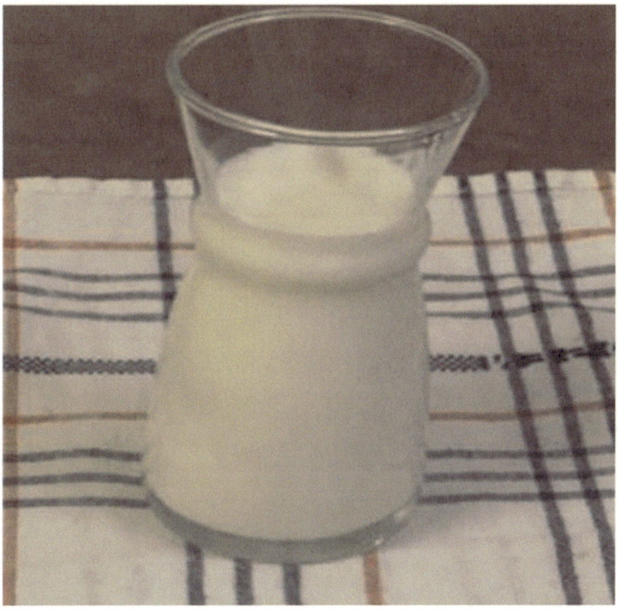

Figure 6.
Milk as storage media.

2.4 Splinting

After replantation, the treatment of choice is splinting [2]. By definition, splinting is an assembly to protect, stabilize, and immobilize loosened, fractured, replanted, and traumatized teeth [3]. Also splinting is defined by American Association of Endodontists as "a rigid or flexible device or compound used to support, protect, or immobilize teeth that have been loosened, replanted, fractured, or subjected to certain endodontic procedures" [36].

To allow immobilization of the teeth during the initial period, it is mandatory using the so-called splint which is essential for the repair of periodontal ligament [37]. The use of semirigid splint is more indicated than the rigid one, considering that the long period of splinting is not recommended due to its expected complications namely substitutive resorption or ankylosis [38, 39]. One of the adverse healing outcomes of splinting is that forceful placement of the splint may cause additional trauma to the already affected pulp of the avulsed tooth [40].

2.4.1 Types of splints

Many different splinting techniques have been described [41]:

Wire-composite splint, orthodontic splint, titanium trauma splint (TTS) splint, resin splint, Kevlar/fiberglass splint (fiberglass), self-etching and bonding material, and suture splint.

Kahler et al. also described splint types [42]:

- Composite and wire splints.
- Composite and fishing line splints.

- Orthodontic wire and bracket splint 0.3–0.4 mm in diameter.
- Fiber splints (polyethylene or Kevlar fiber mesh).
- Titanium trauma splint (TTS).
- Arch bar splints.
- Wire ligature splints.
- Composite splints.

Semirigid/flexible (physiologic) [43]:

- Orthodontic brackets and arches.
- Wire and composite splints.
- Fiber splints.
- Titanium trauma splints (TTS).

In cases of associated alveolar or jawbone fracture, a more rigid splint is indicated and should be left in place for about 4 weeks.

Cap splints and orthodontic bands were associated with a greater frequency of pulp necrosis and pulp canal obliteration when compared with acid etch resin splints and no splinting [44].

These splinting techniques were used prior to the development of a passively

- applied acid etch resin technique and are no longer recommended [20]
- according to the recent guidline, 2020 [20].

Stabilize the tooth for 2 weeks using a passive flexible splint such as wire of a diameter up to 0.016″ or 0.4 mm bonded to the tooth and adjacent teeth. Keep the composite and bonding agents away from the gingival tissues and proximal areas. Second option is nylon fishing line (0.13–0.25 mm) which can be used to create a flexible splint, using composite to bond it to the teeth. Nylon (fishing line) splints are not recommended for children with mixed dentition, since the status of the other teeth may result in instability or loss of such splint.

2.4.2 Management of the soft tissues and surrounding alveolar bone

Tooth-supporting tissue injuries and lip injuries may be associated with avulsion [45].

Soft tissue tearing of the socket gingiva associated with avulsed tooth should be noted [46].

There are three benefits may be gained from the tight stitching of such tearing [47]:

1. Stop of the bleeding.
2. Avoid the penetration of microorganism into periodontium.
3. Allow the primary healing of the wound.

In addition to the soft tissue, the socket itself needs to be manipulated before replantation of the root, if the alveolar bone has collapsed, attempts should be made to reconstruct its wall [48].

2.5 In clinic treatment

2.5.1 Root canal treatment in avulsed teeth

2.5.1.1 Closed apex

It is mandatory to initiate root canal treatment within 2 weeks of tooth replantation [20, 22]. Root canal treatment should start with intracanal medication; calcium hydroxide or antibiotic-corticosteroid paste dressing for 2 weeks up to 1 month or 6 weeks [49, 50] is followed by root canal filling.

2.5.1.2 Open apex

No root canal treatment is performed at first, but a close follow-up is needed to detect any clinical or radiographic signs of pulp necrosis. The aim is to re-establish blood supply of open apices and maintain root development which could happen spontaneously after replantation.

Radiographic and clinical examination is indicted after 2 weeks, 4 weeks, 6–8 weeks, 3 months, 6 months, 1 year, and yearly thereafter for at least 5 years. If there is any sign of external infection-related root resorption, endodontics intervention is advised whether it is apexification, root canal treatment, or regenerative endodontic procedures (REPs) [20, 22, 48].

2.5.2 Regenerative/revitalization procedures and avulsions

REPs have been proposed based on translational studies. In 2016, American Association of Endodontists and European Society of Endodontology have proposed clinical considerations and position statement; respectively, discussing REPs [51]. In avulsion injuries, REPs are only indicated in cases of immature root with open apex and signs of pulp necrosis. The clinical protocol is the same that have been proposed previously in the mentioned guidelines. A recent report implemented this approach to treat avulsed tooth and showed successful outcome with a 30-month follow-up [52]. The key is using biocompatible materials that would recruit stem cells to build hard tissue barriers and allow physiological growth of roots. Biocompatible materials could be MTA or tricalcium silicate cements, e.g. bioceramicsm that revealed successful outcomes in several reports [53].

3. Adjunctive therapy

3.1 Antibiotic use

Antibiotics given at the time of replantation to prevent the infection may occur due to tooth contamination or may be present in the storage media. Also, it can be prescribed prior to endodontic treatment. It is theoretically effective in preventing bacterial invasion of the necrotic pulp and; further, it may prevent the inflammatory resorption (**Figure** 7) [54].

In all cases, appropriate dosage for the patient's age and weight should be calculated.

Amoxicillin or penicillin remains the first choice due to their effectiveness on oral flora and low incidence of side effects. Alternative antibiotics should be considered for patients with an allergy to penicillin [55].

The effectiveness of tetracycline administered immediately after avulsion and replantation has been demonstrated in animal study [56, 57]. Specifically, doxycycline is an appropriate antibiotic to use because of its antimicrobial, anti-inflammatory, and anti-resorptive effects. But still doxycycline exerted no effect on the occurrence of complete pulp revascularization in replanted teeth [58]. Tetracycline or doxycycline is generally not recommended for patients under 12 years of age to avoid the risk of discoloration of permanent teeth [20, 56, 57].

3.1.1 Indications of antibiotics in patients with avulsed tooth

By searching the literature so far, there are some indications of antibiotic prescribed for the patient with avulsed tooth (**Figure 8**).

1. Replanted tooth with possibly contaminated root and/or storage media [20, 54] for medically compromised patient.

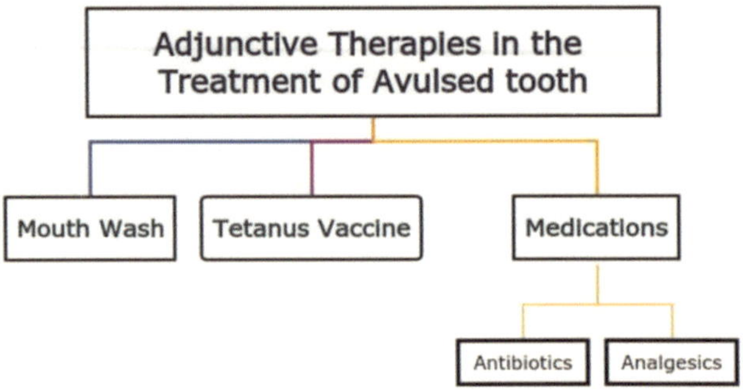

Figure 7.
Adjunctive therapies in the treatment of avulsed tooth.

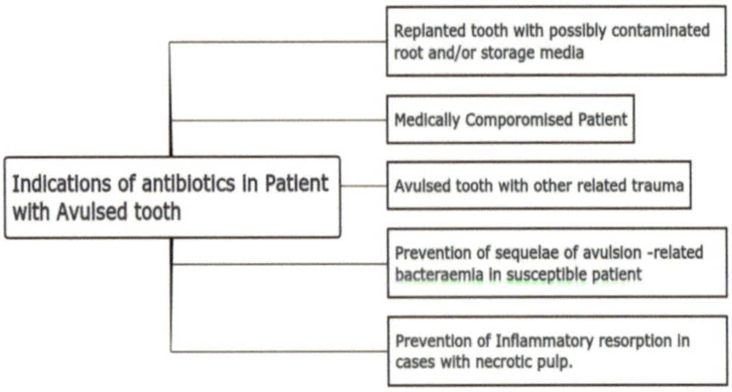

Figure 8.
Indication of antibiotics in patient with avulsed tooth.

2. Avulsed tooth with other related trauma [20].

3. Prevention of sequalae of avulsion-related bacteremia in the susceptible patients [59].

4. Prevention of inflammatory resorption in cases with necrotic pulp (tetracycline with its antimicrobial and anti-resorptive effect) [58].

3.2 Analgesic

Prescription of analgesic is case-dependent; accordingly, it should be assessed individually. The use of stronger pain killer is unlikely [20, 48].

3.3 Mouth wash

Chlorhexidine (CHX) is a commonly used antiseptic mouthwash and is available over the counter (OTC); the use of adjunctive short-term of CHX can enhance oral hygiene by managing dental plaque [60].

The recent recommendation is to use a chlorhexidine (0.12%) mouth rinse twice a day for 2 weeks (during the entire period of splinting).

3.4 Tetanus vaccine

The possibility of environmental contamination of the injury can justify the administration of tetanus vaccine [19].

The patient should be sent to a physician for consultation regarding a tetanus booster within 48 h of the initial visit [20].

4. Alternative treatment

4.1 Decoronation

In cases of severe replacement resorption (RR) and ankylosis, decoronation can be considered as an alternative treatment with good clinical outcomes for children and adolescents to the age when an appropriate implant is possible. If carried out at the right time; it helps to preserve the bucco-palatal dimensions of the alveolar bone and at the same time allows for vertical bone growth. This enables for future implant insertion without the need for the costly and invasive procedure of alveolar ridge augmentation. However, this approach still needs solid studies to verify it [61, 62].

Timing of the decoronation is crucial and should be planned for each individual case with regard to the patient's age, growth intensity, and growth pattern. In young patients, it is advantageous to retain an ankylosed tooth, if possible, to act as a space maintainer. However, it is very necessary to intervene before the effect of infraposition causes significant arrested alveolar bone growth that makes a final prosthetic solution difficult. When ankylosis is diagnosed before the age of 10 years, there is a high risk of severe infraposition, and the tooth should be carefully monitored every 6 months. There is also a risk of severe infraposition during the pubertal growth spurt which varies in time from one person to another and thus needs also careful monitoring [63].

Clinically, the procedure is simple. Under local anesthesia and a full-thickness flap, the crown of the ankylosed tooth is sectioned earlier the cementoenamel junction. The root is cleaned with a K-file and washed with saline, and the canal is allowed to fill with blood and then the flap is repositioned. Subsequently, esthetics is maintained using an adhesive bridge [62].

4.2 Autotransplantation

Autotransplantation of an immature maxillary premolar to replace an ankylosed tooth is considered a highly successful alternative technique and is particularly indicated when crowding requires extraction of a premolar. To achieve pulpal revascularization and successful periodontal healing of the donor tooth, the ideal root should develop to three-fourths of the complete root length. In such cases, the whole root of the ankylosed tooth must be extracted, and a premolar will be transplanted in its place. The transplant tooth with its sound periodontal ligament will induce new bone formation, have continued root development, and even maintain its vitality. An esthetic restoration and orthodontic treatment will follow the transplant [64, 65].

4.3 Partial prosthesis/dental implant

4.3.1 Prognosis and outcomes

The long-term prognosis of replanted avulsed teeth shows great variability; the observed outcomes are greatly heterogeneous ranging from healing without symptoms to inflammation and rapid tooth loss. Many studies had shown a relatively low survival rate of replanted avulsed teeth, compared to other types of traumata, ranging from 50% to 83.3% [66]. Under favorable conditions, replanted teeth may be retained for 5 or 10 years and even few of them for a lifetime. However, some may fail very soon after replantation.

4.3.2 Factors associated with unfavorable outcomes and low survival rate [65]:

- Delayed replantation
- Unphysiological storage
- Teeth with open apices

After replantation of the tooth, the prognosis commonly remains uncertain. Replacement resorption and inflammatory resorption are probable adverse outcomes in comparison with the more favorable functional healing (FH): [66]

- **Functional healing**

The damaged tissues including the cementum and dentin are being resorbed by multinuclear giant cells. In regions with minor damage, the ruptured periodontal fibers are being rebuilt (regeneration). In case of small resorption cavities, the denuded root surface is being recolonized by neighboring cementoblasts and these deposit the cementum in which the new periodontal fibers are anchored. This process represents healing with physiologic function (functional healing, FH) [66, 67].

- **Inflammatory (infection-related) root resorption**

Root surfaces affected by the trauma are quickly colonized by multinuclear giant cells. If these cells are continuously stimulated by microbial products from an infected root canal, not adequately treated, infection-related resorption (IRR, formerly named inflammatory resorption) will result. Provided the tooth is still restorable, adequate endodontic treatment might stop the progression of IRR.

- **Replacement resorption (ankylosis) (Figure 9)**

Replacement resorption is a special form of root resorption, and it follows serious luxation or avulsion injury. It is a common sequela of delayed replantation and/or dry storage. Due to excessive drying before replantation, the damaged periodontal ligament cells will start an inflammatory response over extended areas on the root surface. The resulting large resorption cavities may not be entirely covered by the cementoblasts in time. Regenerating alveolar bone will be attached directly onto the root surface. In time, through physiologic bone remodeling, the root cementum and dentin will be replaced by bone; a process termed replacement resorption (RR) or ankylosis-related root resorption [65–67].

If revascularization does not occur or appropriate endodontic therapy is not performed after tooth replantation, pulpal necrosis will occur. The combination of microbes in the root canal and the external surface of the root results in aggressive resorption and can lead to rapid tooth loss [20, 65].

In a growing patient and/or tooth with open apices, the ankylosed tooth shows severe and progressive infraocclusion. The alveolar bone will stop advancing in a coronal direction with the rest of the jaw leaving a big bone defect when the tooth is eventually lost causing major esthetic and functional challenges when it is time for the final replacement [48, 67].

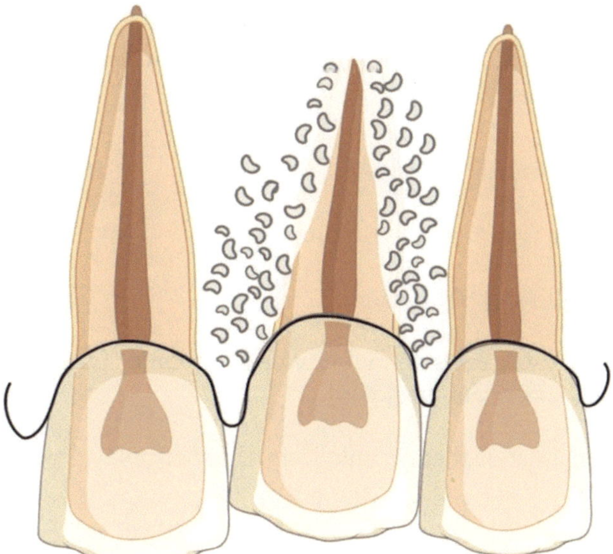

Figure 9.
Replacement root resorption (ankylosis).

5. Follow-up

Mature replanted teeth need clinical and radiographic monitoring at 2 weeks (with splint removal), 4 weeks, 3 months, 6 months, 1 year, and hence yearly for at least 5 years. For teeth with open apices where spontaneous pulp revascularization might occur, clinical and radiographic monitoring should be more frequent due to the high risk of infection-related (inflammatory) and/or ankylosis-related (replacement) root resorption. Therefore, replanted teeth with open apices should have clinical and radiographic monitoring at 2 weeks (with splint removal), 1 month, 2 months, 3 months, 6 months, 1 year, and hence yearly for at least 5 years [20].

Evaluation may include the following outcomes:

5.1 Favorable outcomes

The replanted tooth is

- Asymptomatic, functional,
- normal mobility,
- no sensitivity to percussion,
- normal percussion sound,
- no radiolucencies and no radiographic evidence of root resorption. The lamina dura appears normal.
- In addition, for teeth with open apices, radiographic evidence of continued root formation and tooth eruption.

Pulp canal obliteration is expected and can be recognized radiographically sometime during the first year after the trauma.

5.2 Unfavorable outcomes

- Patient may or may not have symptoms.
- Presence of swelling or sinus tract.
- The tooth may have excessive mobility or no mobility (ankylosis) with high-pitched (metallic) percussion sound.
- In case of open apex, if there is ankylosis, the tooth may gradually become infrapositioned.
- Presence of radiolucencies.
- Radiographic evidence of infection-related (inflammatory) resorption, ankylosis-related (replacement) resorption, or both.

- Or absence of continued root formation (in case of open apex).
- When ankylosis occurs in a growing patient, infraposition of the tooth is highly likely to create disturbances in alveolar and facial growth over the short, medium, and long term.

6. Avulsion of primary teeth

A relatively recent meta-analysis showed trauma of primary dentition to be as common as 22.7% [68] with variable prevalence of avulsion from 7 to 13% [69]. In general, avulsed primary teeth should not be replanted (according to the recommendations of the IADT) [19]. Nevertheless, there are case reports with varying degrees of success after replantation of primary teeth, whereas others reported negative results to the replanted primary tooth and its permanent successor. One systematic review concluded that here is a lack of high-quality studies to support this approach [69].

Such a severe injury to the primary tooth may have negative impact on the development and/or eruption of its permanent successor. Premature loss of avulsed primary teeth might sometimes lead to space loss, masticatory, speech, and esthetic problems; this may also cause negative impact on their behavior, pschological, and social well-being. Removable or fixed appliances present valid treatment options to minimize space loss and improve esthetics when necessary. Furthermore, movement of the tooth during avulsion and the proximity between the primary tooth and the germ of its developing successor may interfere with its further growth and maturation leading to the occurrence of enamel defects and tooth malformations. The risk of sequelae in the permanent successor after avulsion of primary teeth is higher when the injury occurs in young children (<2 years), when the trauma is of greater magnitude such as when more teeth are involved and lower jaw is affected [70, 71].

Sequelae to the permanent successor include (**Figure 10**) [70]:

1. Malformations
    - crown dilaceration,
    - root dilaceration,
    - root angulation,
    - root duplication,
    - odontoma-like malformation,
    - arrest of root formation,
    - sequestration of the permanent tooth germ.
2. Enamel defects
    - white/cream or yellow/brown demarcated opacities,

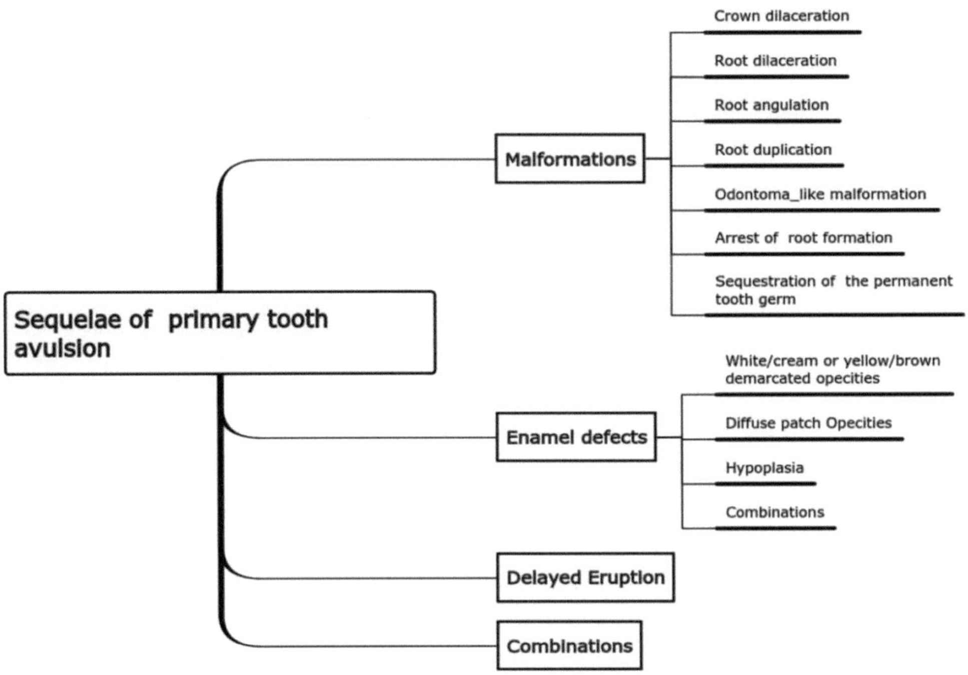

Figure 10.
Sequelae of primary tooth avulsion.

- diffuse patchy opacities.,
- hypoplasia,
- combinations of these.

3. Delayed eruption
4. Combinations

7. The role of teledentistry in the treatment of avulsed teeth

Teledentistry can be used to monitor those traumatic injuries cases remotely. Teledentistry combines dentistry and telecommunications simultaneously with clinical information and images over remote distances for dental consultation and treatment planning [72].

In cases of traumatic injuries and avulsions specifically, initial emergency instructions could be delivered on phones till obtaining emergency healthcare services is possible. This helps in calming patients or patients' guardians and maintains the first actions of replanting teeth or storing it in proper storage medium according to the recommendations. Teledentistry is also used at times of follow-up to report symptoms or other complications. It is mainly essential when specialty dentist is not available, yet their consultation, supervision, and valuable support could be used by the dental team in managing such cases [73]. A report showed that around 60% of patients contacted the telemedical center during the so-called "out of office hours" for dental trauma injuries. This percentage signifies the importance of having proper teledental channels addressing these incidents.

8. Discussion

Tooth avulsion is the complete displacement of the tooth from its socket in the dental arch.

In this chapter, we tried to gather the scattered information about tooth avulsion. Despite the rich published literature, but still a lot of researches are needed to reach evidence-based conclusions.

Although the tooth avulsion is the topic of concern in general dentistry, we tried to write this perceived paper in the specialist's manner to reflect more light on many related details.

Causes of tooth avulsion are divided into those for deciduous dentition and other for permanent dentition which are differ from each in their pattern and severity of the trauma [11–17].

Epidemiology has shown a reduction of cases during COVID-19 era. This was explained by patients' perceived fear of acquiring viral infections and thus hesitancy to reach out to emergency centers [8–10].

Avulsion treatment outcomes are very dependent on the first-aid measure as well as the agility to seek dental treatment.

For the management, put it as two phases may let the whole picture organized and well determined by specific time (at the time of trauma) the first phase and the other which are at the clinic.

The storage media (milk, HBSS, saliva, or saline) are discussed in detail regarding the characteristic of each. Nevertheless, researches are still looking for an ideal medium; some materials such as propolis and egg white are very promising. However, the quality of evidence is considered low [74]; on the other hand, teeth splinting is discussed generally as well as specifically for the avulsed teeth (with and without alveolar bone fracture) [20].

The literature regarding the adjunctive therapies for the teeth avulsion showed the role of these therapies; in this chapter, we considered them concisely with stress upon the indications for each [19, 20, 48, 60].

Criteria of successful treatment is widely discussed which is depending on both clinical and radiographic features.

Alternative treatments for the avulsed tooth in cases of the failure of aforementioned treatment are decoronation, autotransplantation, partial prosthesis, and dental implant [61–65].

The key of optimum outcomes in avulsions cases rely on both radiographical and clinical follow-ups. This signifies the importance of teledentistry and its role in addressing such incidents [72].

The main adverse outcome of tooth replantation is replacement root resorption (ankylosis). It implies possible risks of infraocclusion, impairment of alveolar bone growth, and tooth loss. The risk increases dramatically with delayed replantation [20].

9. Conclusion

Tooth avulsion is one of few emergencies in dentistry; prevalence differs from area to area according to the cause and gender. Replantation, immediate or delayed is the treatment of choice for the avulsed permanent tooth still immediate and proper replantation is important for long term good prognosis. Many factors may determine the outcome and use of antibiotic; although it is questionable, it is indicated in certain conditions. Although there is no strong evidence for their effect on healing, storage media is one of the factors for the preservation of the vitality of the tooth. It is used according to its availability at the trauma site. There are two stages in the treatment: emergency treatment and definitive treatment; even so, there is no grantee for the success of the treatment. Any avulsed tooth may be followed by complications, either immediately or lately. Despite the recommendation for the manager of the avulsed teeth, still not all recommendation can be applied for every avulsed tooth. Accordingly, any tooth has got special related factors which would determine the treatment plan after studying them carefully.

As a result, immediate and proper replantation is important for long-term good prognosis.

Conflict of interest

The authors declare no conflict of interest.

Acronyms and abbreviations

IADT	International Association of Dental Traumatology
FH	functional healing
IRR	inflammatory root resorption
RR	replacement resorption
PPE	personal protective equipment
HBSS	Hanks' Balanced Salt Solution
PDL	periodontal ligament
AGPs	aerosol-generating procedures
SAT	systemic antibiotic therapy
CHX	chlorohexidine
OTC	over counterpart
TTS	titanium trauma splints

Author details

Manal Abdalla Eltahir[1*], Randa Fath Elrahman Ibrahim[2] and Hanan Alharbi[3]

1 Oral and Maxillofacial Surgery and Diagnostic Science, College of Dentistry, Qassim University, Qassim, Saudi Arabia

2 College of Dentistry, Qassim University, Qassim, Saudi Arabia

3 Department of Conservative Sciences, Division of Endodontics, College of Dentistry, Qassim University, Qassim, Saudi Arabia

*Address all correspondence to: manltahir@yahoo.com

IntechOpen

© 2022 The Author(s). Licensee IntechOpen. This chapter is distributed under the terms of the Creative Commons Attribution License (http://creativecommons.org/licenses/by/3.0), which permits unrestricted use, distribution, and reproduction in any medium, provided the original work is properly cited.

References

[1] Emerich K, Czerwinska M, Ordyniec-Kwasnica I. Immediate self-replantation of an avulsed permanent mandibular incisor—A case report. Dental Traumatology. 2010;**26**(5):443-446

[2] Flores MT, Andersson L, Andreasen JO, Bakland LK, Malmgren B, Barnett F, et al. Guidelines for the management of traumatic dental injuries. II. Avulsion of permanent teeth. Dental Traumatology. 2007;**23**(3):130-136

[3] Andreasen JO, Andreasen FM, Andersson L. Textbook and Color Atlas of Traumatic Injuries to the Teeth. Wiley-Blackwell; 2019

[4] Benmansour A. Treatment of complete traumatic avulsion of an incisor tooth in adults. Medecine et Sante Tropicales. 2013;**23**(2):128-131

[5] Hicks RW, Green R, Van Wicklin SA. Dental avulsions: Review and recommendations. The Nurse Practitioner. 2016;**41**(6):58-62

[6] Trope M. Avulsion and replantation. Refuat Hapeh Vehashinayim. 1993; **19**(2):6-15

[7] I. P. Condutas endodônticas em dentes reimplantados. Espelho Clínico: São Caetano do Sul. 2001;**4**(24):8-9

[8] Woolley J, Djemal S. Traumatic dental injuries during the COVID-19 pandemic. Primary Dental Journal. 2021; **10**(1):28-32

[9] Hakeem FF, Alshahrani SM, Ghobain MA, Albabtain I, Aldibasi O, Alghnam S. The impact of COVID-19 lockdown on injuries in Saudi Arabia: Results from a level-I trauma center. Frontiers in Public Health. 2021;**9**: 704294

[10] Yang J, Yang G, Jin R, Song G, Yuan G. Changes in paediatric dental clinic after reopening during COVID-19 pandemic in Wuhan: A retrospective study. BMJ Open. 2022;**12**(1):e048430

[11] Andreasen JO, Andreasen FM, Andersson L. Textbook and Color Atlas of Traumatic Injuries to the Teeth. Copenhagen, Denmark: Mosby; 1994

[12] Brin I, Ben-Bassat Y, Heling I, Brezniak N. Profile of an orthodontic patient at risk of dental trauma. Endodontics & Dental Traumatology. 2000;**16**(3):111-115

[13] Kaba AD, Marechaux SC. A fourteen-year follow-up study of traumatic injuries to the permanent dentition. ASDC Journal of Dentistry for Children. 1989;**56**(6):417-425

[14] Bak NB. Accidental tooth avulsion during tonsillectomy. Ugeskrift for Laeger. 2010;**172**(21):1611-1612

[15] Tapashetti SA, Mahale P, Sattur A. Iatrogenic avulsion of a tooth—an endodontic mishap caused by rubber dam clamp—A case report. International Journal of Scientific Research. 2018;**7**(2): 460-461

[16] Yasny JS. Perioperative dental considerations for the anesthesiologist. Anesthesia and Analgesia. 2009;**108**(5): 1564-1573

[17] Kaur A, Kumar V, Logani A. Accidental avulsion of a recently traumatised maxillary anterior tooth during rubber dam application. BMJ Case Report. 2021;**14**(8)

[18] Andersson L, Andreasen JO, Day P, Heithersay G, Trope M, Diangelis AJ, et al. International Association of Dental

Traumatology guidelines for the management of traumatic dental injuries: 2. Avulsion of permanent teeth. Dental Traumatology. 2012;**28**(2):88-96

[19] Day PF, Flores MT, O'Connell AC, Abbott PV, Tsilingaridis G, Fouad AF, et al. International Association of Dental Traumatology guidelines for the management of traumatic dental injuries: 3. Injuries in the primary dentition. Dental Traumatology. 2020;**36**(4):343-359

[20] Fouad AF, Abbott PV, Tsilingaridis G, Cohenca N, Lauridsen E, Bourguignon C, et al. International Association of Dental Traumatology guidelines for the management of traumatic dental injuries: 2. Avulsion of permanent teeth. Dental Traumatology. 2020;**36**(4):331-342

[21] Levin L, Day PF, Hicks L, O'Connell A, Fouad AF, Bourguignon C, et al. International Association of Dental Traumatology guidelines for the management of traumatic dental injuries: General introduction. Dental Traumatology. 2020;**36**(4):309-313

[22] Krastl G, Weiger R, Filippi A, Van Waes H, Ebeleseder K, Ree M, et al. European Society of Endodontology position statement: Endodontic management of traumatized permanent teeth. International Endodontic Journal. 2021;**54**(9):1473-1481

[23] Paediatric DTUaBSo, Dentistry. Permanent Dentition Acute Management of Traumatic Injuries and Follow-up Care during the COVID-19 Pandemic. 2020

[24] Soares Ade J, Gomes BP, Zaia AA, Ferraz CC, de Souza-Filho FJ. Relationship between clinical-radiographic evaluation and outcome of teeth replantation. Dental Traumatology. 2008;**24**(2):183-188

[25] Andreasen JO. Effect of extra-alveolar period and storage media upon periodontal and pulpal healing after replantation of mature permanent incisors in monkeys. International Journal of Oral Surgery. 1981;**10**(1):43-53

[26] Glendor U, Halling A, Andersson L, Eilert-Petersson E. Incidence of traumatic tooth injuries in children and adolescents in the county of Vastmanland, Sweden. Sweden Dental Journal. 1996;**20**(1–2):15-28

[27] Cohenca SK, Eidlitz D, Nuni E, Moshonov J. New treatment protocols for avulsed teeth. Refuat Hapeh Vehashinayim. 2004;**21**:48-53

[28] Bezerra SRSBR, Arruda IMS, Requejo LSL, Carneiro SCDAS. Reimplante dental: Estágio atual. Revista da Faculdade de Odontologia de Pernambuco. 1992;**12**(12):29-33

[29] De Brier N, Borra V, Singletary EM, Zideman DA, De Buck E, et al. Storage of an avulsed tooth prior to replantation: A systematic review and meta-analysis. Dental Traumatology. 2020;**36**(5):453-476

[30] Adnan S, Lone MM, Khan FR, Hussain SM, Nagi SE. Which is the most recommended medium for the storage and transport of avulsed teeth? A systematic review. Dental Traumatology. 2018;**34**(2):59-70

[31] Is Khinda V, Kaur G, Kallar S, Khurana H. Clinical and practical implications of storage media used for tooth avulsion. International Journal of Clinical Pediatric Dental. 2017;**10**(2):158-165

[32] Hasan MR, Takebe H, Shalehin N, Obara N, Saito T, Irie K. Effects of tooth storage media on periodontal ligament preservation. Dental Traumatology. 2017;**33**(5):383-392

[33] de Paula Reis MV, Moura CC, Soares PB, Leoni GB, Souza-Neto MD, Barbosa DZ, et al. Histologic and micro-computed tomographic analyses of replanted teeth stored in different kind of media. Journal of Endodontia. 2014; **40**(5):665-669

[34] Souza BDM, Garcia LFR, Bortoluzzi EA, Felippe WT, Felippe MCS. Effects of several storage media on viability and proliferation capacity of periodontal ligament cells. European Archives of Paediatric Dentistry. 2020;**21**(1):53-59

[35] Poi WR, Sonoda CK, Martins CM, Melo ME, Pellizzer EP, de Mendonca MR, et al. Storage media for avulsed teeth: A literature review. Brazilian Dental Journal. 2013;**24**(5):437-445

[36] Endodontists. AAo: An Annotated Glossary of Terms Used in Endodontics. 7th ed. Chicago: American Association of Endodontists; 2003

[37] Veras SRA, Bem JSP, de Almeida ECB, Lins C. Dental splints: Types and time of immobilization post tooth avulsion. Journal of Istanbul University Faculty of Dentistry. 2017;**51**(3 Suppl 1): S69-S75

[38] Lin S, Emodi O, Abu E-NI. Splinting of an injured tooth as part of emergency treatment. Dental Traumatology. 2008; **24**(3):370-372

[39] Yoon H, Song M. Long-term retention of avulsed maxillary incisors with replacement root resorption: A 9-year follow-up. Case Report Dental. 2021;**2021**:8872859

[40] Emshoff R, Moschen I, Strobl H. Adverse outcomes of dental trauma splinting as related to displacement injury and pulpal blood flow level. Dental Traumatology. 2008;**24**(1):32-37

[41] Brown CL, Mackie IC. Splinting of traumatized teeth in children. Dental Update. 2003;**30**(2):78-82

[42] Kahler B, Hu JY, Marriot-Smith CS, Heithersay GS. Splinting of teeth following trauma: A review and a new splinting recommendation. Australian Dental Journal. 2016;**61**(Suppl. 1):59-73

[43] Hadziabdic N. The basics of splinting in dentoalveolar traumatology. In: Almasri M, Kummoona R, editors. Maxillofacial Surgery and Craniofacial Deformity: Practices and Updates. London: IntechOpen; 2020

[44] Kahler B, Heithersay GS. An evidence-based appraisal of splinting luxated, avulsed and root-fractured teeth. Dental Traumatology. 2008;**24**(1): 2-10

[45] Andreasen JOAaFM. Essentials of Traumatic Injuries to the Teeth: A Step-By-Step Treatment Guide. 2nd ed. Conpenhagen, Denmark: Munksgaard; 2001

[46] Trope M. Clinical management of the avulsed tooth: Present strategies and future directions. Dental Traumatology. 2002;**18**(1):1-11

[47] Ram D, Cohenca N. Therapeutic protocols for avulsed permanent teeth: Review and clinical update. Pediatric Dentistry. 2004;**26**(3):251-255

[48] Trope M. Avulsion of permanent teeth: Theory to practice. Dental Traumatology. 2011;**27**(4):281-294

[49] Day PF, Gregg TA, Ashley P, Welbury RR, Cole BO, High AS, et al. Periodontal healing following avulsion and replantation of teeth: A multi-Centre randomized controlled trial to compare two root canal medicaments. Dental Traumatology. 2012;**28**(1):55-64

[50] Bryson EC, Levin L, Banchs F, Abbott PV, Trope M. Effect of immediate intracanal placement of Ledermix paste (R) on healing of replanted dog teeth after extended dry times. Dental Traumatology. 2002;**18**(6):316-321

[51] Galler KM, Krastl G, Simon S, Van Gorp G, Meschi N, Vahedi B, et al. European Society of Endodontology position statement: Revitalization procedures. International Endodontic Journal. 2016;**49**(8):717-723

[52] Lu J, Liu H, Lu Z, Kahler B, Lin LM. Regenerative endodontic procedures for traumatized immature permanent teeth with severe external root resorption and root perforation. Journal of Endodontia. 2020;**46**(11):1610-1615

[53] Hargreaves KM, Diogenes A, Teixeira FB. Treatment options: Biological basis of regenerative endodontic procedures. Journal of Endodontia. 2013;**39**(3 Suppl):S30-S43

[54] Hammarström L, Blomlöf L, Feiglin B, Andersson L, Lindskog S. Replantation of teeth and antibiotic treatment. Endodontics & Dental Traumatology. 1986;**2**(2):51-57

[55] Sae-Lim V, Wang CY, Choi GW, Trope M. The effect of systemic tetracycline on resorption of dried replanted dogs' teeth. Endodontics & Dental Traumatology. 1998;**14**(3): 127-132

[56] Tsilingaridis G, Malmgren B, Skutberg C, Malmgren O. The effect of topical treatment with doxycycline compared to saline on 66 avulsed permanent teeth–a retrospective case-control study. Dental Traumatology. 2015;**31**(3):171-176

[57] Meng M, Chen Y, Ren H, Zhang Q, Chen S, Zhou X, et al. Effect of tetracyclines on pulpal and periodontal healing after tooth replantation: A systematic review of human and animal studies. BMC Oral Health. 2021;**21**(1):289

[58] Hamanaka EF, Poi WR, Brandini DA, Panzarini SR. Use of systemic antibiotic therapy after the replantation of avulsed permanent teeth: A literature review. Brazil Dental Science. 2017;**20**(1)

[59] del Planells P, Barra Soto MJ, Santa Eulalia Troisfontaines E. Antibiotic prophylaxis in pediatric odontology. An update. Medicina Oral Patologia Oral Cirugia Bucal. 2006;**11**(4):E352

[60] Brookes ZLS, Bescos R, Belfield LA, Ali K, Roberts A. Current uses of chlorhexidine for management of oral disease: A narrative review. Journal of Dentistry. 2020;**103**:103497

[61] Cohenca N, Stabholz A. Decoronation—A conservative method to treat ankylosed teeth for preservation of alveolar ridge prior to permanent prosthetic reconstruction: Literature review and case presentation. Dental Traumatology. 2007;**23**(2):87-94

[62] Sala M, Mendoza-Mendoza A, Yanez-Vico RM. Decoronation: An alternative treatment for replacement root resorption. Case Report Dental. 2017;**2017**:2826948

[63] Malmgren B. Ridge preservation/ decoronation. Journal of Endodontia. 2013;**39**(3 Suppl):S67-S72

[64] Abella Sans F, Ribas March F, Zubizarreta-Macho A, Boschini L, Roig Cayon M, Duran-Sindreu TF. Guided autotransplant of a first premolar to replace a maxillary ankylosed incisor using a custom-designed osteotome. Journal of the American Dental Association. 2022;**153**(3):265-272

[65] Petrovic B, Markovic D, Peric T, Blagojevic D. Factors related to treatment and outcomes of avulsed teeth. Dental Traumatology. 2010;**26**(1):52-59

[66] Muller DD, Bissinger R, Reymus M, Bucher K, Hickel R, Kuhnisch J. Survival and complication analyses of avulsed and replanted permanent teeth. Scientific Reports. 2020;**10**(1):2841

[67] Pohl Y, Filippi A, Kirschner H. Results after replantation of avulsed permanent teeth. II. Periodontal healing and the role of physiologic storage and antiresorptive-regenerative therapy. Dental Traumatology. 2005;**21**(2):93-101

[68] Petti S, Glendor U, Andersson L. World traumatic dental injury prevalence and incidence, a meta-analysis-one billion living people have had traumatic dental injuries. Dental Traumatology. 2018;**34**(2):71-86

[69] Martins-Junior PA, Franco FA, de Barcelos RV, Marques LS, Ramos-Jorge ML. Replantation of avulsed primary teeth: A systematic review. International Journal of Paediatric Dentistry. 2014;**24**(2):77-83

[70] Del Negro B, Lauridsen E, Mendes FM, Andreasen JO, Wanderley MT, Hermann NV. Impact of avulsion of the primary incisors on the occurrence of sequelae in the permanent teeth: A retrospective cohort study. Community Dentistry and Oral Epidemiology. 2021

[71] Lenzi MM, da Silva Fidalgo TK, Luiz RR, Maia LC. Trauma in primary teeth and its effect on the development of permanent successors: A controlled study. Acta Odontologica Scandinavica. 2019;**77**(1):76-81

[72] Jampani ND, Nutalapati R, Dontula BS, Boyapati R. Applications of teledentistry: A literature review and update. Journal of International Society of Preventive and Community Dentist. 2011;**1**(2):37-44

[73] Lienert N, Zitzmann NU, Filippi A, Weiger R, Krastl G. Teledental consultations related to trauma in a Swiss telemedical center: A retrospective survey. Dental Traumatology. 2010; **26**(3):223-227

[74] Day PF, Duggal M, Nazzal H. Interventions for treating traumatised permanent front teeth: Avulsed (knocked out) and replanted. Cochrane Database of Systematic Reviews. 2019;**2**: CD006542

Chapter 5

Perspective Chapter: Splinting of Traumatized Teeth

Eswari Ramassamy

Abstract

Repositioning or replantation followed by stabilization with splint is the standard management of traumatized teeth. Numerous types of splints are being used and each type has its own advantages and disadvantages. Knowledge on the different types of splints and its effect on dental tissues so as to aid in the clinical decision on the type of splint to be used for managing a particular type of traumatic dental injury and its fixation period are important. Therefore, this chapter aims in explaining the different methods of splinting along with its advantages and disadvantages of each type along with the standard recommendation for duration of splinting.

Keywords: splinting, flexible splints, rigid splints, traumatized teeth, wire composite splints

1. Introduction

Splinting is recommended in the management of traumatic dental injuries which requires repositioning and stabilization of the luxated teeth. Earlier, the management of luxated teeth was similar to the management of fractures of Jaws, which are arch bars with wires and cap splints. But due to their negative effect on periodontal structures along with the advent of adhesive materials, a wide range of splints are being developed [1, 2]. A splint is "An apparatus used to support, protect or immobilize teeth that have been loosened, replanted, fractured or subjected to certain endodontic surgical procedures" [3]. The aim of this chapter is to enumerate the ideal requirements of splints, types and description of each types of splints and International Association of Dental Traumatology (IADT) recommendations of splinting duration and types.

2. Ideal requirements of splints

1. The splint design must allow direct intraoral application without any laboratory support

2. The materials used for the splint must be easily available

3. The application and removal of the splint must be easy and should not damage the dentition or the surrounding tissues

4. A splinting technique must be applicable for all types of situations like patients with missing tooth, unerupted tooth or clinically short or conical crowns.

5. Throughout the splinting time period, the splint must be able to stabilize the tooth in its correct position and provide proper stabilization.

6. The splint should be passive without exerting untoward forces on the injured teeth.

7. It should be versatile that is it could be applied as rigid, semi-rigid or flexible splint.

8. Once placed, it should neither interfere with occlusion or occlusal movements nor impinge the gingival tissues.

9. Should allow easy maintenance of oral hygiene, thus not predisposing to caries and periodontal problems

10. Should permit diagnostic procedures like pulp testing to be performed and also provide access for performing endodontic procedures.

But, all the splinting techniques do not satisfy all the requirements mentioned above [1, 4, 5].

3. Classification of splints

Splints can be classified as
Rigid splints
Semi-rigid splints/Flexible splints

3.1 Rigid splints

Rigid splints are those splints which does not allow physiologic movement of the repositioned teeth [2].

Eg: Erich arch bars, Acrylic cap splint, Schuchardt splint, Interdental wiring methods like figure-eight wiring & loop wiring.

In case of arch bar splints (**Figure 1**) and the interdental wiring methods, the ligature wires used in these splints tend to become loose with time and come to rest on the marginal gingiva. This could cause gingival irritation and inflammation as it becomes the site for plaque deposition. The patient's inability to maintain good oral hygiene around the wires could worsen the condition [4, 6]. These splints also cause physical damage to gingiva and cementum surface when removed after the splinting period [7]. If these ligature wires, when positioned apical to the cervical prominence while splinting especially in a mobile tooth, they tend to elevate the tooth slowly making the cemento-enamel junction lose its integrity [4, 6].

Schuchardt splint was initially designed for splinting of luxation injuries. But its extreme rigidity and difficulty in adapting to the arch form accounts for its high thickness of 2 mm diameter bar made of aluminum-brass alloy. Acrylic cap splint is cemented on uninjured teeth when used for luxation injuries provides too much rigidity [6].

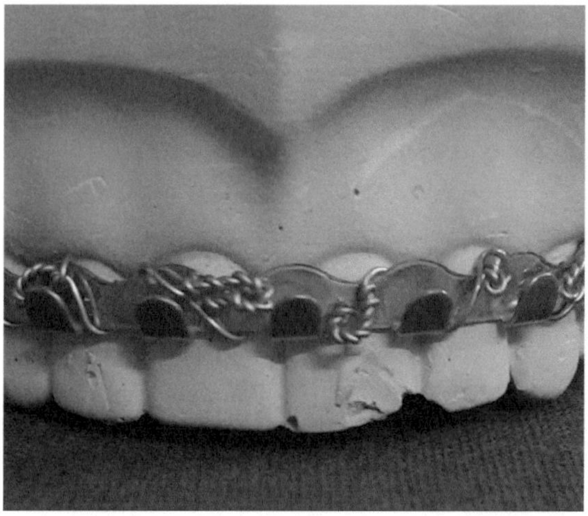

Figure 1.
Arch bar splint.

In addition to these disadvantages, there is high incidence of pulp necrosis, external root resorption and ankylosis of the repositioned teeth when rigid splints are applied [2, 8].

For the above reasons, the usage of rigid splints is restricted only for stabilizing jaw fractures.

3.2 Semi-rigid/flexible splints

Flexible splints are those splints which allow functional movement of the stabilized teeth [4]. Studies conducted on animals had shown that normal masticatory stimulation can lower the incidence of ankylosis which led to the development of flexible splints so as to allow the functional movement of the traumatized and stabilized teeth [9].

Many varieties of flexible splints are being introduced. Most of these splints make use of the acid etch technique.

3.2.1 Composite and wire splints

Flexible wire composite splint (**Figure 2**) uses a wire of 0.3–0.4 mm in diameter bonded onto the labial surface of the teeth with composite [4]. Rigidity of the splint increases with increase in the thickness of wire or by adding composite in the interdental space [1]. Rigidity also increases with increase in the length of the wire splint [10].

The main advantage of this splint is that the materials used for the construction of this splint are routinely available in all dental clinics. Other advantages are it is well accepted by the patients, does not cause any injuries to the supporting structures and easy maintenance of oral hygiene. But a major disadvantage is that it can cause potential damage to enamel while removing [1].

3.2.2 Other alternatives

Many splints are being constructed using other materials as an alternative to wire.

a. Nylon/Fishing Line splint (**Figure 3**) – In this splint a thin nylon/Fishing line is used instead of wire. The advantages of this splint is that it is atraumatic to

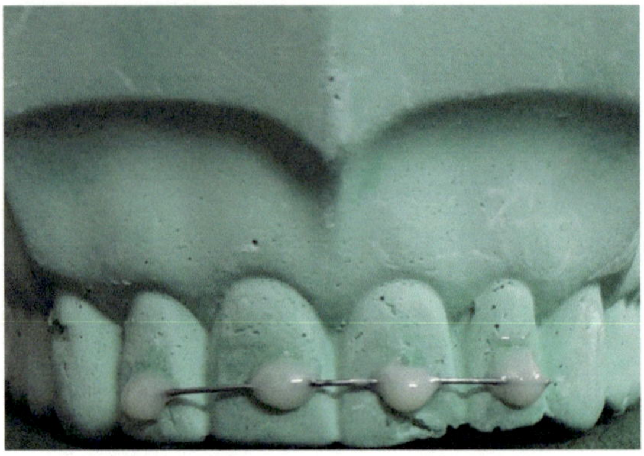

Figure 2.
Wire composite splint.

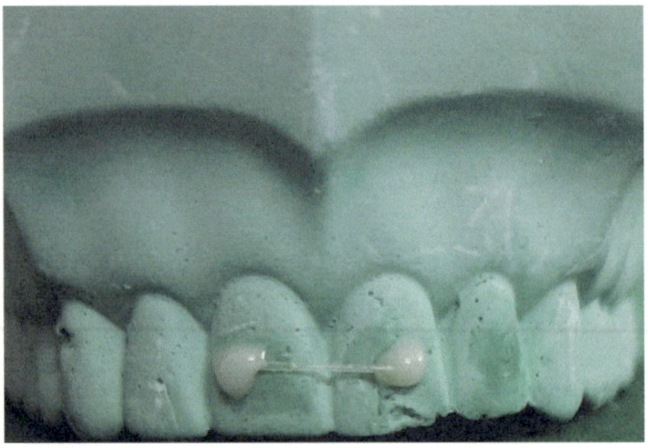

Figure 3.
Nylon line splint.

supporting structures, relatively esthetic, easy to maintain oral hygiene, inexpensive and comfortable for patient [11]. The main disadvantage is that it is slightly difficult to position the nylon line as it is thin. This problem can be overcome by fixing the nylon line and light curing the composite one tooth at a time and thus it is slightly time consuming [12].

b. Power chain (**Figure 4**): Power chain is made of rubber and is used in orthodontics for traction purposes. The advantages of power chain is that it's an easily available, inexpensive material with good esthetics and comfort to the patient. It is very flexible and has holes into which composite can be applied without flowing out and thus reduce the bulk of composite around the splint. Care must be taken not to activate the elastic and it must be used in a passive state. The disadvantage is similar to nylon line as it has to be fixed one tooth at a time to avoid it from slipping [12, 13].

c. Waxed dental floss and flexible orthodontic wires are also successfully used instead of stainless steel wires [6].

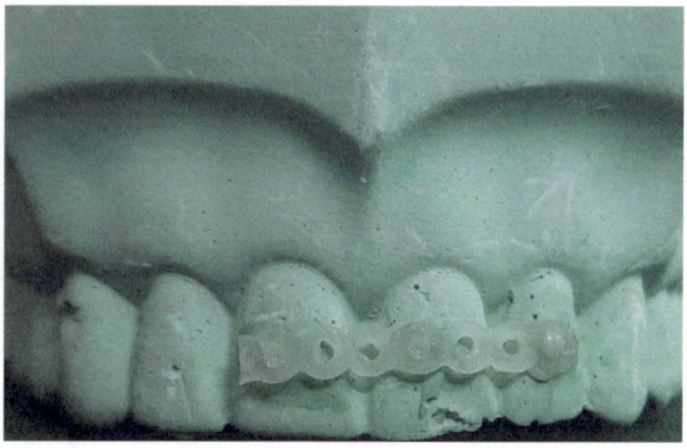

Figure 4.
Power chain splint.

3.2.3 Suture splint

It is the simplest form used as temporary splinting of traumatized deciduous teeth or partially erupted permanent teeth in a situation where the child is difficult to manage. It is a temporary splint because it is retained only for 3 to 4 days until the child becomes more receptive to a definitive treatment. A suture is placed over the incisal edge from palatal gingiva to the labial gingiva. (**Figure 5**) It prevents the tooth from extruding. But the biggest disadvantage of this splint is that sometimes the incisal edge has to be grooved to hold the suture material in position [1, 5].

3.2.4 Orthodontic splint

It requires the orthodontic materials like brackets and wires (**Figure 6**). The brackets are bonded to the teeth and are connected by 0.014 NiTi flexible wire [4].

It is indicated in a few clinical conditions like:

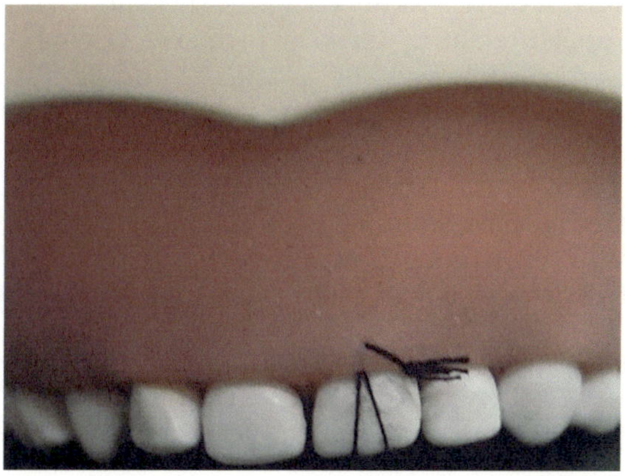

Figure 5.
Suture splint.

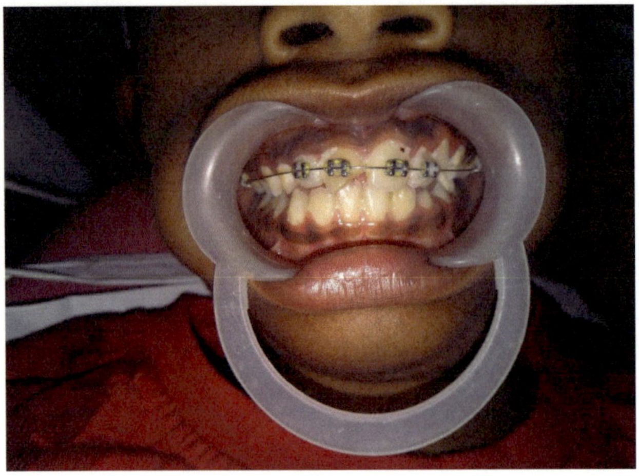

Figure 6.
Orthodontic wire splint.

i. severely malpositioned teeth which makes the placement of wire-composite splint difficult.

ii. In case of intrusive luxation, where repositioning of the tooth is to done [14].

The main advantage of this splint is that it is the least traumatic technique for repositioning tooth with intrusive luxation injury [14]. However, when used in other situations except intrusive luxation, care must be taken to reduce orthodontic forces that disturbs the healing of the luxated tooth [15].

It is known through studies that splints constructed with orthodontic materials always generate some amount of force over the teeth, but these forces could be reduced with certain conditions like the form of arch wire, type of cross section of the wire and the type of ligature used [16]. Hence, it is recommended that only trained clinician in handling orthodontic materials can utilize this splint properly. This becomes a major disadvantage of this splint [17]. Other disadvantages are the requirement of materials which are not commonly available in clinics and irritation to the lips and buccal mucosa and discomfort to the patient especially at the beginning of the treatment, which can be reduced by lubricating the lips [18].

3.2.5 Fiber-reinforced composite splints

These splints use fibers which are attached to the teeth either by unfilled resin or with composite [4].

The commercially available fibers are:

- polyethylene fibers eg. Ribbond (**Figure 7**)
- Glass fibers eg. Fiber-splint and quartz splint
- Kevlar fibers [17]

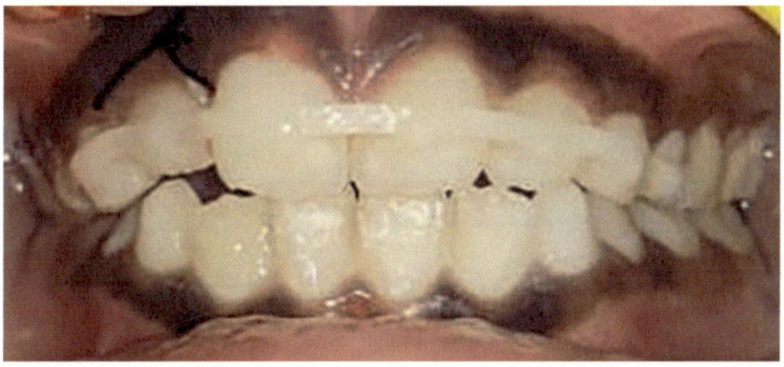

Figure 7.
Ribbond splint.

Fiber splints are esthetically acceptable and it is easy to apply and remove. It does not cause any trauma to surrounding structures and maintenance of oral hygiene is easy. Fiber splints are associated with highest frequency of healing outcomes [19].

3.2.6 Titanium trauma splint (TTS)

This splint was developed by von Arx in collaboration with Medartis AG, Basel, Switzerland. The objective behind developing this splint was to optimize the splinting techniques, (i.e) ease of application and removal from the dental surgeon's aspect and increase in comfort and easy maintenance of oral hygiene from the patient's aspect.

It is a pre-fabricated splint made of titanium of 0.2 mm thickness and 2.8 mm width. Due to its least thickness, it is operator friendly, it does not require any special pliers or other instruments to manipulate; it can be easily adapted onto the arch by fingers. It is available in two different lengths 52 mm and 100 mm and it could be cut to the desired length.

Its unique design with a rhomboid mesh structure makes the splint more flexible without subjecting the splinted teeth to any orthodontic forces. Yet another advantage is that it could be easily secured to the teeth. The rhomboid openings are in the size of 1.8x2.8 mm and hence only a small area of bonding is needed with the tooth. It does not require a bulk composite around the splint; only a thin layer of flowable composite is required.

While removing the splint, the composite can be ground down to the level of TTS and the splint can be "peeled-off" easily from the tooth with a hemostat. Any remnant composite can be removed with easily with a curett and tooth surface can be polished [20]. The only disadvantage of this splint is its high cost [4].

3.2.7 Resin splint

This splint is applied with resin materials like Protemp and Luxatemp, which are used in temprorary prosthetic restorations and for lining prefabricated crowns. Luxatemp is dual cured; by both chemical and light cured, while Protemp is chemically cured material [1]. The resin materials are available in syringe forms and can be directly applied to the labial aspects of the crowns of the teeth to be splinted. Once the material is set/cured, any sharp edges can be removed to prevent irritation to the surrounding soft tissues [21].

The advantages are these materials do not exert any force on tooth during application and are acceptable esthetically and hygienically. They are not indicated when the adjacent are not fully erupted and difficult in case of any edentulous area. The main disadvantage is that they tend to fracture easily and care must be taken during removal. [1].

4. Splinting type and duration

4.1 For permanent dentition

Experiments and studies demonstrated that rigid immobilization for longer duration of time increased the risk of pulp necrosis, external root resorption and ankylosis. The International Association of Dental Traumatology (IADT) has formulated guidelines for the management of traumatic dental injuries. Based on current evidences, short-term, passive and flexible splints are recommended for splinting luxated, avulsed and root-fractured teeth. For alveolar bone fractures, splinting of teeth may be used for bone segment immobilization. Splinting duration depends on the type of dental injury. The duration of splinting for Permanent Dentition as given by IADT 2020 is given in **Table 1** [22].

S. No.	Types of Dental Injuries	Duration of splinting		
		2 Weeks	4 Weeks	4 Months
1	Subluxation	✓ (if splinted)		
2	Extrusion	✓		
3	Lateral Luxation		✓	
3	Intrusion		✓	
4	Avulsion	✓		
5	Root Fracture (apical third, Mid-third)		✓	
6	Root fracture (cervical fracture)			✓
7	Alveolar fracture		✓	

Table 1.
IADT guidelines for splinting duration of permanent dentition.

S. No.	Types of Dental Injuries	Duration of splinting		
		2 Weeks	4 Weeks	4 Months
1	Lateral Luxation		✓ (If splinting required)	
2	Root Fracture		✓ (If splinting required)	
3	Alveolar fracture		✓	

Table 2.
IADT guidelines for splinting duration of primary dentition.

4.2 For primary dentition

According to IADT guidelines, splinting of primary dentition is recommended only in case of alveolar bone fractures. Root fractures and lateral luxations may occasionally require splinting. Only flexible splints are used including alveolar fracture where the splint is stabilized on adjacent uninjured teeth for 4 weeks. (IADT guidelines) The duration of splinting for Permanent Dentition as given by IADT 2020 is given in **Table 2** [22].

5. Removal of splint

One of the important requirement of a splint is that it should be applied and removed easily without causing any damage to the enamel surface. The resin-based materials cause iatrogenic enamel damage while removing them is a major concern. Various techniques are employed for removing the remnant composite material used for retaining the splints from the enamel surface. They are hand instruments like scalers and pliers, burs, abrasive discs, rubber wheels and cups. In an experimental study conducted to assess the surface roughness of enamel after employing various methods to remove the material, it was noted that Soflex discs and 16-blade tungsten carbide bur cause least damage to the enamel [17, 23].

6. Emergency splinting

Patients with multiple injuries as in road traffic accidents, often sustain dental injuries. Traumatic dental injuries not being life-threatening, emergency rooms not being equipped to manage traumatic dental injuries, inadequacy of knowledge and skill of medical personal handling the patients are the reasons for either delaying/ignoring the management of traumatic dental injuries [24, 25]. In such emergency situations, an easy to perform splinting technique is "criss-cross" pattern suture splints which can be rapidly placed by any medical personal. This splint can be placed with 2/0 silk suture material with a horizontal locking mattress design to keep the reimplanted tooth in position until the patient could be mobilized to Dental Department for more definitive management. The advantage of this technique is that it is a quick method which could be performed by any medical personal when the patient is treated under General Anesthesia for other injuries and does not delay the general treatment procedures.

The criss-cross pattern splint is given by the following steps:

Step 1 – the first bite (point 1 in **Figure 8**) is taken at the base of the distal interdental papilla on the labial side of the tooth to be repositioned and crossed over the incisal edge towards the mesial-palatal aspect.

Step 2 – suture then penetrates the base of the mesial interdental papilla (point 2 in **Figure 8**) on the palatal side and emerges out at the base of the distal interdental papilla on the palatal aspect (point 3 in **Figure 8**).

Step 3 – the suture then crosses over the incisal edge to pierce the base of the mesial interdental papilla on the labial aspect (point 4 in **Figure 8**).

Step 4 – from point 4, the suture retraces the path underneath the previous suture upto the criss-cross point (point 5 in **Figure 9**) on the labial aspect and winds around the point 5 to pierce at mid buccal region (point 6 in **Figure 9**) on the labial aspect.

Step 5 – knot is placed between point 1 and 6 (**Figure 9**) [24].

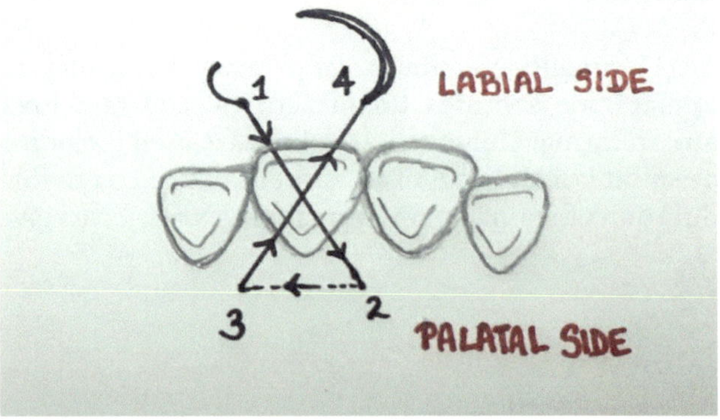

Figure 8.
Criss-cross splint.

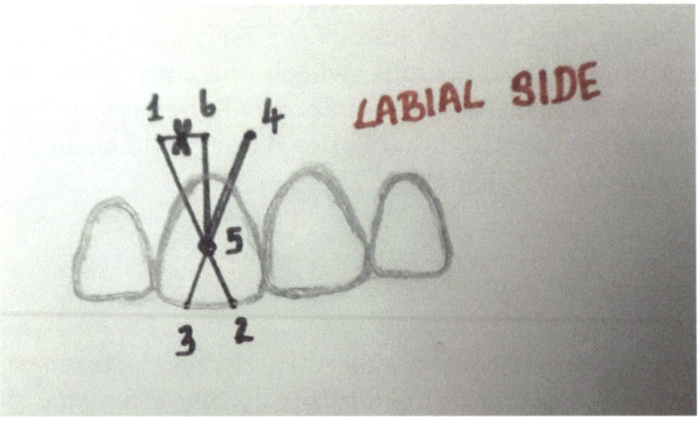

Figure 9.
Criss-cross splint.

7. Home-care instructions to parents

Post-treatment maintenance of good oral hygiene is the key to uneventful healing of the injured tissues. Therefore, parents/caregivers must be sensitized about the importance of maintaining good oral hygiene and also taught the methods to maintain it. Most important instructions to be given are:

1. To avoid their children from participating in contact sports

2. To give only soft diet for a minimum of 2 weeks

3. To brush the teeth only with a soft brush after each meal

4. To use 0.12% chlorhexidine mouth rinse twice a day for 2 weeks

5. Strict adherence to follow-up schedule [26].

8. Conclusion

To summarize, splinting is important for stabilizing the luxated teeth; use of semi-rigid/flexible splints is mandatory as it allows functional movements of the tooth and short-term immobilization is recommended as longer period of splinting is associated with complications.

Author details

Eswari Ramassamy
Department of Pediatric and Preventive Dentistry, Indira Gandhi Institute of Dental Sciences, Sri Balaji Vidyapeeth (Deemed to be University), Puducherry, India

*Address all correspondence to: eswari80ashok@gmail.com

IntechOpen

© 2023 The Author(s). Licensee IntechOpen. This chapter is distributed under the terms of the Creative Commons Attribution License (http://creativecommons.org/licenses/by/3.0), which permits unrestricted use, distribution, and reproduction in any medium, provided the original work is properly cited.

References

[1] Andreasen JO, Oikainen KS. Splinting of traumatized teeth. In: Andreasen JO, Andreasen FM, Andreasen L, editors. Textbook and Color Atlas of Traumatic Injuries to the Teeth. 5th ed. Blackwell Munksgaard: Wiley; 2019. pp. 962-971

[2] Goswami M, Eranhikkal A. Management of Traumatic Dental Injuries Using Different Types of splints: A case series. International Journal of Clinical Pediatric Dentistry. 2020;**13**(2):199-202. DOI: 10.5005/jp-journals-10005-1746

[3] American Association of Endodontists. Glossary of Endodontic Terms. 8th edn. Available at: http://www.nxtbook.com/.nxtbooks/aae/endodonticglossary/index.php.

[4] Kahler B, Hu JY, Marriot-Smith CS, Heithersay GS. Splinting of teeth following trauma: A review and a new splinting recommendation. Australian Dental Journal. 2016;**61**(1):59-73. DOI: 10.1111/adj.12398

[5] Neaverth EJ, Georig AC. Technique and rationale for splinting. Journal of the American Dental Association (1939). 1980;**100**:56-63. DOI: 10.14219/jada.archive.1980.0026

[6] Reynolds JS, Reynolds MT, Powers MP. Diagnosis and management of dentoalveolar inuries. In: Fonesca RJ, Barber HD, Walker RV, Powers MP, Frost DE, editors. Oral & Maxillofacial Trauma. 4th ed. Missouri: Elseveir Saunders; 2013. pp. 248-292

[7] Kahler B, Heithersay GS. An evidence-based appraisal of splinting luxated, avulsed and root-fractured teeth. Dental Traumatology. 2008;**24**(1):2-10. DOI: 10.1111/j.1600-9657.2006.00480.x

[8] Oikarinen K. Tooth splinting: A review of the literature and consideration of the versatility of a wire-composite splint. Endodontics & Dental Traumatology. 1990;**6**:237-250. DOI: 10.1111/j.1600-9657.1990.tb00426.x

[9] Andersson L, Lindskog S, Blomlof L, Hedstrom K-G, Hammarstrom L. Effect of masticatory stimulation on dentoalveolar ankylosis after experimental tooth replantation. Endodontics & Dental Traumatology. 1985;**1**:13-16. DOI: 10.1111/j.1600-9657.1985.tb00552.x

[10] Berthold C, Auer FJ, Potapov S, Petschelt A. Influence of wire extension and type on splint rigidity–evaluation by a dynamic and a static measuring method. Dental Traumatology. 2011;**27**:422-431. DOI: 10.1111/j.1600-9657.2011.01033.x

[11] Antrim DD, Ostrowski JS. A functional splint for traumatized teeth. Journal of Endodontia. 1982;**8**(7):328-331. DOI: 10.1016/S0099-2399(82)80284-7

[12] Ben Hassan MW, Andersson L, Lucas PW. Stiffness characteristics of splints for fixation of traumatized teeth. Dental Traumatology. 2016;**32**(2):140-145. DOI: 10.1111/edt.12234

[13] Sobczak-Zagalska H, Emerich K. Assessment of a power chain as a new dental trauma splint and its comparison with two commonly used splinting materials. Applied Sciences. 2020;**10**: 1-12. DOI: 10.3390/app10238398

[14] Ebrahim FH, Kulkarni G. Fixed orthodontic appliances in the management of severe dental trauma in mixed dentition: A case report. Journal

of the Canadian Dental Association. 2013;**79**:d131

[15] Prevost J, Louis P, Vadot J, Granjon Y. A study of forces originating from orthodontic appliances for splinting of teeth. Endodontics & Dental Traumatology. 1994;**10**:179-184. DOI: 10.1111/j.1600-9657.1994.tb00683.x

[16] Prévost J, Granjon Y. An in vitro study of the passivity of splints in dental trauma. Journal of Dentistry. 1998;**26**(1):39-45. DOI: 10.1016/s0300-5712(96)00069-3

[17] Sobczak-Zagalska H, Emerich K. Best splinting methods in case of dental injury-a literature review. The Journal of Clinical Pediatric Dentistry. 2020;**44**(2):71-78. DOI: 10.17796/1053-4625-44.2.1

[18] Filippi A, von Arx T, Lussi A. Comfort and discomfort of dental trauma splints - a comparison of a new device (TTS) with three commonly used splinting techniques. Dental Traumatology. 2002;**18**(5):275-280. DOI: 10.1034/j.1600-9657.2002.00121.x

[19] Andreasen JO, Andreasen FM, Mejàre I, Cvek M. Healing of 400 intra-alveolar root fractures. 2. Effect of treatment factors such as treatment delay, repositioning, splinting type and period and antibiotics. Dental Traumatology. 2004;**20**(4):203-211. DOI: 10.1111/j.1600-9657.2004.00278.x

[20] von Arx T, Filippi A, Buser D. Splinting of traumatized teeth with a new device: TTS (titanium trauma splint). Dental Traumatology. 2001;**17**(4):180-184. DOI: 10.1034/j.1600-9657.2001.170408.x

[21] Baar EH, Yarshansky OH, ben Yehuda A. Intracoronal incisal splint. The Journal of Prosthetic Dentistry. 1993;**70**:491-492

[22] Bourguignon C, Cohenca N, Lauridsen E, et al. International Association of Dental Traumatology guidelines for the management of traumatic dental injuries: 1. Fractures and luxations. Dental Traumatology. 2020;**36**(4):314-330. DOI: 10.1111/edt.12578

[23] Cehreli ZC, Lakshmipathy M, Yazici R. Effect of different splint removal techniques on the surface roughness of human enamel: A three-dimensional optical profilometry analysis. Dental Traumatology. 2008;**24**(2):177-182. DOI: 10.1111/j.1600-9657.2007.00491.x

[24] Lin S, Emodi O, Abu E-NI. Splinting of an injured tooth as part of emergency treatment. Dental Traumatology. 2008;**24**(3):370-372. DOI: 10.1111/j.1600-9657.2007.00530.x

[25] Díaz J, Bustos L, Herrera S, Sepulveda J. Knowledge of the management of paediatric dental traumas by non-dental professionals in emergency rooms in South Araucanía, Temuco, Chile. Dental Traumatology. 2009;**25**(6):611-619. DOI: 10.1111/j.1600-9657.2009.00835.x

[26] Fouad AF, Abbott PV, Tsilingaridis G, et al. International Association of Dental Traumatology guidelines for the management of traumatic dental injuries: 2. Avulsion of Permanent Teeth. Dental Traumatology. 2020;**36**(4):331-342. DOI: 10.1111/edt.12573

Chapter 6

Perspective Chapter: Orbital Reconstruction and Orbital Volume

Yousry Eldek, Heba Sleem, Mohamad Katamesh and Fahmy Hasanin

Abstract

Orbital fractures are common presentation in the head and neck trauma centers. They can result in functional and esthetic problems. The primary goal in the repair of the orbital fractures is to restore the orbital shape and volume, free the incarcerated or prolapsed orbital tissue from the fracture defect, and span the bony defect with reconstructive implant material. Titanium mesh was very appropriate reconstructive material for anatomic reconstruction. The orbit has a special complex geometry which makes perfect anatomic reconstruction very difficult. The manual process of fitting and adapting the implant within the orbit is time consuming and operator dependent. The advanced techniques in maxillofacial imaging and computer assisted techniques resulted in improvement in the implant design for management of orbital fractures. The current study was made to review the accuracy of adapting the titanium mesh using STL model versus conventional technique for restoring the orbital volume in management of orbital floor fracture.

Keywords: orbital reconstruction, orbital volume, titanium mesh, STL model, computer assisted surgery

1. Introduction

Orbital fractures are one of the most common fractures of the midface and result in significant complications such as enopthalmos, diplopia, restriction of gaze, and dystopia [1]. Orbital reconstruction aims to restore the normal orbital volume and architecture and reduce the herniated orbital tissues to prevent the compications [2]. The choice of the implant material depends on many factors such as: size of the defect, involvement of many walls, adaptation to internal contours, restoration of accurate volume, presence of adjacent sinus cavity, prevention of displacement, restriction of ocular motility, risk of further trauma, and early versus late repair [3].

Avashia et al. reviewed the materials used for orbital reconstruction and classified it into biological materials and manufactured materials. Biologic materials include autografts, allogarfts, xenografts. Manufactured materials include resorbable materials as polymers and nonresorbable materials as porous polyethylene, bioactive glass, silastic rubber, titanium, teflon, nylon, and other materials. Avashia et al. reported no consensus for any material as the optimal choice for orbital floor reconstruction [4].

Many surgical techniques have been adopted and evaluated for correction of orbital volume. Topography of the orbital floor (S shape in sagittal plane) is one of the difficult factors during insertion and manipulation of reconstructive material. However there is a continuous search and study for the best method to achieve accuracy, feasibility, and reliability for restoration of the orbit [5].

2. Titanium implant

Literature review revealed the use of many surgical approaches and many implant materials for orbital reconstruction. Titanium mesh was very appropriate reconstructive material for anatomic reconstruction [6]. Titanium implants are considered as an established implant material to reconstruct the orbital and craniofacial skeleton. There are many forms and shapes of titanium mesh and different thickness and sizes [7].

Titanium mesh is the most commonly used reconstructive material for orbital reconstruction [8]. Intra-operative manual bending and adaptation to the titanium mesh after exposure and reduction of fractured segments is a traditional or conventional technique. However, this leads to more dissection, multiple trials, and longer operative time especially in comminuted fractures. This technique makes the reconstruction process a subject of interpersonal variation because the manipulation and bending of the implant material depends on the operator experience [9].

Titanium meshes have high biocompatible properties. They are easily molded to fit simple and complex orbital defects. They can provide a strong support without change in the shapes or locations over time. They can be fixed to adjacent bone. They have many good characters such as: availability, easy sterilization, and a well-recognized osseointegration. Titanium has a high corrosion resistance because of the spontaneously forming thin oxide layers on the surface. This guarantees its passive behavior to avoid toxic or allergic reactions [4].

In 2009, **Lee and Nunery** revealed that the use of titanium mesh in the orbital floor can lead to fibrous adhesion around the implant resulting in diplopia or restricted eye movement after orbital floor repair by 2 months. It is a rare complication which requires replacing the titanium mesh with another implant. They considered the titanium itself caused fibrous adhesion and named it "orbital adherence syndrome" [10]. However, in 2013, **Kersey et al.** revealed in their study that the fracture can result in rupture or splitting through the periorbita, causing fibrous adhesion due to inadequate separation between the orbital contents and the bone or the implant and this complication can ocuur occur with or without the titanium implant [11].

3. Computer assisted surgery

The orbit has a special complex geometry, so the perfect anatomic reconstruction is very difficult. The process of fitting and adapting the implant in the orbit is time consuming and operator dependent. The narrow field in addition to the complex anatomy of the orbit make the orbital reconstruction difficult and almost impossible to achieve "true-to-original" 3D shape [12].

The management of the orbital fractures has changed over the years. The advanced techniques for maxillofacial imaging and computer assisted techniques lead to an improvement in the implant design for orbital reconstruction [13].

Over the last 2 decades, there was great and rapid improvement in the computed tomography which has added a third dimension to the imaging of complex cranio-maxillofacial deformity. This development has significantly decreased the degree of inaccuracy that is inherent in any clinical assessment. Three dimensional (3D) reconstruction from volume data collected from helical CT is now an established technique in craniomaxillofacial surgery to provide animated screen images and accurate reproduction of the hard and/or soft tissues with models [14].

The development of computer assisted surgeries represents a new technology and a turn point in the field of craniofacial reconstruction. Some of the computer assisted techniques are used for virtual reconstruction of the fractured orbit and rapid prototyping. STL model was used for adapting and contouring the orbital mesh to allow accurate orbital volume, decrease operative time, decrease hospital costs, strengthen the surgical skills, and improve patient outcomes [15–17].

Lim et al. found that the direct intraoperative trimming and adaptation may take long operative time depending on the extension of the defect and experience of the surgeon when compared with STL models [18]. On the other hand, preoperative rapid prototyping reduces the intraoperative time, risk of orbital mesh malposition, poor anatomical contour, and trauma to soft tissue because of multiple insertions during trimming and adaptation of the titanium mesh [19].

Rapid prototyping is a new technique characterized by rapidly and accurately preparing solid bodies with complex shapes, so it has a promising and extensive application in the medical fields [20]. Since its introduction into craniomaxillofacial surgery in the 1990s, it has been used for the treatment of various medical problems, such as orbital hypertelorism, craniosynostosis, facial asymmetry, craniomaxillofacial defects, maxillofacial implants, orthognathic surgery, tumor surgery [21].

Rapid prototyping is a three dimensional (3D) printing process which involves an additive manufacturing technology which offers an expedient and accurate reproduction of an osseous anatomy. The intact orbit was mirrored onto the fractured one to create virtual model. The virtual model data were converted to STL (Standard Triangulation Language or Standard Tessellation Language) format to form a solid physical orbital model using a 3D printer and computer-aided manufacturing machines. STL model was used to adapt and contour the orbital mesh to allow accurate orbital volume, decrease risks and time consuming, and help improve postoperative results [18, 21].

In 1986, **Hull** introduced the stereolithography apparatus (SLA) technique to create an accurate, hardened, three dimensiona; acrylic models from CT data [22, 23]. In 1990, the first stereolithographic patient model was built. It represented an actual three- dimensional model to reproduce the anatomy of a patient based on CT images taken during that patient's examination [24].

In 1998, **Perry et al.** reported that 3D models of the facial skeleton differ in their accuracy, reproducibility and cost. The early attempts to build and form models from CT scans were stacked polystyrene slices where each of which represented a corresponding slice from an axial scan. Since then model building has developed into 2 distinct processes: computer aided manufacture (CAM) and stereolithography. In the computer aided manufacture (CAM) technique, the models are milled by computer guidance from different materials as soft expanded polyurethane and titanium alloy. It is considered as a removal process by an expensive milling machine. Stereolithography is a computer controlled construction process including 0.25 mm layer by layer polymerization of LASER curable liquid resin which are built on top of each other. It is accurate, slow and expensive technique [14].

In 1999, **Holck et al.** described the benefits of the sterolithography (SLA) modeling system for planning the surgery for bony orbital pathology. They reported that the SLA models were beneficial preoperatively for evaluating the dimensions of the bony defects and surgical planning. Intraoperatively, SLA models facilitated the surgical rehabilitation of the orbit leading to postoperative satisfactory results [24].

In 2006, **Metzger et al.** measured the accuracy of a technique for making individual preformed titanium meshes for orbital fractures. The study included 5 patients with unilateral orbital fractures and the patients underwent preoperative CT scans of 1 mm thickness followed by surgical planning using surgical planning software, then stereolithographic models were built after using the mirroring tool from unaffected side on affected side. Titanium meshes were then adapted manually on the STL models and sterilized. Intra-operatively, the meshes were positioned with the aid of navigation tools to ensure correct placement of the mesh as on the template by using reference points. Postoperative CT scans were obtained to compare the actual position of the titanium mesh implant to the planned position of the orbital floor. They reported accurate reproduction of the planned surgery [25].

In 2006, **Schon et al.** used individually preformed implants to reconstruct an extensive orbital floor fractures in 19 patients. The orbital floor and walls were studied by preoperative diagnostic CT scan data. The form of the virtual reconstructed orbit was printed into a model for the orbital cavity by a template machine. They reported that the orbital reconstruction using a preformed implants is less time consuming, more accurate, and less invasive in comparison to free hand efforts for the restoration of the orbital fractures using titanium mesh and calvarial grafts [26].

In 2010, **Zhang et al.** studied 21 patients with delayed treatment of unilateral impure fracture of the orbit and post-traumatic enophthalmos. They used anatomically adaptive titanium mesh depending on computer-aided design and computer-aided manufacturing techniques (CAD/CAM). After exposure to orbital floor defect and reduction to the herniated soft tissue, the titanium mesh was placed to restore the internal orbit. Measurements were taken to evaluate the change in the degree of enophthalmos and orbital volume before and after surgery. They found that this method was useful to some degree to decrease the expanded orbital volume and correct post-traumatic enophthalmos [27].

In 2012, **He et al.** made a retrospective review of a consecutive clinical case series. 64 patients from 2008 to 2010 were diagnosed with delayed orbitozygomatic fractures with enophthalmos. Traditional surgery and computer-assisted treatment (navigation and 3D models) were used for zygoma reduction. They found that computer-assisted surgery can improve the treatment results [28].

In 2016, **Oh et al.** made a study to use individualized prebent titanium-Medpor mesh implants and stereolithographic modeling in a series of patients who underwent orbital wall reconstruction. They obtained good results and concluded that orbital reconstruction can be optimized by using individually manufactured rapid prototype skull model and premolded synthetic scaffold by computer-aid of mirroring-reconstruction of 3-dimensional images and 3-dimensional printing techniques [29].

In 2020, Sigron et al. made a study to compare the efficacy of the intraoperative bending of titanium mesh with the efficacy of pre-contoured "hybrid" patient-specific titanium mesh using 3D-printed anatomical models as bending guides for the surgical repair of isolated orbital floor fractures. They concluded that t the use of 3D-printed orbital models leads to a more accurate reconstruction and a time reduction during surgery [30].

4. Orbital volume measurement

Orbital volume measurement after maxillofacial trauma reveals a significant data for evaluating the severity of the injury and prevention of possible complications caused by enophthalmos [31]. The Volume of the orbit is the space formed by the size and position of the orbital walls [32].

In 1873 in France, **Gayat** may have been the first to publish orbital volume data [33]. He used lead pellets to fill the orbital cavity of 11 skulls and poured them into a graduated cylinder to determine the orbital volume. He found the average of the orbital volume approximately equal to 29 cm^3. After **Gayat**, some authors used alternative methods for measurement on corpses using silicone, water, glass beads or sand were used [34].

During the 20th century, OVM for living patients became possible with the development of medical imaging techniques. The first OVM for a living patient was performed in the 1960's with manual evaluation of roentgenographic images [33].

With the advent of tomodensitometry, volume measurement of irregular objects became possible. In 1985, **Forbes et al.** transferred the data from CT scan images to special program to calculate the volume of the orbital structures. The software counted the number of pixels to calculate the volume according to the number of slices and special formulas [35].

Manual segmentation for OVM (planimetry methods) is considered to be the most common method for this purpose. It depends on the summation of the manually delineated areas obtained from a CT images [36]. The operator manually delineates the boundaries of the orbital bone cavity on a series of CT slices. The boundaries are defined by the operator and not by standard charts. This can represent a source of errors with low reproducibility. Planimetry method is extremely time-consuming to be accurate but its advantage lies in its availability on all standard medical imaging softwares [37].

Automatic methods for OVM contains automatic segmentation of the orbital cavity which can be undertaken using a function integrated within software. This method relies on atlas segmentation [38]. Semi-automatic method for OVM is defined as a method using volumetric built-in functionality in software, combined with manual adjustments. Various semi-automatic methods are available, depending on the software used. The are some softwares which are considered as different methods described in the literature for OVM [37].

Several studies have shown a correlation between an increased OV and enophthalmos. Using planimetry, **Whitehouse et al**. showed that enophthalmos increased by 0.8 mm per 1 cm^3 of OV expansion [39]. In 1993, **Charteris et al**. proposed that the amount of increase in the orbital volume may determine the need for surgical intervention [40].

Some authors consider the OV as a predictive of long-term symptoms, while other authors did not find a significant correlation between an increased OV and enophthalmos [41]. Choi et al. showed that the OV cannot be considered as a reliable measure to estimate the size of enophthalmos because of inter-individual variations in the OV [42].

The use of intraoperative navigation during the orbital surgery according to data from CT scans or MRI assisted in implementation of preoperative plan, volume measurement, and protecting the vital structures [38]. In the recently published studies, administration of CT images was recommended as the standard method to determine the volume of the orbital cavity in living patients [34]. However, there is no consensus concerning the gold standard for orbital volume measurement [43].

The difference in the volume of bony orbit can reach 0–8% between the right and left orbit when measured in the same person [35, 44], and up to 22% between subjects [32]. This normal difference can be considered as a protective factor for the surgeon, allowing him some malleability in the work for not insisting to achieve the ideal OV and reflecting the great tolerance in orbital volumetric restoration. A perfect symmetry between the 2 orbits is not necessary, and a variation of around 10–20% of the volume between the 2 orbits may involve no or only minor imperceptible facial irregularity. This minor difference may lead to a satisfactory result for the patient and the surgeon [44].

Stereolithography (SLA) technology developed into many types such as powder bed fusion, fused deposition modeling (FDM), selective laser sintering (SLS) for 3D printing which is known as additive manufacturing or desktop fabrication. Some metals as titanium, silver, gold, steel, and stainless steel can be used as raw materials for 3D printing. However, the plastics are most commonly used such as: acrylonitrile butadiene styrene (ABS) or "Lego" plastic material, polylactic acid (PLA) which is readily available in soft and hard grades, polyvinyl alcohol (PVA), and polycarbonate (PC). ABS materials are sturdy, strong, and providing more structural integrity than PLA which is less expensive, more biocompatible, and providing more precise prints [45–48].

5. Conclusion

Both techniques conventional technique and STL model for titanium mesh adaptation lead to significant correction of the orbital volume. Conventional technique is still a valid and cheap method among the attractive new techniques. STL technique is helpful in the cases presented with massive orbital disruption and/or malunion. It offers less operative time and less tissue manipulation.

DOI: http://dx.doi.org/10.5772/intechopen.106369

Author details

Yousry Eldek[1]*, Heba Sleem[2], Mohamad Katamesh[2] and Fahmy Hasanin[3]

1 Oral and Maxillofacial Specialist, Nasser Institute Hospital, Cairo, Egypt

2 Faculty of Dentistry, Professor of Oral and Maxillofacial Surgery, Ain Shams University, Cairo, Egypt

3 Faculty of Dentisry, Professor of Oral and Maxillofacial Surgery, Cairo University, Cairo, Egypt

*Address all correspondence to: usridk@gmail.com

IntechOpen

© 2022 The Author(s). Licensee IntechOpen. This chapter is distributed under the terms of the Creative Commons Attribution License (http://creativecommons.org/licenses/by/3.0), which permits unrestricted use, distribution, and reproduction in any medium, provided the original work is properly cited.

References

[1] Potter JK, Iii EE. Biomaterials for Reconstruction of the Internal Orbit. Journal of Oral and Maxillofacial Surgery. 2004;**62**(10):1280-1297

[2] Ellis E 3rd, Tan Y. Assessment of internal orbital reconstructions for pure blowout fractures: Cranial bone grafts versus titanium mesh. Journal of Oral and Maxillofacial Surgery. 2003;**61**(4):442-453

[3] Dubois L, Steenen SA, Gooris PJJ, Bos RRM, Controversies AGB. Controversies in orbital reconstruction — III. Biomaterials for orbital reconstruction: A review with clinical recommendations. International Journal of Oral and Maxillofacial Surgery. 2015;**45**(1):41-50

[4] Avashia YJ, Sastry A, Fan KL, Mir HS, Thaller SR, Dmd Þ. Materials used for reconstruction after orbital floor fracture. The Journal of Craniofacial Surgery. 2012;**23**(7 Suppl. 1):1991-1997

[5] Scolozzi P, Momjian A, Heuberger J. Computer-aided volumetric comparison of reconstructed orbits for blow-out fractures with nonpreformed versus 3-dimensionally preformed titanium mesh plates: A preliminary study. Journal of Computer Assisted Tomography. 2010;**34**(1):98-104

[6] Singh M, Mamatha NS, Kedarnath NS, Kumar RS, Vijayanand S, Haidry N. Reconstruction of the orbital floor using titanium mesh: A study of three cases. International Journal of Medical Reviews and Case Reports. 2014;**1**:1-3

[7] Yi W-S, Xu X-L, Ma J-R, Ou X-R. Reconstruction of complex orbital fracture with titanium implants. International Journal of Ophthalmology. 2012;**5**(4):488-492

[8] Liss J, Stefko ST, Chung WL. Orbital surgery: State of the art. Oral and Maxillofacial Surgery Clinics. 2010;**22**(1):59-71

[9] Cleveland PW, Smith JE. Complications of facial trauma of the fronto-orbital region. Facial Plastic Surgery. 2017;**33**(06):581-590

[10] Bae H, Lee H, Nunery WR. Orbital adherence syndrome secondary to titanium implant material. Ophthalmic Plastic & Reconstructive Surgery. 2009;**25**(1):33-36

[11] Kersey TL, Ng SGJ, Rosser P, Sloan B, Hart R. Orbital adherence with titanium mesh floor implants: A review of 10 cases. Orbit. 2013;**32**(1):8-11

[12] Elgalal MT, Kozakiewicz M, Olszycki MB. Custom implant design and surgical pre-planning using rapid prototyping and anatomical models for the repair of orbital floor fractures; 2009. Available from: https://posterng.netkey.at/esr/viewing/index.php?module=viewing_poster&task=viewsection&pi=40353&ti=122509&si=688&searchkey=#poster

[13] Vargo J, Townsend J, Sullivan S, Detamore M, Andrews B. Modern applications of computer bioengineering in maxillofacial surgery: Image guided surgical navigation and CAD/CAM custom implants. Journal of Computer Engineering & Information Technology. 2017;**6**:2-5

[14] Perry M, Banks P, Richards R, Friedman EP, Shaw P. The use of computer-generated three-dimensional models in orbital reconstruction. The

British Journal of Oral & Maxillofacial Surgery. 1998;**36**(4):275-284

[15] Hoang D, Perrault D, Stevanovic M, Ghiassi A. Surgical applications of three-dimensional printing: A review of the current literature & how to get started. Annals of Translational Medicine. 2016;**4**(23):456

[16] Olszewski R. Three-dimensional rapid prototyping models in cranio-maxillofacial surgery: Systematic review and new clinical applications. Proceedings of the Belgian Royal Academies of Medicine. 2013;**2**(1):43-47

[17] Li WZ. Application of computer-aided three-dimensional skull model with rapid prototyping technique in repair of zygomatico-orbito-maxillary complex fracture. International Journal of Medical Robotics and Computer Assisted Surgery. 2009;**5**:158-163

[18] Lim CGT, Campbell FDI, Clucas DM, Mech N. Rapid prototyping Technology in Orbital Floor Reconstruction: Application in three patients. 2014;**1**(212):143-146

[19] Scolozzi P. Computer-aided volume measurement of posttraumatic orbits reconstructed with AO titanium mesh plates: Accuracy and reliability. Ophthalmic Plast Reconstr Surg. 2008;**24**(5):383-389

[20] Peng Q, Tang Z, Liu O, Peng Z. Rapid prototyping-assisted maxillofacial reconstruction. Annals of Medicine. 2015;**47**(3):186-208

[21] Bill JS et al. Stereolithography in oral and maxillofacial operation planning. International Journal of Oral and Maxillofacial Surgery. 1995;**24**(1):98-103

[22] Schmitt SM, Chance DA. Fabrication of titanium implant-retained restorations with nontraditional machining techniques. The International Journal of Prosthodontics. Jul-Aug 1995;**8**(4):332-336. PMID: 7575975

[23] Holck DE, Boyd EM, Ng J, Mauffray RO. Benefits of stereolithography in orbital reconstruction. Ophthalmology. 1999;**106**(6):1214-1218

[24] Nayar S, Bhuminathan S, Bhat WM. Rapid prototyping and stereolithography in dentistry. Journal of Pharmacy & Bioallied Sciences. 2015;7(Suppl. 1):S216

[25] Metzger MC, Schön R, Schulze D, Carvalho C, Gutwald R, Schmelzeisen R. Individual preformed titanium meshes for orbital fractures. Oral Surgery, Oral Medicine, Oral Pathology and Oral Radiology. 2006;**102**:442-447

[26] Schön R, Metzger MC, Zizelmann C, Weyer N, Schmelzeisen R. Individually preformed titanium mesh implants for a true-to-original repair of orbital fractures. International Journal of Oral and Maxillofacial Surgery. 2006;**35**(11):990-995

[27] Zhang Y, He Y, Zhang ZY, An JG. Evaluation of the application of computer-aided shape-adapted fabricated titanium mesh for mirroring-reconstructing orbital walls in cases of late post-traumatic enophthalmos. Journal of Oral and Maxillofacial Surgery. 2010;**68**(9):2070-2075

[28] He D et al. Orbitozygomatic fractures with enophthalmos: Analysis of 64 cases treated late. Journal of Oral and Maxillofacial Surgery. 2012;**70**(3):562-576

[29] Oh TS, Jeong WS, Chang TJ, Koh KS, Choi J-W. Customized orbital wall reconstruction using three-dimensionally printed rapid prototype model in patients with orbital wall

fracture. The Journal of Craniofacial Surgery. 2016;**27**(8):2020-2024

[30] Sigron GR et al. Three-dimensional analysis of isolated orbital floor fractures pre-and post-reconstruction with standard titanium meshes and 'hybrid' patient-specific implants. Journal of Clinical Medicine. 2020;**9**(5):1579

[31] Deveci M, Öztürk S, Şengezer M, Pabuşcu Y. Measurement of orbital volume by a 3-dimensional software program: An experimental study. Journal of Oral and Maxillofacial Surgery. 2000;**58**(6):645-648

[32] Parsons GS, Mathog RH. Orbital wall and volume relationships. Archives of Otorhinolaryngology-Head & Neck Surgery. 1988;**114**(7):743-747

[33] Curtin H, Fay A. Comparison of methodologies in volumetric Orbitometry. Ophthalmic Plast Reconstr Surg. 2013;**29**(6):431-436

[34] Mottini M, Wolf CA, Jafari SMS, Katsoulis K, Schaller B. Stereographic measurement of orbital volume, a digital reproducible evaluation method. British Journal of Ophthalmology. 2017;**101**:1-5

[35] Forbes G, Gehring DG, Gorman CA, Brennan MD, Jackson IT. Volume measurements of normal orbital structures by computed tomographic analysis. American Journal of Neuroradiology. 1985;**6**(3):419-424

[36] Bontzos G et al. Ex vivo orbital volumetry using stereology and CT imaging: A comparison with manual planimetry. European Radiology. 2019;**29**(3):1365-1374

[37] Sentucq C et al. Overview of tools for the measurement of the orbital volume and their applications to orbital surgery. Journal of Plastic, Reconstructive & Aesthetic Surgery. 2021;**74**(3): 581-591

[38] Jansen J, Schreurs R, Dubois L, Maal TJJ, Gooris PJJ, Becking AG. Orbital volume analysis: Validation of a semi-automatic software segmentation method. International Journal of Computer Assisted Radiology and Surgery. 2016;**11**:11-18

[39] Whitehouse RW, Batterbury M, Jackson A, Noble JL. Prediction of enophthalmos by computed tomography after' blow out' orbital fracture. British Journal of Ophthalmology. 1994;**78**(8):618-620

[40] Charteris DG, Chan C, Whitehouse RW, Noble JL, Eye MR, Chan C. Orbital volume measurement in the management of pure blowout fractures of the orbital floor. British Journal of Ophthalmology. 1993;**77**(2):100-102

[41] Schönegg D et al. Correlation between increased orbital volume and enophthalmos and diplopia in patients with fractures of the orbital floor or the medial orbital wall. Journal of Cranio-Maxillofacial Surgery. 2018;**46**(9):1544-1549

[42] Choi SH, Kang DH, Gu JH. The correlation between the orbital volume ratio and enophthalmos in unoperated blowout fractures. Archives of Plastic Surgery. 2016;**43**(6):518

[43] Kwon J, Barrera JE, Jung T-Y, Most SP. Measurements of orbital volume change using computed tomography in isolated orbital blowout fractures. Archives of Facial Plastic Surgery. 2009;**11**(6):395-398

[44] Andrades P et al. Degrees of tolerance in post-traumatic orbital volume correction: The role of

prefabricated mesh. Journal of Oral and Maxillofacial Surgery. 2009;**67**(11):2404-2411

[45] Ngo TD, Kashani A, Imbalzano G, Nguyen KTQ, Hui D. Additive manufacturing (3D printing): A review of materials, methods, applications and challenges. Composites. Part B, Engineering. 2018;**143**:172-196

[46] Thomas GP. Materials Used In 3D Printing and Additive Manufacturing. AzOM. 2013. Available from: http//www.azom.com/article. aspx,

[47] Hesse B. ABS or PLA: Which 3D Printing Filament Should You Use? 2015. Retrieved from: https://www.digitaltrends.com/cool-tech/abs-vs-pla-3d-printing-materials-comparison/

[48] Tappa K, Jammalamadaka U. Novel biomaterials used in medical 3D printing techniques. Journal of Functional Biomaterials. 2018;**9**(1):17

Chapter 7

Perspective Chapter: Trauma from Occlusion – Practical Management Guidelines

Prashanth Shetty, Shweta Hegde, Shubham Chelkar, Rahul Chaturvedi, Shruti Pochhi, Aakanksha Shrivastava, Dudala Lakshmi, Shreya Mukherjee, Pankaj Bajaj and Shahzada Asif Raza

Abstract

Occlusal trauma is trauma to the periodontium from functional or parafunctional force's causing damage to the teeth and its attachment apparatus by exceeding its adaptive and reparative capacities. Occlusal instability is a common cause for trauma from occlusion, resulting in numerous complications. It often leads to interference which reflexively shifts or slides the jaw forward on one or both the side to find a spot where most teeth come together. This action protects the teeth from injury caused by chewing on just one tooth. Overtime, this shift can cause a whole host of problems from TMJ pain, post restorative complications, headache, tooth sensitivity, recession, broken and loss of teeth and orofacial pain. These occlusal interferences and bite discrepancies are treatable with minimally invasive dentistry. Occlusal equilibration is a therapy that is used when the cause of trauma is due to occlusal instability. This involves the reshaping of the teeth where the improper biting surfaces are located. The key lies in decoding the cause, but often treatment is only directed towards the effects. Only a thorough evaluation and occlusal analysis will lead to a definitive diagnosis that will help in better anticipation of the damages.

Keywords: occlusal trauma, occlusal instability, occlusal interferences, occlusal analysis, biometric analysis, occlusal equilibration

1. Introduction

Ideal occlusion is characterized by simultaneous contacting of all teeth at maximum intercuspation, with an equal intensity force on right and left side of the arch. This helps to preserve all the physiological components of the stomatognathic system namely the occlusion, the attachment apparatus, TMJ and the neuromusculature in harmony as they are closely interrelated. When the functional or parafunctional occlusal forces exceeds the capacity for adaptation and repair of one tooth or group of teeth and its attachment, limited or progressive injury occurs. This is called occlusal trauma. In the presence of interference, the jaw will reflexively shift and slide forward on one or both the side to find a spot where most teeth come together. An unstable occlusion is a common cause for numerous post restoration complications. Overtime, this may cause a whole host of problems from TMJ pain, headache to sensitivity, recession, broken and lost teeth and Orofacial Pain.

Establishing a stable and harmonious occlusion goes a long way in preventing the deterioration of the dentition and its associated structures [1]. Trauma from occlusion is a clinical finding often ignored by the dentist as it is not a part of the chief complaint. The key lies in decoding the cause, but most often treatment is only directed towards the effects. Only a thorough evaluation and occlusal analysis will lead to a definite diagnosis. A good diagnosis helps in better anticipation of the direction the damages will take.

Digital occlusal analysis is a powerful tool which provides the dentists with an objective reproducible data. These occlusal technologies along with a biometric approach will allow for an accurate diagnosis treatment and reevaluation of the inter relationship between teeth, muscles & joints [2].

2. Terminologies used with trauma from occlusion

2.1 Trauma from occlusion

Occlusal trauma was defined as "An injury to the attachment apparatus as a result of excessive occlusal force" "Glossary of Periodontics terms" (American Academy of Periodontology 1986), [3].

2.2 Occlusal interferences

Any contact that inhibits the remaining occluding surfaces from achieving stable and harmonious contacts.

2.3 Occlusal adjustment

Reshaping of the occlusal surfaces of teeth by grinding to create harmonious contact relationships between the upper and lower teeth, or orthodontic movement of the teeth to create more harmonious contact relationship.

2.4 Fremitus

A palpable or visible movement of a tooth when subjected to occlusal forces (also known as functional mobility).

2.5 Premature occlusal contact

A condition of tooth contact that diverts the mandible from a normal path of closure.

3. Classification

3.1 Glickman's classification (1953)

3.1.1 According to duration of cause

I. Acute trauma from occlusion:

This type of trauma is caused because of abrupt occlusal impact, like due to biting on a tough object or high restorations or prosthetic appliances. The clinical signs and symptoms of the condition include tooth pain and sensitivity to percussion, fremitus, tooth mobility and once the cause is removed, symptoms subside and complete healing takes place [4–7].

II. Chronic trauma from occlusion:

When abnormal occlusal forces are exerted on the tooth-supporting structures for a longer duration of time, chronic trauma from occlusion occur. It is more significant than the acute condition because it results in progressive changes in occlusion clinically seen as tooth migration, tooth wear and extrusion of teeth [4–7].

3.1.2 According to nature of cause

I. Primary trauma from occlusion:

It refers to the injury resulting from excessive occlusal forces applied to a tooth or teeth with adequate support

II. Secondary trauma from occlusion:

It refers to the injury resulting from normal occlusal forces applied to a tooth or teeth with inadequate support.

3.2 Box's classification

3.2.1 Physiologic occlusion

Box defined it as a condition, in which the systems of forces acting upon the tooth during the occlusion are in a state of equilibrium, and they do not and cannot change the normal relationship existing between the tooth and its supporting structures [8].

3.2.2 Traumatic occlusion

The damage produced in the periodontium is due to the overstress produced by the occlusion (**Table 1**).

Precipitating factor	Magnitude of force Director of the principle PDL fibers Duration of the force application Frequency of the force application	
Predisposing factor	**Intrinsic**	**Extrinsic**
	Orientation of the long axis of the teeth Morphological characterization of the tooth Morphology of the alveolar process (quality & quantity of the bone)	Local factors like plaque Long span fixed partial denture supported on few teeth Inappropriate bone resection Parafunctional habits Other factors, including overhanging filling, poorly contoured restoration Food impaction etc.

Table 1.
Etiology of trauma from occlusion.

4. Pathophysiology of trauma from occlusion

Excessive occlusal force
↓
Soft tissue change
Traumatic v shaped gingival crescent
Stillman's cleft (indentations in the gingival margin generally on one side of tooth)
McCall's festoons (Buccal Bone dehiscence)
Absence of stippling – Edema secondary to trauma
↓
Alteration in occlusal forces
↓
Hard tissue change
Occlusal wearing pattern of tooth not attributed to any abnormality in patient diet
↓
Tooth mobility, migration, shifting & tilting of tooth
↓
Discomfort on eating
↓
Sensitivity of teeth
↓
Hypertonicity of muscle
↓
Mandibular deviation

5. Stages of tissue response to excessive occlusal forces

Excessive force of occlusion causes the tissue to respond in three stages Injury, repair and adaptive remodeling of periodontium.

5.1 Stage 1: injury

Soft tissue injury is the immediate result of excessive occlusal forces. The magnitude of forces varies from slightly excessive, greater then excessive or severely high.

The centre of rotation of a single rooted tooth lies at the junction of middle and apical third of the tooth and is located near the furcation area of the multirooted teeth.

When excessive occlusal forces are subjected to teeth they rotate around the fulcrum of rotation. This rotation in the tooth socket creates areas of presser and tension on the opposite side of the fulcrum. When the force is unidirectional, these are created on the opposite surface, whereas in the case of jiggling forces these areas may co – exist on the same surface.

Effect of excessive occlusal forces on the periodontium.

Slightly excessive forces- simulates bone resorption in area of presser, causing the widening of periodontal ligament space. Elongation of PDL fibers takes place in the areas of tension.

Greater than slightly excessive forces- caused marked changes in the tooth supporting structures producing areas of hyalinization and necrose when excessive compressive forces are produced from trauma from occlusion.

Severely high occlusal force- results in thrombosis, hemorrhage, tearing & widening of pdl space and undermined bone resorption. If the forces are removed, or tooth moves away the periodontium is completely repaired.

5.2 Stage 2: repair

Takes place when the damage tissue is replaced by new connective tissue and cells. This is a well-regulated mechanism and the healing process is directly or indirectly facilitated by the extracellular matrix and certain inflammatory mediators. The activity is increased during TFO & the body tries to reinforce the trabeculae within the new bone by a process known as buttressing bone formation. When it occurs in the buccal and lingual surface of the alveolar bone it is known as peripheral buttressing and central buttressing when this process occurs within the bone this helps to bear increased occlusal load. There is a shelf-life thickening of the bone on the labial or lingual surface of the alveolar bone is referred to as lipping.

5.3 Stage 3: adaptive remodeling of the periodontium

Establishes a structural relationship in such a way that the forces of occlusion are no longer harmful to the periodontium, and the repair process can keep pace with the destructive occlusal forces.

Tooth mobility is an important clinical sign when TFO is increase it occurs in two phases the initial phase there is an increase in the width of the PDL and reduction of the number of the periodontal fibers leading to alveolar bone resorption.

The second phase results in the permanent widening of the PDL space which occurs after the repair of the traumatic lesion as an adaptation to the increased forces.

6. Is traumatic occlusion reversible?

If excessive occlusal forces are neutralized, healing takes place. The presence of plaque may however impair healing so resolution of inflammation should be first initiated. Injury caused by TFO is reversible but there may or may not be complete restoration of the supporting structures of the tooth.

7. Examination, evaluation, diagnosis and prognosis of trauma from occlusion

Clinical history of the patient and clinical examination are the cornerstones of correct diagnosis of TFO.

7.1 Clinical features of occlusal trauma

1. No periodontitis
2. Tooth wear (mild faceting or marked attrition)
3. Fractures of the enamel or restorations
4. Occlusal interferences (either from the retruded contact position to intercuspal position (ICP) or in lateral excursions/protrusive movements)
5. Ridging of buccal mucosa
6. Indentations in lateral border of the tongue
7. Reddening of the tip of the tongue.

7.2 Tooth mobility

Miller's Index (1938) is most often used to classify tooth mobility. Normal physiological movement vary between 10 μm and 150 μm and is not detectable on examination.

Class 0 – Within physiologic range when force is applied.

Class I – Mobility more the physiologic range.

Class II – Tooth moves upto 1 mm or more laterally (mesiodistal/buccolingual). Inability to vertically depress the tooth (apicocoronally).

Class III – Tooth can be moved 1 mm or more laterally (labiolingually or mesiodistally). Tooth can be depressed in a vertical direction.

7.3 Fremitus test

TFO can clinically detected using this test. The movement or vibratory pattern is measured when the teeth are placed in contacting positions and during lateral and protrusive movements.

In this test the vibratory movement of the tooth/teeth is identified and graded by placing dampened index finger along the labial surfaces of maxillary teeth.

The patient is asked to tap the teeth together in MIP and then grind systematically in lateral and protrusive movements.

Classification system used:

Class I fremitus: Mild movements/vibration detected.

Class II fremitus: No visible movements/easily palpable vibration.

Class III fremitus: Movements are visible to the naked eye.

7.4 Radiographic signs

I. Widening of the PDL space, often with thickening of the lamina dura along the lateral aspect of the root in the apical region and in bifurcation areas

II. Irregular widening of the periodontal ligament space.

III. Vertical rather than horizontal destruction of the interdental septum, with the formation of infrabony defects

IV. Bone sclerosis in the periapical area or in the interdental bone crest.

V. Radiolucency and condensation of the alveolar bone

VI. In advanced stages of TFO inflammatory root resorption is seen.

VII. Increase in periapical bone density around a vital tooth on a radiograph indicative of a type of Sclerosing Osteitis and a positive clinical sign of TFO helps guide us to a correct diagnosis and treatment plan.

Radiographical Features

1. Hypercementosis.

2. Secondary dentin laid down in the pulp chamber.

8. Occlusal trauma and implants

Osseointegration of implants is a direct structural and functional connection between ordered living bone and the surface of a load carrying implant.

Functional load enhances the integration when the load is adequately distributed. Occlusal overload however adversely affects implant stability. Strain is the key factor in controlling bone remodeling. Strain is created when any object is subjected to external stress. Stress in the oral environment is the occlusal overload. Mechano-receptors present in the bone play a major role in initiating bone remodeling. When implant restorations are subject to TFO, stress of a higher level are imposed at the interface. This initiates resorption of bone and may lead to failure of implants.

Crestal bone loss observed around implants occurs mainly because of the difference in modulus of elasticity of the implant and bone. As the modulus of elasticity of titanium is 5–10 times greater than that of the cortical bone. In osseointegrated implants stresses are concentrated at the crestal bone level. Thus, any sustained overload on the implant restoration may lead to implant instability.

9. Our present understanding of trauma from occlusion

Periodontal health depends on the normal occlusal forces. Any increase in the functional demand the periodontium accommodates by thickening of the lamina dura and reinforcement of bony trabeculae.

When the functional demand of the tooth cannot be met, tissue injury results. If the stimulus is chronic and noxious widening of the PDL space is seen at the expense of bone resorption. This has a cushioning effect which enables the tooth to bear the excess forces.

Many concepts still needs to be clarified about trauma from occlusion. However, the following conclusions can be drawn from the present data.

Presently there is no evidence that suggests that gingivitis or periodontitis is caused by trauma from occlusion or can accelerate the progression of gingivitis to periodontitis.

PDL is a dynamic tissue and has the ability to adapt to increased forces of occlusion by widening of the periodontal ligament & crestal bone resorption. But when the excessive forces are removed, the periodontium & the tooth comeback to their normal state of function.

Trauma from occlusion may be considered a co factor which can increase the rate of progression of an existing periodontal disease.

As a rule the first line of treatment should be to resolve inflammation by elimination of local factors by scaling & root planning.

An important component to ensure smooth function & comfort of the patient is occlusal therapy.

10. Treatment of trauma from occlusion

10.1 Treatment plan: systematic approach

I. Make the patient aware, accept and own the problem and make them partners on the road to co-discovery and co-treatment in order to achieve functional, esthetic and biological goals.

II. Identify bacterial risk, periodontal charting, habits evaluation, fremitus test, pathological wear, mobility and migration.

III. Evaluation of functional disharmony in the Masticatory apparatus (R.O.M, Load test, JVA, EMG, occlusal scan, TMJ Doppler Auscultation, Muscle palpation. Evaluate the 5 requirements of occlusal stability by Dawson's Academy. Evaluate TMJ- for Piper's classification.

IV. Assess the complete records- clinical, radiographic, photographic, diagnostic models,

Mount cast with facebow transfer at the first point of contact, protrusive and centric records are taken to program the articulator.

Treatment Planning can be done with the help of

a. Two-dimensional wax up or

b. 3-dimensional digital wax up

10.2 Treatment options

Different treatment options can be planned for the same diagnosis. The option taken will be determined by several patient related factors and occlusal analysis. The treatment of TFO involves removal of the excessive occlusal forces and bringing the tooth/teeth in a comfortable position. Many treatment modalities have been advised to treat TFO. These include,

I. Occlusal adjustments and occlusal equilibration

II. Management of parafunctional habits.

III. Biometric management of trauma from occlusion.

IV. Orthodontic tooth movement.

V. Occlusal reconstruction.

VI. Extraction of selected teeth.

10.3 Occlusal adjustments and occlusal equilibration

10.3.1 Occlusal equilibration

"It is a controlled destruction of tooth surface aimed at reducing the biological price the dentition will eventually pay if not done. Establishing a stable and harmonious occlusion goes a long way in preventing the deterioration of the dentition and its associated structures. This can be achieved by occlusal equilibration, which is a minimally invasive therapy involving reshaping of the teeth when improper biting forces are located.

10.3.2 Steps in occlusal equilibration

1. Mock Equilibration in the Articulator.

   The centric and eccentric interference are marked and eliminated in a sequence. Establishing of a harmonious and optimum anterior guidance to the new envelop of function. Developing the guidance with a wax up after customizing the anterior guidance table. This establishes a tentative blue print of the procedures and amount of reduction to be carried out on the identified teeth.

2. Occlusal adjustment is done directly in the mouth with a Kois Deprogrammer (**Figure 1**) with an anterior ramp at pre-establishing vertical dimension and centric relation.

10.3.3 Occlusal equilibration can be done in 4 steps

1. Find the first point of contact with a 200 μm horse shoe paper.

2. Remove the clinical contact, continue with the equilibration (40 μm paper).

3. Obtain equal intensity contact from canine backward (8 μm paper).

4. Chewing pathway adjustment is done with 200 μm paper.

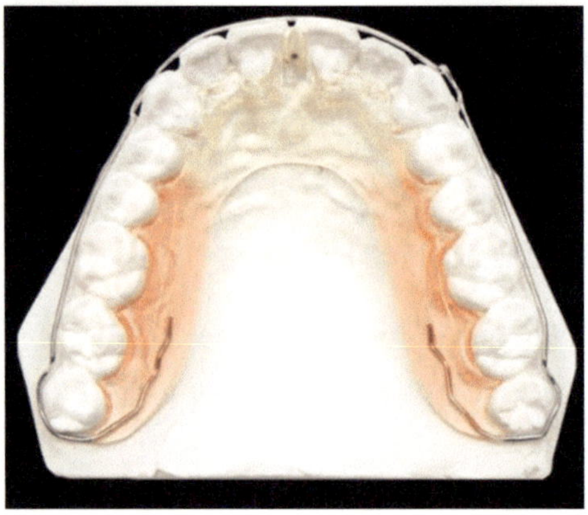

Figure 1.
Kois deprogrammer. SOURCE- https://www.koiscenter.com/kois-center-a-new-standard/kois-center-research/kois-deprogrammer/.

10.3.4 Grinding rules to be followed

1. Narrow the stamp cusps before reshaping the fossa.
2. Do not shorten the stamp cusp.
3. Always adjust centric interferences first.
4. Eliminate all posterior incline contacts & preserve only the cusp tip.

10.3.5 Occlusal reduction

i. Centric relation interferences (interference to the arc of closure)

   a. Retrusive interference

   b. Centric slide – MUDL

ii. Selective Reduction of tooth structure that interferes with the lateral excursions, deflective interferences (Line of closure) lateral interferences Patient is guided to left and right eccentric positions.

   a. BULL- Balancing interference

   b. LUBL- Working interference

iii. Elimination of all posterior tooth structure that interferes with the protrusive excursions (Protrusive interferences) –

   DUML- The patient is guided to centric and asked to slide forward and back

iv. PATHWAY ADJUSTMENT

Harmonization of anterior guidance to the envelop of function at an erect posture and asked to chew on 200-micron paper.

a. Stable holding contacts on Central incisor (anterior teeth at the cervical ⅕th of the tooth)- Anterior retained stops (MIP)

b. All contact anterior to this is removed.

c. Equalize the contact to get as many teeth into contact as possible without striking the inclines. Optimum guidance is when anterior teeth does not interfere with the Chewing pathway.

- Finally, the patient is asked to chop-Chop in centric and grind in all direction with an 8-micron paper in the mouth.

- End result should be one good heavy contact on all the teeth from canine backwards on the functional cusp and opposing fossa. With light contact on 2nd molar and no contact on the incisors, verify dots in the back and lines in the front.

- End with a clench test- Patient is asked to close the mouth and squeeze firmly and checked for comfort. In teeth/muscle/TMJ if there is a bilateral smooth simultaneous, uniform harmonious jaw function with no instability in the joint.

- Completed with a Shim Stock contact test.

- Finished and polished to a smooth finish with a polishing paste.

- A maintenance protocol also needs to be followed every 2 weeks, for a month requiring constant checkup (**Figure 2**).

10.4 Management of parafunctional habits

Parafunctional habit is a repetitive behavior that targets oral structures occlusal wear, fractured cusps, clenching/bruxism, obstructive sleep apnea are common signs of parafunctional activity. They can occur consciously when awake or at night and have been linked to stress & anxiety.

Management begins with creating a cognitive and behavioral awareness. Use of hard acrylic splints which are correctly adjusted for occlusion, helps protect the teeth and relax the muscles.

Localized occlusal interference splint and orthotic devices help in management of dental arch malrelationship.

10.5 Biometric management of trauma from occlusion

A biometric approach includes the jaw vibrational analysis (JVA) (**Figure 3**) of the TMJ, EMG (**Figure 4**) of the muscles and digital occlusal scan (**Figure 5**) of the teeth.

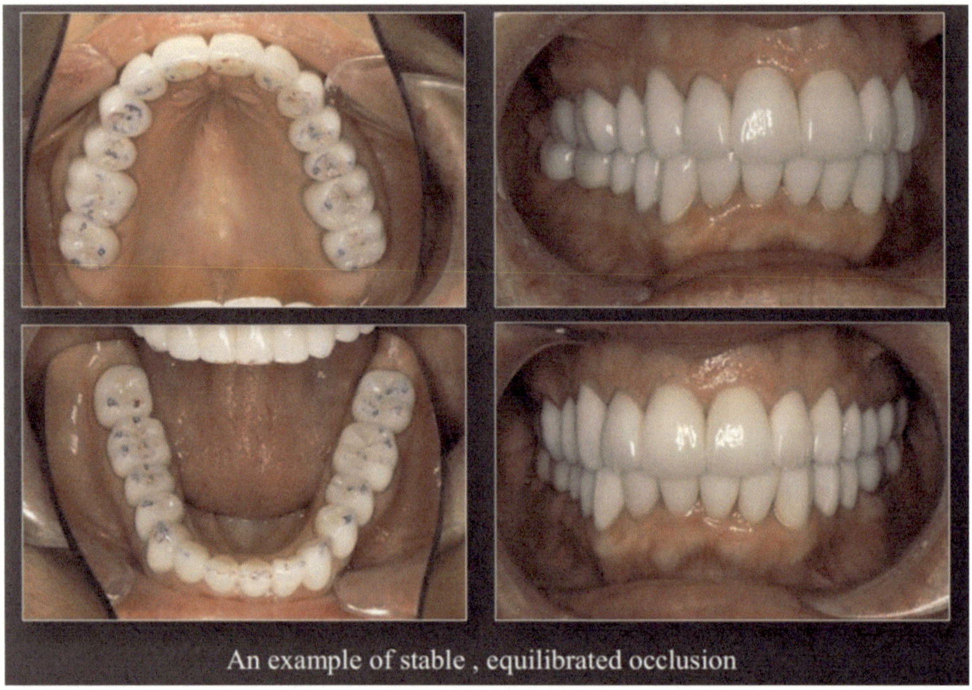

Figure 2.
Equilibrated occlusion.

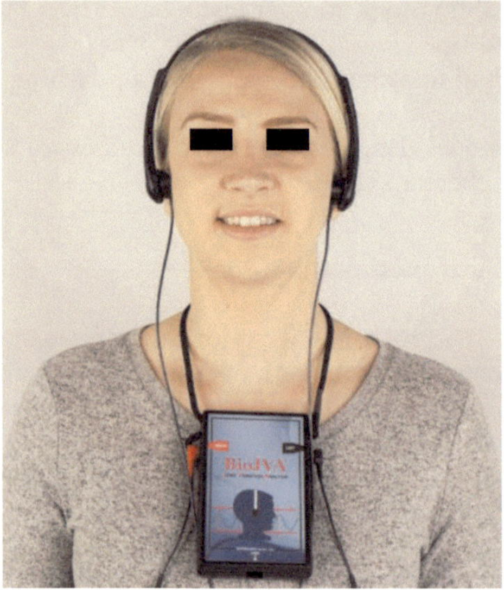

Figure 3.
Jaw vibrational analysis [JVA]. SOURCE- https://www.bioresearchinc.com/joint-vibration-analysis/.

Harmony in the muscle, joint, teeth & restorations are closely interrelated, the biometric approach gives the critical information needed to create this harmony,

Advanced computerized systems are now able to give objective, reproducible data allowing for accurate diagnosis, treatment and re-evaluation of occlusal condition.

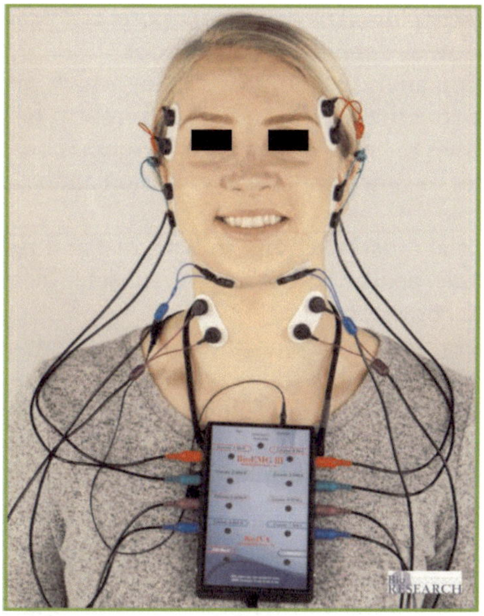

Figure 4.
Electromyograph [EMG]. SOURCE- https://www.bioresearchinc.com/emg-bioresearch/.

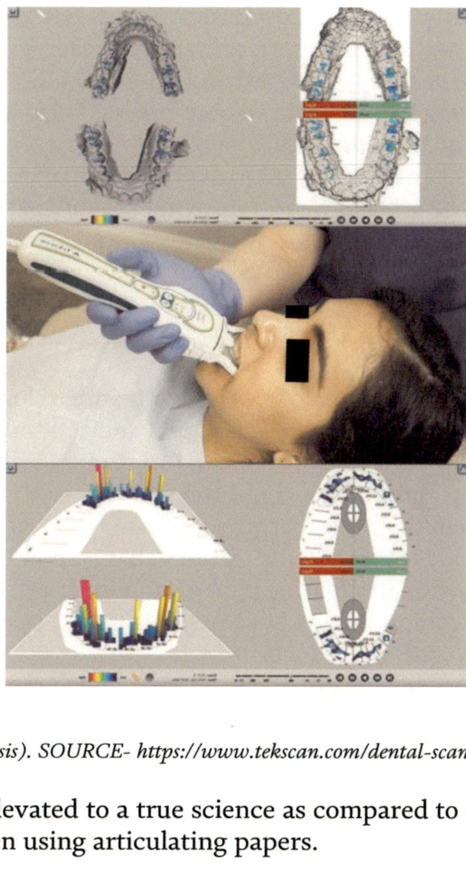

Figure 5.
T-scan (digital occlusal analysis). SOURCE- https://www.tekscan.com/dental-scan-t-scan.

Occlusion analysis is elevated to a true science as compared to subjective analytical methods followed when using articulating papers.

When used pro-actively clinicians can detect potential problem early thus preventing the progression of debilitating conditions.

Step 1. – Joint vibration analysis is an instrument which produces virtual image of the recordings by measuring the wavelength of different types of vibration and patterns of friction. It is shown to be 98% specific in diagnosis of joint pathology. It can be paired with other devices to synchronize the vibration analysis with jaw tracking and EMG recording.

Step 2- The Craniofacial muscle activity in both rest and function is recorded using the EMG to determine the specific activity of the muscles of mastication, timed exactly with the occlusal contact forces.

EMG studies help improve muscle coordination, and reduce incoordination and hyperactivity. Electric activity in the muscle quiets down almost immediately after a clench is released, whereas with occlusal disharmony muscle activity is prolonged even after the teeth are separated. Electromyography helps measure specific muscle activity, allowing treatment to be biologically based instead of just spatially driven.

Step 3- Digital Occlusal Scans- gives a functional picture of the mouth which helps establish the dynamic occlusion that balances both force and time. The role of occlusion is often overlooked, minimized or ignored in dental practice due to difficulty in understanding the concepts. Occlusal scans can be used along with tenets of both popular school of thoughts regarding occlusion by coordinating the timing and activity of individual muscle as well as canine protected occlusion.

When used simultaneously with a link software between EMG and occlusal scan it will help improve the patient's overall occlusion. This is because the scan software shows the exact timing and specific tooth contact and loads in conjunction with muscle activity. The use of disocclusal time reduction (DTR) therapy can reduce the time taken for disocclusion from MIP to Canine rise, and also help reduce interference that disrupt the harmony of tooth muscle joint complex.

Digital scans also help analyze and address the causes of occlusal discrepancy instead of just treating the effects. Thus, removing potential triggers from any muscle based clinical pathologies creating harmony synergy and symmetry in the stomatognathic system [2].

10.6 Orthodontic tooth movement

Tooth malposition are prime cause for Trauma from Occlusion. Orthodontic therapy (**Figure 6**) has a big role to play in prevention and treatment of malposition. The teeth should be moved to a position which will improve its stability and long-term prognosis by eliminating abnormal occlusal forces. Early detection of occlusal trauma and correction can help mitigate the harmful occlusal forces and help prevent damage to the teeth and the periodontium. Investigations that help aid this include visual inspection of occlusion with articulating paper, mobility assessment, full mouth radiographs and use of computer aided occlusal evaluation system. The assessment should be made both in static and functional excursions.

Orthodontic treatment may itself create occlusal interferences, these are temporary and do not last long. The reasons are usually related to inappropriate tooth position, occlusal morphology and overload in excursive movements. These interferences if present should be allowed to settle down over a duration of time by natural accommodation and assessed over a period of time. A through occlusal analysis should always be performed before and after completion of orthodontic treatment.

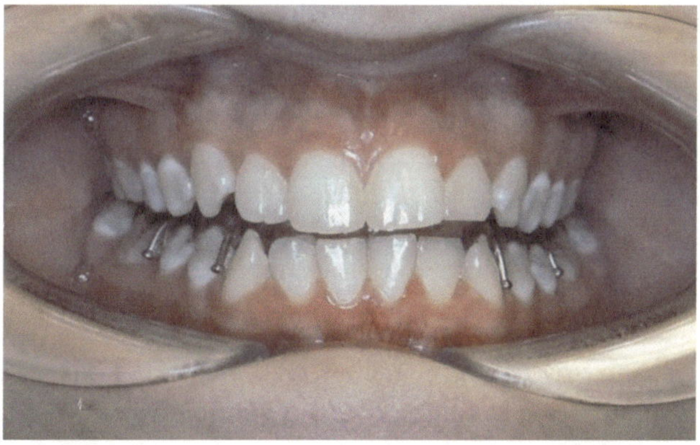

Figure 6.
Orthotic appliances. SOURCE- https://drandrewwilloughby.com/smile-gallery/neuromuscular-orthotics-for-treatment-of-tmj-dysfunction/.

10.7 Occlusal reconstruction

Redesigning of the complete occlusal scheme is done when no other means of occlusal equilibration can be achieved. This is done by fabrication, crowns, fixed partial and implant supported prosthesis and requires a thorough understanding of occlusion and then extensively on an appropriate articulated cast and is then replicated in the patient's mouth.

The chewing and biting surfaces of teeth are in balance and proper alignment. Thus, the pressure on individual teeth is lessen there by making them less susceptible to trauma. Thereby improving the normal functioning of the mouth.

A thorough examination and a differential diagnosis procedure is essential to restore the health of the articulating system restore individual tooth to its best anatomic position. This requires an integrated approach including (using) all disciplines of dentistry, to support, manage, limit and lessen the wear and destruction of the element of the masticatory apparatus and restore a healthy physical support.

10.8 Surgical management

Extraction of tooth that interferes with occlusion is a rarely used option. In certain situations, extraction of the selective teeth with poor prognosis with extensive periodontal involvement is done to improve the prognosis of the remaining teeth. This helps achieve a proper true position and alignment of the remaining teeth and immediate structures and the total articulating system.

11. Discussion

Trauma from occlusion is a term often used but least understood. It refers to tooth/tissue injury due to distorted occlusion and/or occlusal forces. The damaging forces may affect the tooth, its supporting structures and immediate structures that may extend to involve the articulating system. A lack of awareness often leads to the cascading consequences in the masticatory system.

This is mostly to do with difficulty in decoding the cause as a result management is only directed at the effects. Treatment approach needs to include through evaluation of occlusion, understanding of occlusal instability and early diagnosis of changes in the supporting structures.

11.1 Periodontal management

Any occlusal force which goes beyond the adaptive capacity of the underlying tissues leads to damage to the periodontal structures. The current understanding of the role of TFO is it can amplify not cause localized loss of attachment.

Trauma from occlusion is reversible but attachment loss may not be. The development of pockets and recession are not a direct consequence of TFO. The development of pockets and recession are not a direct consequence of TFO but due to other etiological factors & plaque and calculus. When diagnosing the periodontal condition, his/her unique susceptibility, history and site specificity, specific to the direction of the force to a particular tooth [6, 9].

Management is directed towards intercepting any pathological process or to eliminate conditions conducive to disease or injury by looking for risk factors early help manage with minimal treatment. This is done by containing inflammation and instituting proper plaque control measures including supra/sub gingival debridement. If mobility persists teeth should be stabilized with fixed splints only after the traumatic occlusal forces are eliminated. If TFO is left untreated the chances of periodontal disease increases greatly [10].

Occlusal instability is a trigger to a host of adverse consequences leading to occlusal disharmony. Failure to replace missing teeth, malocclusion and improperly aligned teeth to each other produces irregular and less repeatable chewing strokes. The chewing is shorter and slower and may also have an irregular pathway. Mandibular deviation may result in order to avoid deflective contacts. This manifests as pain in the jaw muscles, and a host of adverse consequences in the masticatory apparatus. Occlusal equilibration is the widely used option of treatment, in which the chewing and biting surfaces of the teeth is either selectively reduced or restored to achieve the ideal occlusion [11].

Analysis of the direction of the stress in the centric closure versus that of eccentric closure discloses on the important causes of pathologic wear of teeth and the resultant effect on the supporting structures. Objective treatment plan should restore a harmonious cuspal relationship within physiologic limit and harmonize the jaw in centric at peace with the neuromusculature. This allows the jaw to function where it is comfortable and not restricted [12].

The goal is to confine all excursive contacts on to the anterior teeth, removing any posterior interferences if any that trigger and activates the muscle hyperactivity that prevents the turning off of the elevator muscle activity. The role of occlusion is often overlooked minimized or ignored in general dental practice. As many dentists find it difficult to understand concepts and when, where and how to incorporate occlusal technologies in to the practice [1].

Biometric approach gives clinician a powerful objective tool for incorporating occlusal analysis leading to improved clinical results and fewer failures in prosthetic restorations and orthodontic tooth repositioning. It connects the biological markers with the patient's occlusion and gives critical information that is required to create harmony between teeth, muscles and jaw [2].

Prevention, Interception and correction are terms synonymous with orthodontic, should also be integrated into management of TFO. Malposition of teeth are prime

DOI: http://dx.doi.org/10.5772/intechopen.105960

reasons for development of damaging forces, orthodontics is the ideal means of correcting these teeth irregularities. Early diagnosis and repositioning of teeth to an ideal occlusion in static and dynamic function allows for proper anatomical alignment of opposing teeth and the arches. Adapting a comprehensive individualized treatment approach after assessing the effects on each element of the masticatory apparatus will lead to a better outcome.

If parafunctional habits are involved, habit counseling, cognitive and behavioral awareness therapy needs to be instituted. The habits can lead gradually weaved off, if needed the help of permissive or stabilizing splints can be used. This may be followed by a restorative management.

12. Conclusion

The key to understand trauma from occlusion is to understand how the brain finds the teeth, it finds the teeth by the best of fit. The jaw should be allowed to close into maximum intercuspal position without any interference and not force itself in, So better the fit into MIP the healthier the occlusion. The chewing pathway is as important as the anterior guidance which does not interferes with the pathway. Occlusion is unique to each individual so is the pathway. A systemic approach in the sequence of treatment selected and planned will help in improving the long-term prognosis and rehabilitation of patients by establishing the occlusion which is in harmony with the envelope of function. An inter disciplinary treatment approach with digital occlusal analysis will go a long way in developing neuro-occluso-muscular harmony.

Acknowledgements

We would like to acknowledge and appreciate the support and facilities provided by Triveni Institute of Dental Sciences Hospital and Research Centre Bilaspur, Chhattisgarh, India and thank them sincerely for the same.

Nomenclature

TFO	Trauma from occlusion
TMJ	Temporomandibular joint
MIP	Maximum intercuspal position
EMG	Electromyography
JVA	Joint Vibrational Analysis
PDL	Periodontal Ligament
ICP	Intercuspal position
ROM	range of movement
μm	micron (measurement unit)

Author details

Prashanth Shetty*, Shweta Hegde, Shubham Chelkar, Rahul Chaturvedi, Shruti Pochhi, Aakanksha Shrivastava, Dudala Lakshmi, Shreya Mukherjee, Pankaj Bajaj and Shahzada Asif Raza
Triveni Institute of Dental Sciences Hospital and Research Centre, Bilaspur, India

*Address all correspondence to: dr.prashanths@gmail.com

IntechOpen

© 2022 The Author(s). Licensee IntechOpen. This chapter is distributed under the terms of the Creative Commons Attribution License (http://creativecommons.org/licenses/by/3.0), which permits unrestricted use, distribution, and reproduction in any medium, provided the original work is properly cited.

References

[1] Dawson PE. Functional occlusion: From TMJ to smile design. Journal of Indian Prosthodont Society. 2007; **7**:49

[2] Becker RM. Biometrics role in occlusion. Compendium of Continuing Education in Dentistry. 2009;**29**(1):1-7

[3] American Academy of Periodontology. Glossary of Periodontal Terms. 4th ed. 2001. p. 35

[4] Glickman I, Smulow J. The combined effects of inflammation and trauma from occlusion in periodontics. International Dental Journal. 1969;**19**:393

[5] Glickman I, Sumlow JB. Effect of excessive occlusal forces upon the pathway of gingival inflammation in human. Journal of Periodontology. 1965; **36**:141-147

[6] Glickman I, Smulow JB. Further observations on the effects of trauma from occlusion in humans. Journal of Periodontology. 1967;**38**:280-293

[7] Glickman I, Smulow JB. Adaptive alterations in the periodontium of the rhesus monkey in chronic trauma from occlusion. Journal of Periodontology. 1968;**39**:101-105

[8] Box HK. Traumatic occlusion and traumatogenic occlusion. Oral Health. 1930;**20**:642-646

[9] Leonard HJ. The occlusal factor in periodontal disease. Journal of Periodontology. 1946;**17**:80-91

[10] Jin LJ, Cao CF. Clinical diagnosis of trauma from occlusion and its relation with severity of periodontitis. Journal of clinical periodontology. 1992;**19**(2): 92-97

[11] Shefter GJ, McFall WT Jr. Occlusal relations and periodontal status in human adults. Journal of Periodontology. 1986;**57**:1-6

[12] Singh DK, Jalaluddin M, Rajeev R. Trauma from occlusion: The overstrain of the supporting structures of the teeth. Indian Journal of Dental Sciences. 2017; **9**:126-132

Chapter 8

Perspective Chapter: Dental and Orofacial Trauma Impacts on Oral-Health-Related—Quality of Life in Children – Low- and Middle-Income Countries

Yolanda Malele-Kolisa, Nazia Khan, Mpho Primrose Molete, Maphefo Desiree Thekiso and Mzubanzi Mabongo

Abstract

Orofacial trauma including traumatic dental injuries is a public health problem and has the potential to adversely affect the quality of life in children. These injuries include hard and soft tissue. Quality of life is impacted when the health and oral health of the children and their parents and family are affected. Oral health includes the ability to speak, smile, smell, taste, chew, swallow, and convey emotions through facial expressions with confidence. Poor oral health conditions include dental injuries from trauma, result in pain, soreness, discomfort, and embarrassment during routine daily activities. Traumatic dental injuries contribute to the aesthetic, functional, psychological, social, and economic distress lowering self-image and negatively impacting the quality of life among children, and their families in both developed and low- and middle-income countries. It is important to appreciate the impacts of dental trauma on children and their families more so in areas of low income as these areas have a higher propensity of above average oral-related quality of life impacts. Necessary dental management and treatment should be performed as soon as possible consequent to injury to relieve pain and discomfort, restore function, uplift appearance, and self-esteem, and enhance social well-being. This holistic management approach will improve treatment outcomes and ultimately enhance the quality-of-life post-dental injury.

Keywords: dental trauma, pain, health-related quality of life, children, low-middle income countries

1. Introduction

Dental Trauma or Traumatic Dental Injuries (TDI) refer to injury in the oral cavity involving the hard, soft tissues and periodontium such as the gingiva, periodontal ligament, alveolar bone, and cementum. Although there is some classification to the type of traumatic injuries, the traumas can occur in various combinations and be associated with some facial or bodily injury [1]. A severe form of trauma in children is that of orofacial fractures, these types of fractures cause significant morbidity, and mortality in children, and may have a devastating impact on their quality of life [2]. Dental trauma account for 5% of all bodily injuries in all ages and children are most affected; furthermore, 1 in 5 children have experienced an injury to their anterior teeth before leaving school [1].

1.1 Epidemiology

The global prevalence of dental trauma among children is approximately 17.5%–22.0% and is found to be higher in America as compared to the rest of the world. In South America it is 34,1%, followed by Europe, 26%, then Africa 16.7% and then Asia (8.91%) [1, 3]. Frequent causes of dental trauma is falling at home, followed by school and sports injuries. The greatest incidence of trauma in children occur in the primary teeth at the ages of 2–3 years old when toddlers are developing their motor skills as they learn to walk [4]. The incidence rate of primary teeth traumatic injuries is 2.75 and that of permanent teeth injuries is 2.72, yet often little emphasis is given to the management of primary teeth as it is assumed that the teeth will eventually exfoliate and require no care. However, we need to be mindful of the consequential effects that lead to developmental disturbances of underlying permanent teeth that result from pre-mature loss of primary teeth [1].

In primary teeth the prevalence of TDI has been found to be approximately 24.4% with boys more prone to injuries (30%) than girls (26.8%). Most occurred at home (72%) followed by at school. Children with incompetent lip closures are also found to be most vulnerable (49.4%), followed by those with increased overjet (44.1%) and increased open bite (33.3%) [3]. Globally the prevalence of primary teeth trauma in Southeast Asia is 27%, followed by America 26.5%, Eastern Mediterranean and Africa at 22.7%; then the lowest being Europe at 14.2%. Moreover, prevalence of TDI on permanent teeth of 12-year-olds, globally is 18.1%.

Severe extensive trauma as orofacial fractures not only affect the oral cavity but also the facial and head and neck regions as well. Such fractures commonly affect adults with less than 15% affecting children [5]. These traumas are a substantial public health problem as they cause significant morbidity, mortality in children, and may have a devastating impact emotionally, physically and functionally on children [2]. These trauma's result from motor vehicle accidents, falls, violence, and sports injuries. When they do affect children, they can also cause possible concussion and brain injury [6]. These consequences can have long lasting impact on the social and cognitive functioning of a child. Type of fractures that were associated with concussion reported by a USA study, included orbital fracture (54.8%); nasal fracture (28.8%); skull fracture (25.6%); maxillary fracture (23.7%).

A systematic review assessing 27 studies consisting of 403,339 patients around the world found that in terms of the pattern of aetiology in maxillofacial fractures globally, Road Traffic accidents (RTA) accounted for the highest cause (34%). This is followed by falls (31%); violence (11%) and sports injuries (4%). RTA are found to be highest (over 40%) in Africa and Asia. Falls are more prevalent in Europe especially among school children and violence is more prevalent in North America [7]. One would expect the traumatic dental impact on oral related quality of life literature to be readily available.

In South Africa, study reviewing 87 children under the age of 13 with facial fractures admitted at the Red Cross trauma unit in Cape Town between2006 and 2014 found that over half of the children (n = 49) had injuries that were caused by motor vehicle accidents particularly when children were unrestrained in the car. Of the motor-vehicle collision (n = 25 were passengers and (n = 24) were pedestrians. Other injuries were caused by falls (n = 20); assaults (n = 8); and (n = 7) reported as others [8]. In Johannesburg a study undertaken at the Chris Hani Baragwanath paediatric trauma unit indicated the prevalence of head injuries to be as high as 45.7%, this was followed by mouth injuries (26.6%) [7]. The dental injury experienced involved largely maxillary and mandibular incisors and canines. In addition, teeth displacement, intrusion, mobility, fracture avulsion and pulp injury were prevalent [9]. In a separate study aimed at describing the nature of injuries sustained by patients attending the trauma unit at Chris Hani Baragwanath Academic Hospital, over three months in 2017; the injuries sustained by the children less than five years were found to be 12.35% [10]. The prevalence of orofacial and dental trauma is significant in the LMIC. Moreover, the severity of trauma seems to me more than the primary anterior dentition but more severe head injuries where one study it was as high as 45,7% [7] and mouth approximately 27% [7]. The impact of these traumas on health-related quality of life warrants a more attention.

1.1.1 *Factors related to the occurrence of TDI and Oro-facial injuries in low- and middle-income counties*

The prevalence of orofacial trauma has increased over the years in many LMIC because of interpersonal violence, motor vehicle accidents and wars. Particularly among the adult population [11]. Having said that, most dental injuries studies in LMIC are focused on the adult population and very little studies have been undertaken on the child population.

The few studies that have been looked at show that there are similarities between LMIC and high income countries in terms of demographic characteristics of male children being more affected and the most common places of injury being the home environment [12].

A study conducted in India in 2015 looking at association between TDI, Obesity and socio-economic status among 6- and 13-year-old, found that the injuries were more prevalent among overweight and obese children. Furthermore, children from low socio-economic status had a higher likelihood of experiencing dental trauma than children from medium and upper socio-economic status [13].

Of concern is the studies of child orofacial trauma in LMIC being linked to physical child abuse and fatalities [14]. Physical Child abuse is defined by the WHO as an experience that results in actual or potential physical harm of a child from a parent or person in a position of responsibility, power and trust [15]. In South Africa two of the most recent studies on physical child abuse among children in a Cape Town children's hospital found the following; injuries to the face occurred in 59% of child abuse cases and that most of the times, the lips were traumatised (54%) [16]. The second study assessed autopsy reports of 1809 children under the age of 9 years old between (1998–2004). They found that 2.62% of the fatalities were attributed to physical child abuse among children aged 1 month and 11 years old. The main cause of the children's death being head injuries [17].

2. Rationale

The pattern of trauma in children described depict that the condition is a dental public health problem as reflected by the prevalence, the rising incidence and the economic burden that Low-Middle Income (LMIC) countries have to bear in managing and treating such cases. These conditions have a severe impact on individual children, families, and society generally especially due to its long-term consequences. Therefore, acknowledging the public health impacts of dental trauma and, understanding the health-related quality of life impacts is necessary for holistic management of the problem. Oral-health-related quality of life is context reliant, and it is used increasingly as a person-reported outcome measure in oral health research. More so that environment, economic, society, culture and age, may influence health, illness and quality of life [18].

3. Objectives

The objectives of this chapter are to:

- Outline the epidemiology of traumatic injuries among children affecting orofacial area in LMIC's.
- Describe the concept of oral-health-related quality of life.
- Discuss the effects of dental trauma on oral-health-related quality of life in children and families in LMIC's.
- Give a brief report on the management of the traumas

4. Methods

An extensive literature search was conducted on the health research databases, PubMed, CINAHL, EBSCOhost, and Google Scholar and this generated current literature for comprehensive information on the epidemiology of dental trauma, management and the oral-health-related quality of life impacts.

5. Health-related quality of life and Oral-health-related quality of life

Health related quality of life (HRQoL) evolves from the general concept of quality of life [19], which the latter implies general satisfaction with life. Gururatana and colleagues [20] have labelled HRQoL as a multi-dimensional construct comprising the physical, emotional and social aspects relating to illness and its treatment [20]. Thus HRQoL can be summarised as a functional effect of sickness, illness and the related treatment as perceived by the patient [19]. A goal for overall oral health should include measure of oral health-related-quality-of-life as oral health is a predictor of health and wellbeing [21]. Oral-health-related quality of life (OHRQoL) is thus, explained simply and loosely as the 'impact of oral conditions on daily functioning' [22].

The dental profession has for many years used clinical indices to measure oral health and disease outcomes which only provide one facet of child oral health [23, 24]. As much as clinical indices have measured oral conditions well, they do not take into account the children's and family's subjective perspective and the impact of oral problems on their day-to-day life [25]. Thus, OHRQoL is a patient reported outcome used to assess the outcome of oral diseases on patients' overall wellbeing.

5.1 Conceptual framework

The health-related quality of life relationships model by Ferrans et al. [26] in **Figure 1**; shows the relationships between the individual and environmental characteristics and an oral disease/condition (dental trauma) and how all the elements namely *biological functions, symptoms, functional status, general health perceptions* influence overall health-related quality of life [26].

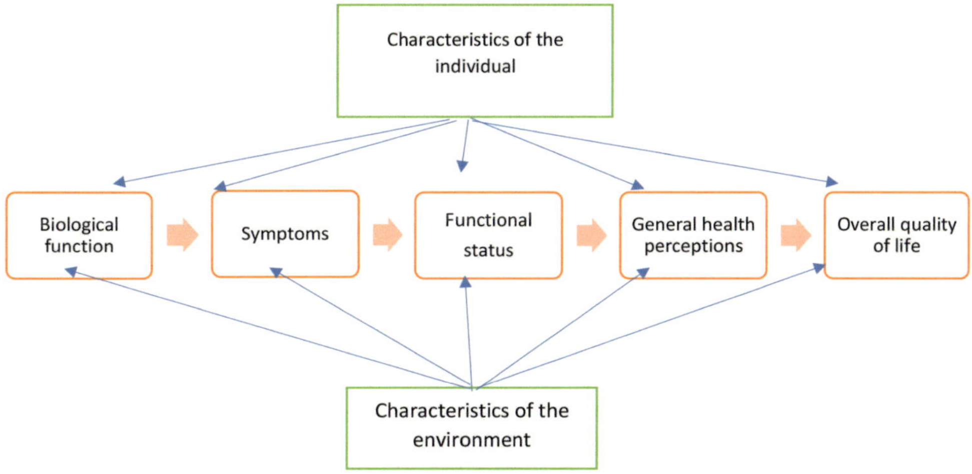

Figure 1.
A conceptual framework of health-related quality of life and its determinants. Source: Ferrans et al., 2005 (Ferrans CE, Zerwic JJ, Wilbur JE, Larson JL. Conceptual model of health-related quality of life. Journal of Nursing Scholarship. 2005;37(4):336–42.) [26].

Children OHRQoL Tool	Year published	Validated
Family Impact Scale (FIS) [27]; PART OF Child Oral Health Quality of Life Questionnaire (COHQOL)	2002	Yes
Parental/Caregiver Perceptions Questionnaire (P-CPQ) [28]; PART OF Child Oral Health Quality of Life Questionnaire (COHQOL)	2003	Yes
Child Perceptions Questionnaire (CPQ_{6-7}); (CPQ_{8-10}), and (CPQ_{11-14}) ([29, 30]; PART OF Child Oral Health Quality of Life Questionnaire (COHQOL)	2004–2006	Yes
Child-Oral Impacts On Daily Performances (COIDP) [23];	2004	Yes
Early Childhood Oral Health Impact Scale (ECOHIS) [31];	2007	Yes
Child Oral Health Impact Profile(COHIP) [32].	2007	Yes
Infant Toddler Quality of Life Questionnaire (ITQOL,) [33].	2008	Yes
PedsQL-Oral Health Scale [34].	2009	Yes
Paediatric Oral-Health-Related Quality Of Life (POQL) [35].	2011	Yes
Scale of Oral Health Outcomes (SOHO) [36].	2012	Yes
Child Health Utility 9D Index [37].	2014	Yes

Table 1.
Synopsis of Children's Oral health related quality life tools.

5.2 Measurement of oral health-related quality of life

Dental trauma invariably has the result of extreme pain and hampers daily activities, and it negatively affects normal growth; a crooked bite causing reduced self-esteem and cognitive development, may impair speech, school performance, and is costly to manage. Objective measures of disease are important, they might give insight into the impact of oral diseases on quality of life. It is for this reason that we summarise the patient-based tools available to measure subjectively, the impacts of oral diseases on children and adolescents using objective measures in **Table 1**. The environment and the culture are aspects of the society that determines how health is perceived, experienced and conceptualised by communities according to Traebert and colleagues [38]. Thus, the conceptualisation of health-related quality of life is a social construct, additionally health related quality of life is measured objectively using the tools seeking subject inputs from subjects. These measures can be applied daily in facilities or practices to assess and report these impacts of oral diseases to evaluate dental management of oral trauma. These validated tools are often used to assess the effect or impact of any oral condition or oral disease.

6. Impact of dental trauma on oral health related quality of life

6.1 Physical impact of dental trauma

Traumatic injuries do not only affect facial aesthetics, but also normal masticatory function, making it difficult for the child to chew. Dental problems that cause chewing to be painful affect the intake of dietary fibre and some nutrient-rich foods; significantly lowering serum levels of beta carotene, folate, and vitamin C [39]. Furthermore, trauma to anterior teeth can result in difficulties experienced in the pronunciation of words or phrases. For example, if upper incisor teeth are missing, the pronunciation of the v and f becomes indistinct [40]. Further literature indicates that if the lower incisors are missing, which may be trauma related, the sounds such as 'z', 'sh', and 'ch', will become defective [40] and 's' sound more complicated. Such situations lead to serious speech problems resulting in the child becoming annoyed or feeling reluctant to verbally interact with his/her classmates. The above highlights the strong correlation between teeth and speech.

6.2 Psychological impact of dental trauma

The psychological and social sequelae of dental trauma are a common finding causing the impairment of the child's social functioning, emotional balance, and well-being [41]. The unexpected nature of the traumatic dental injury, accompanied by emotional distress, physical impairment, and accompanying pain often contribute to a lasting memory of the traumatic experience. The memory issue is significant for a paediatric patient, who will have to endure the additional stress of transportation, emergency diagnostic procedures, and treatment [41] and even be triggered by such memories.

Emotionally the child may become an introvert and he/she may be reluctant to smile and find it difficult to adapt to everyday life [40]. This hurts their self-esteem and confidence. The self-esteem associated with oral health decreases as the teeth appear less attractive [42].

Overall, dental injuries are the most serious dental condition experienced by children [40]. Therefore, it is of utmost importance that treatment is sought as soon as possible after the onset of injury, allowing for favourable treatment outcomes [43] and enhanced quality of life, to be as close to normal/pre-trauma as possible.

6.3 Social impact of dental trauma: Effects on family

Families and households in Low Middle-Income Countries (LMIC's) are subjected to poverty with published literature demonstrating that family income and deprivation level are a potential risk factor to TDI's [33]. Dental traumas impact the quality of life of not just the child, but the whole family [34]. The assessment of OHRQoL in younger children may be challenging due to children's limited understanding of what is being evaluated [35]. Thus, more often the parental or family perception is important in providing evidence of the impact of TDI's on children and family OHRQoL.

In LMIC's parents of low-income households are often required to work long hours resulting in decreased family time, thus TDI's on the teeth and mouth can result in considerable psychological stress and social costs on the OHRQoL of parents due to pain experienced by children and high absenteeism from work [36]. Furthermore, illiteracy levels among adults are high in LMIC's resulting in parents with low education lacking specific TDI's prevention skills to transfer to their children [37].

Severe dental trauma is associated with a higher impact on the OHRQoL family function, as parents expand greater attention on the injured child due to the severity of the lesion. Family daily activities can be negatively affected in severe trauma cases as the children experience more physical and psychological discomfort, limited functionality and more financial resources are required for rehabilitation of the child [44]. The severity of caries on teeth with TDI's have a higher impact on family OHRQoL more so that complicated trauma cases may involve fractured dentine or dentine/pulp [45] resulting in parents feeling more distressed immediately after the injury and after the TDI treatment [41]. TDI's on older children in LIC's has a significant lower impact on the parents/family OHRQoL because older children are more independent needing less parental intervention and supervision than younger children [42].

7. Factors related to oral health-related quality of life outcomes on the child with dental trauma

Treatment of traumatic dental injuries reduces the OHRQoL of the children and adolescents [46]. Management of dental trauma involve multiple dental specialties including pedodontics, endodontics, orthodontics, oral medicine and periodontology, and oral surgery. This integration is necessary to ensure the correct rehabilitation of the patient [40]. Dental trauma requires special comprehensive examinations and detailed history of the incident to determine the correct diagnosis and to rapidly manage the injuries [40].

As shown in the Fig 1, some factors influence the outcome and a better or worse OHRQoL on the individual and environmental level in LMIC's. At *individual level*, a Brazilian study reported that factors such as parental dental anxiety has a significant correlation with children's OHRQoL because parental dental anxiety is an indicator of the children's oral health, children's dental service utilisation and a major barrier to access dental care [47]. Children who present with dental trauma are generally trauma prone. Nearly half of the children with multiple dental traumas will re-traumatise the same tooth [41]. Also, in LMIC's individual family dynamics such as compliance and cooperation by the patient and the family, starting from the moment of injury is critical [41]. In a Brazilian study, an effective management of dental trauma was shown to require a swift multidisciplinary management with long-term follow-up care [48].

On the *environmental level*, the following health systems aspects such as the availability of the facility and increased waiting time in hospital emergency departments may be responsible for the late presentation of dental trauma patients thus contributing to unfavourable outcomes and a poor OHRQoL scores in a Turkish study [43]. Also related to *health systems* is the issue of collaboration between paediatricians in hospital emergency departments and paediatric dentists will enable urgent and best-possible care for the injured patients ultimately improving prognosis [43]. The mode of treatment such as comprehensive dental treatment on the dental chair or full mouth rehabilitation under general anaesthesia has been associated with considerable improvement in OHRQoL [49] and thus highlights the importance of multidisciplinary care, however this is a great challenge in LMIC's. The factors mentioned above are not exhaustive however is a considerable gap in the paucity of studies conducted in Africa.

In many of the developing countries, majority of households are subjected to poverty. It is thus plausible that a review by Das et al. [50] highlights that the families with a lower socioeconomic status, when the facilities are not sufficient, living conditions with unsafe environments may lead to children to be prone to traumatic injuries. The poor living surroundings, the quality of health care is questionable, therefore the children and families suffer severe impacts on their care and experience a lower OHRQoL.

The success of the dental treatment is not only based on the clinical outcome, but also the psychological impact of treatment [51]. The ability of a treatment to enable a person to improve function (eat, speak,) and socialise without pain, discomfort, or active disease have been indicators of success.

Most literature of the factors on TDIs and OHRQoL are conducted in the developed countries. In LMIC such as Brazil, the impact of restorative treatment only improved the OHRQoL impact of adolescents than the families. This may be due to economic and financial cost passed on to families [50]. Another Brazilian study reported concomitant presence of other conditions such as dental caries, pain, orofacial dysfunction, in addition to dental trauma, impact twofold to the OHRQoL [50]. There is skewness of literature in that majority of studies are conducted in Brazil and few conducted in other LMIC such as Africa when it comes to traumas and OHRQoL. This chapter highlights that more work needs to be conducted in developing countries seeing that countries' economy, environment, and societal aspects have a potential to influence the impact of traumas on the oral health quality of life in societies.

8. Management of traumatic dental injures and orofacial trauma in paediatric patients

Although the incidence of facial trauma in the paediatric population is higher than in the adult population, the incidence of facial fracture is lower in children [52]. The frontal bone is commonly involved, and the type of management is mostly conservative treatment [7] (**Box 1**).

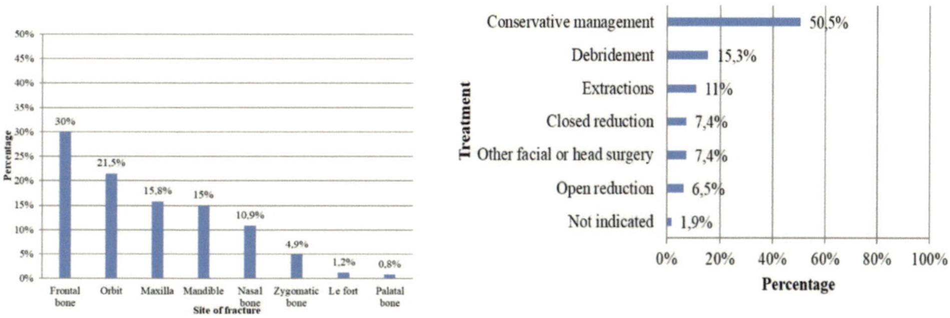

Box 1.
*Source: Fouche and Mabongo 2019. *permission to reproduce image was obtained from both the authors and SADJ.*

8.1 Traumatic dental injuries

8.1.1 Management and treatment

8.1.1.1 Crown fracture: Uncomplicated

The clinical and radiographic findings show a break in enamel or dentin. In this case one would need to restore normal aesthetics and function by restoring and smoothening the tooth margins [53, 54].

8.1.1.2 Crown fracture: complicated

The clinical and radiologic findings reveal a loss of tooth structure and pulp exposure. In primary teeth, management decisions are based on the vitality of the pulp and the life expectancy of the tooth, alternatives could therefore be, pulpotomy, pulpectomy, or extraction. For permanent teeth, the treatment would be, direct pulp capping, pulpotomy, or a complete root canal treatment.

8.1.1.3 Crown and root fracture (uncomplicated or complicated)

Clinical findings usually reveal a mobile coronal fragment attached to the gingiva with or without pulp exposure. In primary teeth, an extraction would be indicated. In permanent teeth, stabilisation of the coronal fragment would be necessary. If you cannot remove the fragment, complete root canal treatment with post-core and crown. If the root component is irreparable, then an extraction would be indicated.

8.1.1.4 Concussion

In this case, clinical findings would reveal a tooth that is tender to pressure and percussion without mobility. There may also be some sulcular bleeding. Management would involve optimising the healing of the periodontal ligament and maintaining the vitality of the pulp.

8.1.1.5 Subluxation

This involves injury to the tooth structures with loosening, however there is no tooth displacement. There may be sulcular bleeding. In primary teeth, the tooth should be observed over 2 weeks, if no healing occurs and the pulp is affected, then an extraction would be indicated. In permanent teeth, the tooth needs to be splinted for 2 weeks and the vitality of the pulp should be closely monitored.

8.1.1.6 Lateral luxation

The periodontal ligament is torn and there may be a fracture of the supporting alveolar bone. The tooth could be displaced palatally or lingually. Often it is locked in that position and not mobile. In primary teeth try to gently reposition the tooth. If it is not possible and the displacement is causing discomfort in the oral cavity, then an extraction would be indicated. In permanent teeth, reposition as soon as you can, and stabilise the tooth for approximately 2–4 weeks. In addition, monitor the vitality of the pulp closely.

8.1.1.7 Intrusive luxation

In this type of luxation, the tooth is driven into the socket compressing the periodontal ligament and crushing the alveolar socket, therefore it appears shortened. In addition, the tooth is not mobile or tender to touch. In primary teeth, the tooth may re-erupt spontaneously, however, if it is found to cause disruption to eruption of a permanent tooth, extraction is indicated. In permanent teeth, the tooth can be repositioned passively or surgically and then stabilised with a splint for up to 4 weeks. During treatment, monitor the vitality of the pulp closely.

8.1.1.8 Extrusive luxation

The tooth is partially displaced axially, and the tooth appears elongated and mobile. In addition, the periodontal ligament is usually torn. For primary teeth, time should be given to allow them to reposition spontaneously. Should the extrusion be severe or there is mobility, an extraction should be indicated. In permanent teeth, repositioning should occur as soon as possible, then it should be stabilised and splinted for 2 weeks.

8.1.1.9 Avulsion

When the tooth is completely displaced out of the socket, primary teeth should not be replanted. In permanent teeth, replanting should occur as soon as possible, and the tooth be splinted for 2 weeks.

8.2 Orofacial trauma

General considerations in the young trauma patient include maintenance of the airway, balance of fluid and electrolyte levels and adequate nutritional intake during treatment. As in adults, the pre-injury skeletal and dentoalveolar anatomy and function are re-established by anatomic reduction of fractures based on the occlusion [55].

Like in adults, paediatric fractures are managed by conservative, closed reduction and open reduction and internal fixation. Children have greater osteogenic potential and faster healing rates than adults Therefore, immobilisation times should be shorter. Surgical interventions usually require two operations under general anaesthesia. For open reduction and internal fixation, care should be taken not to traumatise both root of teeth and dental follicles [46].

i. Conservative Management

In this mode of treatment, the is no active surgical intervention, close observation of the patient, control of pain, and minimal movement of the fractured bone is maintained, this is by restricting the patient to a soft diet in the case of fractured jaws. Un-displaced and minimally displaced fractures of the jaws are best treated by this option in children. Most facial fractures in children are managed by this modality [47].

ii. Closed reduction

This mode of treatment may be compromised by fewer available teeth, lack of stability of primary teeth due to root resorption, and anatomy of the crowns of the teeth available primary teeth and partially erupted permanent teeth making arch stabilisation with Erich arch bars impossible. All these factors make intermaxillary fixation (IMF) more difficult than in adults. Secondly, IMF is not easily tolerated by children, as it restricts mandibular movements causing discomfort and increased anxiety; furthermore, it is detrimental to the child's quality of life, as a liquid diet adversely affects nutritional intake. Lastly, IMF may result in ankylosis of the temporomandibular joint in patients with condylar fractures [46].

iii. Open reduction and Internal fixation

In older children with displaced fractures closed or open reduction and internal fixation (ORIF) may be indicated. ORIF of mandible fractures in children is generally avoided due to the potential damage to developing tooth germs and disruption of the periosteum. The other challenges in children include the small size of the facial bones and the relatively soft bone showing good elasticity. A reduction of the mandibular immobilisation period also contributes to the recovery of joint function and early return to function [46].

The goals for management are to restore function, form, aesthetics, and most importantly in children, to preserve growth and development. Managing paediatric facial fractures is complex because of the continued growth and development of the facial skeleton, [46]. Therefore, management strategies must provide proper stabilisation of fractures to restore facial anatomy, without hindering future bone and soft tissue growth. Many paediatric facial fractures can be managed conservatively owing to the high osteogenic potential of the paediatric skeleton; however, surgical intervention may be necessary for patients with severe facial injuries [56].

9. Conclusions and future directions

Management of dental trauma in both developed and developing countries requires a life-long commitment on behalf of the patient and dentist, especially in a growing patient with a developing facial musculature, oral structures, and dentition. The traumatic injuries affect all communities regardless of countries economy status; however, literature has shown that the severity of traumas such as those leading to head injuries was reported more in the developing countries. Oral trauma among children, their experiences and the impact of the trauma must be, understood by all the multi-disciplinary team of practitioners. There was minimal literature on the impacts of traumatic injuries on OHRQoL in the LMIC areas such as Africa though plenty of Brazilian and some Indian studies were evident. The socio-dental indicators or the tools measuring the patient-based impact of dental and oral trauma, despite being developed in non-African settings, are vital in providing important feedback on how to evaluate the management of trauma and thus should be part of the general protocols for management. Dental practitioners must be cognizant of the non-clinical impacts of orofacial and dental trauma and be familiar with the socio-dental indices to measure patient-based outcomes. It is recommended that more studies are conducted in the LMIC, specifically African countries to highlight the importance of patient-based inputs and evaluation of care related to traumatic dental injuries.

Acknowledgements

The authors would love to acknowledge the supportive research environment within the department of community dentistry and the broader School of Oral Health Sciences at the University of Witwatersrand and the department of maxillofacial surgery, University of Pretoria.

Conflict of interest

The authors declare no conflict of interest.

Author details

Yolanda Malele-Kolisa[1*], Nazia Khan[2], Mpho Primrose Molete[1], Maphefo Desiree Thekiso[1] and Mzubanzi Mabongo[2]

1 Department of Community Dentistry, University of Witwatersrand, South Africa

2 Department of Maxillofacial Surgery, University of Pretoria, South Africa

*Address all correspondence to: yolanda.kolisa@wits.ac.za

IntechOpen

© 2022 The Author(s). Licensee IntechOpen. This chapter is distributed under the terms of the Creative Commons Attribution License (http://creativecommons.org/licenses/by/3.0), which permits unrestricted use, distribution, and reproduction in any medium, provided the original work is properly cited.

References

[1] Petti S, Glendor U, Andersson L. World traumatic dental injury prevalence and incidence, a meta-analysis—One billion living people have had traumatic dental injuries. Dental Traumatology. 2018;**34**(2):71-86

[2] Joachim M, Tuizer M, Araidy S, El-Naaj IA. Pediatric maxillofacial trauma: Epidemilogic study between the years 2012-2015 in Israeli medical center. International Journal of Oral and Maxillofacial Surgery. 2019;**48**:40

[3] Patnana AK, Chugh A, Chugh VK, Kumar P, Vanga NRV, Singh S. The prevalence of traumatic dental injuries in primary teeth: A systematic review and meta-analysis. Dental Traumatology. 2021 Jun;**37**(3):383-399

[4] Azami-Aghdash S, Azar FE, Azar FP, Rezapour A, Moradi-Joo M, Moosavi A, et al. Prevalence, etiology, and types of dental trauma in children and adolescents: Systematic review and meta-analysis. Medical Journal of the Islamic Republic of Iran. 2015;**29**(4):234

[5] Meier JD, Tollefson TT. Pediatric facial trauma. Current Opinion in Otolaryngology & Head and Neck Surgery. 2008 Dec;**16**(6):555-561

[6] Afrooz PN, Grunwaldt LJ, Zanoun RR, Grubbs RK, Saladino RA, Losee JE, et al. Pediatric facial fractures: Occurrence of concussion and relation to fracture patterns. Journal of Craniofacial Surgery. 2012;**23**(5):1270-1273

[7] Barbosa KGN, de Macedo BÍ, d'Avila S, Ferreira RC. Systematic review and meta-analysis to determine the proportion of maxillofacial trauma resulting from different etiologies among children and adolescents. Oral and Maxillofacial Surgery. 2017;**21**(2):131-145

[8] Wong FK, Adams S, Coates TJ, Hudson DA. Pediatric Facial Fractures. The Journal of Craniofacial Surgery. 2016;**27**(1):128-130

[9] Fouche G, Mabongo M. The epidemiology and management of traumatic facial fractures in children seen in a tertiary hospital in Johannesburg. South Africa. South African Dental Journal. 2019;**74**(7):358-363

[10] Khan N. Injury Survey at Chris Hani Baragwanath Academic Hospital, Soweto, South Africa [thesis]. Johannesburg, South Africa: University of the Witwatersrand; 2020. Available from: https://wiredspace.wits.ac.za/bitstream/handle/10539/29745/Dr%20Nazia%20Khan%20final%20research%20report%20october%202019.pdf?sequence=1

[11] Abid A, Maatouk F, Berrezouga L, Azodo C, Uti O, El-Shamy H, et al. Prevalence and severity of oral diseases in the Africa and Middle East region. Advances in Dental Research. 2015;**27**(1):10-17

[12] Dharmani CK, Pathak A, Sidhu HS. Prevalence of traumatic dental injuries to anterior teeth in 8-12-year-old schoolchildren of Patiala City, Punjab, India: An epidemiological study. International Journal of Clinical Pediatric Dentistry. 2019;**12**(1):25

[13] Basha S, Mohammad RN, Swamy HS, Sexena V. Association between traumatic dental injury, obesity, and socioeconomic status in 6-and 13-year-old schoolchildren. Social Work in Public Health. 2015;**30**(4):336-344

[14] Sarkar R, Ozanne-Smith J, Bassed R. Systematic review of the patterns of orofacial injuries in physically abused children and adolescents. Trauma, Violence, & Abuse. 2021;**22**(1):136-146

[15] Meinck F, Steinert JI, Sethi D, Gilbert R, Bellis MA, Mikton C, et al. Measuring and Monitoring National Prevalence of Child Maltreatment: A Practical Handbook. Copenhagen, Denmark: WHO; 2016

[16] Naidoo S. A profile of the oro-facial injuries in child physical abuse at a children's hospital. Child Abuse & Neglect. 2000;**24**(4):521-534

[17] Phillips VM, Van Der Heyde Y. Oro-facial trauma in child abuse fatalities. South African Medical Journal. 2006;**96**(3):213-215

[18] Raymundo de Andrade LH, de Souza RB, Castro GF, Ribeiro de Souza IP. Impact of oral problems on daily activities of HIV-infected children. European Journal of Paediatric Dentistry. 2011;**12**(2):75-80

[19] Juczyński Z. Health-related Guality of life: Theory and measurement. Acta Universitatis Lodziensis Folia Psychologica. 2006;**10**:3-15

[20] Gururatana O, Baker SR, Robinson PG. Determinants of children's oral-health-related quality of life over time. Community Dentistry and Oral Epidemiology. 2014;**42**(3):206-215

[21] Wandera M, Kayondo J, Engebretsen IMS, Okullo I, ÅSTRØM AN. Factors associated with caregivers' perception of children's health and oral health status: A study of 6-to 36-month-olds in Uganda. International Journal of Paediatric Dentistry. 2009;**19**(4):251-262

[22] Locker D, Allen F. What do measures of 'oral health-related quality of life' measure? Community Dentistry and Oral Epidemiology. 2007;**35**(6):401-411

[23] Gherunpong S, Tsakos G, Sheiham A. Developing and evaluating an oral health-related quality of life index for children; the CHILD-OIDP. Community Dental Health. 2004;**21**(2):161-169

[24] Sheiham A. Dental caries affects body weight, growth and quality of life in pre-school children. British Dental Journal. 2006;**201**(10):625-626

[25] Malele-Kolisa Y. Oral-Health-Related Quality of Life and Oral Health Needs of Adolescents Living with HIV in Johannesburg [thesis]. Johannesburg, South Africa: University of the Witwatersrand; 2021. Available from: https://wiredspace.wits.ac.za/handle/10539/32076. [Accessed: April 7, 2022]

[26] Ferrans CE, Zerwic JJ, Wilbur JE, Larson JL. Conceptual model of health-related quality of life. Journal of Nursing Scholarship. 2005;**37**(4):336-342

[27] Locker D, Jokovic A, Stephens M, Kenny D, Tompson B, Guyatt G. Family impact of child oral and oro-facial conditions. Community Dentistry and Oral Epidemiology. 2002;**30**(6):438-448

[28] Jokovic A, Locker D, Stephens M, Kenny D, Tompson B, Guyatt G. Measuring parental perceptions of child oral health-related quality of life. Journal of Public Health Dentistry. 2003;**63**(2):67-72

[29] Jokovic A, Locker D, Tompson B, Guyatt G. Questionnaire for measuring oral health-related quality of life in eight-to ten-year-old children. Pediatric Dentistry. 2004;**26**(6):512-518

[30] Jokovic A, Locker D, Guyatt G. Short forms of the child perceptions questionnaire for 11-14-year-old children

(CPQ 11-14): Development and initial evaluation. Health and Quality of Life Outcomes. 2006;**4**(1):1-9

[31] Pahel BT, Rozier RG, Slade GD. Parental perceptions of children's Oral health: The early childhood Oral health impact scale (ECOHIS). Health and Quality of Life Outcomes. 2007;**5**(1):6

[32] Broder HL, McGrath C, Cisneros GJ. Questionnaire development: Face validity and item impact testing of the child Oral health impact profile. Community Dentistry and Oral Epidemiology. 2007;**35**:8-19

[33] Easton JA, Landgraf JM, Casamassimo PS, Wilson S, Ganzberg S. Evaluation of a generic quality of life instrument for early childhood caries-related pain. Community Dentistry and Oral Epidemiology. 2008;**36**(5):434-440

[34] Steele MM, Steele RG, Varni JW. Reliability and validity of the PedsQL™ oral health scale: Measuring the relationship between child oral health and health-related quality of life. Children's Health Care. 2009;**38**(3):228-244

[35] Huntington NL, Spetter D, Jones JA, Rich SE, Garcia RI, Spiro A 3rd. Development and validation of a measure of pediatric oral health-related quality of life: the POQL. Journal of Public Health Dentistry. 2011;**71**(3):185-193

[36] Tsakos G, Blair YI, Yusuf H, Wright W, Watt RG, Macpherson L. Developing a new self-reported scale of oral health outcomes for 5-year-old children (SOHO-5). Health and Quality of Life Outcomes. 2012;**10**(1):1-8

[37] Foster Page LA, Thomson WM, Marshman Z, Stevens KJ. The potential of the child health utility 9D index as an outcome measure for child dental health. BMC Oral Health. 2014;**14**(1):90

[38] Traebert J, Foster Page LA, Murray Thomson W, Locker D. Differential item functioning related to ethnicity in an oral health-related quality of life measure. International Journal of Paediatric Dentistry. 2010;**20**(6):435-441

[39] Sheiham A, Steele J. Does the condition of the mouth and teeth affect the ability to eat certain foods, nutrient and dietary intake and nutritional status amongst older people? Public Health Nutrition. 2001;**4**(3):797-803

[40] Dascălu IT, Manolea HO, Coleş E, Dăguci C, Bătăiosu M, Andrei CM, et al. The prevalence of crown injuries to frontal teeth at schoolchildren aged 6 to 14 and their effects on the periodontal tissue. Romanian Journal of Morphology and Embryology. 2016;**57** (2 Suppl):729-735

[41] Lee JY, Divaris K. Hidden consequences of dental trauma: The social and psychological effects. Pediatric Dentistry. 2009;**31**(2):96-101

[42] Buldur B, Güvendi ON. Conceptual modelling of the factors affecting oral health-related quality of life in children: A path analysis. International Journal of Paediatric Dentistry. 2020;**30**(2):181-192

[43] Vukovic A, Vukovic R, Markovic D, Soldatovic I, Mandinic Z, Beloica M, et al. After-hours versus office-hours dental injuries in children: Does timing influence outcome? Clinical Pediatrics. 2016;**55**(1):29-35

[44] Pauli LA, Costa F, Dos S, Amaral CC, Ardenghi TM, Demarco FF, et al. Severe traumatic dental injuries and oral health related quality of life of preschool children. RGO-Revista Gaúcha de Odontología. 2020:68. DOI: 10.1590/1981-863720200004820190044. Available from: https://www.scielo.br/j/rgo/a/

FSntRKrQtRhnJXszFVYMc8x/abstract/?lang=en

[45] Sakaryali D, Bani M, Cinar C, Alacam A. Evaluation of the impact of early childhood caries, traumatic dental injury, and malocclusion on oral health-related quality of life for Turkish preschool children and families. Nigerian Journal of Clinical Practice. 2019;**22**(6):817-817

[46] Milani AJ, Castilho T, Assaf AV, Antunes LS, Antunes LAA. Impact of traumatic dental injury treatment on the oral health-related quality of life of children, adolescents, and their family: Systematic review and meta-analysis. Dental Traumatology. 2021;**37**(6):735-748

[47] Goettems ML, Ardenghi TM, Romano AR, Demarco FF, Torriani DD. Influence of maternal dental anxiety on oral health-related quality of life of preschool children. Quality of Life Research. 2011;**20**(6):951-959

[48] Ode W, Lopez V, Wong ML, Schou L, Yu VSH. Understanding patients' and dentists' perspectives in dental trauma management: A mixed-methods study. Dental Traumatology. 2018;**34**(5):320-328

[49] Farsi NJ, Farsi DJ, Aldajani MB, Farsi NM, El-Housseiny AA. Sustainability of improvement in Oral health-related quality of life in children after dental treatment. Patient Preference and Adherence. 2021;**15**:271

[50] Das P, Mishra L, Jena D, Govind S, Panda S, Lapinska B. Oral health-related quality of life in children and adolescents with a traumatic injury of permanent teeth and the impact on their families: A systematic review. International Journal of Environmental Research and Public Health. 2022;**19**(5):3087

[51] Farsi DJ, Farsi NJ, El-Housseiny AA, Turkistani JM, Farsi NM. Impact of dental rehabilitation on Oral health-related quality-of-life in healthy children and those with special health care needs. The Journal of Contemporary Dental Practice. 2018;**19**(4):367-374

[52] Andrew TW, Morbia R, Lorenz HP. Pediatric facial trauma. Clinics in Plastic Surgery. 2019;**46**(2):239-247

[53] Andreasen JO, Andreasen FM, Andersson L. Textbook and Color Atlas of Traumatic Injuries to the Teeth. 4th ed. Oxford: Blackwell Munksgaard; 2007

[54] Council O. Guideline of management of acute dental trauma. American Academy of Pediatric Dentistry Reference Manual. 2011;**34**:2011. Available from: http://www.aapd.org/assets/1/7/g_trauma.pdf

[55] Zimmermann CE, Troulis MJ, Kaban LB. Pediatric facial fractures: Recent advances in prevention, diagnosis and management. International Journal of Oral and Maxillofacial Surgery. 2005;**34**(8):823-833

[56] Dalena MM, Liu FC, Halsey JN, Lee ES, Granick MS. Assessment of panfacial fractures in the pediatric population. Journal of Oral and Maxillofacial Surgery. 2020;**78**(7):1156-1161

Chapter 9

The Impact of Traumatic Dental Injuries on the Mental and Social Well-Being of Children and Adolescents: Recommendations for Patient Management

Aneesa Moolla

Abstract

Traumatic injuries to the oral cavity are frequent during childhood, with a documented rate of more than 30% worldwide. These injuries commonly include the skull and mouth, and thus teeth are frequently impacted. Consequently, the individual ends up in pain accompanied by both esthetic and functional issues. The combination of these factors can have a detrimental impact upon normal functioning of a young individual's lives if the injury is not efficiently treated or managed. This then impacts on the individual's mental health and their quality of life. Not being able to function as part of a society that they are accustomed to, can cause people to withdraw from society and lose self-confidence. The negative psychological effect of traumatic dental injuries is specific to an individual, and as such each patient should be treated holistically with all factors taken into account. There is a dearth in literature around the full psycho-social impacts of traumatic dental injuries. Dentistry as a clinical field is advancing in treatment of such injuries, but there is still a lack of knowledge and awareness regarding the individual experience and how this could be managed going forward in terms in-chair strategies and the involvement of a multi-disciplinary team.

Keywords: traumatic dental injuries, patient management, dental trauma management, child health

1. Introduction

Facial esthetics play an important role in how one perceives one own self and how one is perceived by others. Any detrimental impact caused by trauma that then affects one's physical appearance can lead to distress and anxiety. This in turn can then affect the quality of life of individuals who are impacted.

Globally, the reported prevalence of traumatic dental injuries (TDI) during childhood or adolescence is a common occurrence with up to 30% [1–3] of young

IntechOpen

individuals being impacted. For those affected, these TDIs are painful experiences on a physical level, but they often also influence the emotional and psychosocial well-being of these individuals [4, 5]. Current evidence [6] supports the above notion that children and adolescents who have suffered a traumatic injury to the dentition experience significant negative impacts to their overall well-being.

The psychological, social and emotional impacts of a TDI are unique to each individual which then impacts upon their treatment preferences, coping and eventual recovery. Contemporary dentistry and medicine now recognize the critical prerequisite which is to identify and address these psychosocial aspects as part of a more holistic approach to healthcare. Furthermore, if such traumatic injuries are not effectively and holistically managed, then the affected individuals are shown to be more likely to suffer decreased self-esteem and low feelings of self-worth due to their changed appearance [4]. Quality of life is negatively impacted and often children whose appearance is affected are reluctant to laugh or smile and if there is pain or a fracture then they are also unable to enjoy their food or even brush their teeth properly. This has further consequences for them in terms of their health. This could then impact their lives negatively as they often do not have the coping mechanisms in place to help them navigate these difficult situations. Thus, childhood and adolescence are sensitive developmental periods that may pose complex challenges to the effective management of dental trauma. Dealing with the consequences of childhood trauma is a complex interplay between managing expectations with the hidden impacts of the traumatic event. This eventually influences both patient compliance and cooperation which are key to successful outcomes. Thus, full family collaboration and involvement from the starting point of injury is critical. The emphasis on a team effort being a point of note to be emphasized at all visits. There is also an urgency to engage in consistent monitoring and long-term follow up, especially in the not fully mature patient with a developing dentition. The high probability that there will be psychological impacts stemming from the traumatic event has become a frequent finding with studies [4–6] showing that effects can be seen in the overall negative well-being of the child.

In this chapter we will consider the possible social and psychological consequences of dental trauma in young individuals whilst simultaneously indicating the various management techniques for approaching these dental traumatic injuries in children and adolescents.

2. Psychological impact of dental trauma on children and adolescents

Tooth loss affects many people and can impact individuals severely in that it often leads to hidden consequences that need to be managed strategically and holistically. These hidden consequences at impact affected individuals in varying degrees include psychosocial and emotional impacts. A recent study [4] also indicated that the mental well-being of children is frequently adversely affected following dental trauma and the consequences of such injuries significantly impact the psychosocial and emotional wellbeing of the affected children. This is because whether a tooth was knocked out due to dental trauma or disease, the result is the same: negatively affected oral health and esthetics.

It is common knowledge amongst oral health professionals that not attending to tooth loss can have detrimental effects for oral health wellbeing in any individual. The long term effects include tooth migration, jawbone loss and even the eventual loss of additional remaining teeth. Thus as noted, dental trauma and the physical effects are usually given priority within the clinical context. However, a critical aspect of dental trauma which is linked to the nature or circumstances of the incident itself, is the potential for affected children to consequently experience negative mental health outcomes. Whilst the physical effects of tooth loss are known and documented widely, distinguishing the deeper level emotional effects of the dental trauma can be more challenging.

Evidence also indicates that previous traumatic injuries to a child's dentition impacts negatively on their oral-health-related quality of life [7, 8]. No matter the reason, tooth loss or other types of dental trauma for any individual is almost always a negative experience. Children are particularly vulnerable in these circumstances. A child who has been impacted by dental trauma can go on to develop decreased feelings of self-worth and a lowered self-esteem due to their changed appearance. They may often also experience feelings of sadness, anger, hopelessness and loss of confidence. Affected appearances may also predispose these children to teasing, bullying [9] and torment from other children or peers they come into contact with. This is especially the case for those injuries that have not been effectively or holistically managed.

To this effect, literature around general physical injuries on any part of the body of a child indicates that approximately 50% of all injured children can show signs of post-traumatic stress disorder (PTSD) at six weeks and as late as eight months after the physical injury [10, 11]. In terms of facial esthetics, Kaur et al. found that disappointment with one's own dental esthetics is a strong predictor for negative self-esteem [12]. A myriad of dental issues that include visible tooth loss, visible untreated caries and malaligned teeth influence a person's perceptions of esthetics as well as psychosocial behavior in young people. This then impacts on self-esteem.

It is now almost a decade since the global medical pediatric emergency fraternity called out for improved psychological evaluations and assessments of children impacted by any type of trauma [11]. This was so that management and support guidelines could be duly effected in order to be able to emotionally support those young individuals who are vulnerable and at high risk of developing Post Traumatic Stress Disorder (PTSD). Consequently, it is crucial that oral health professionals are also conscious of the possibility that some children with a traumatic dental injury may experience negative psychological effects due to the mental trauma associated with the distressing incident. The impacts of negative mental health within the dental context may only become obvious at subsequent dental visits through displays of anxiety and disruptive behavior. These factors also need to be further explored. It should also be noted that the affected children have to deal with both the traumatic incident from their own perspective, as well as the secondary emotions and distress from their parents and/or friends.

3. Impact of traumatic injury on social well-being and Oral health related quality of life (QoL) in children and adolescents

Taking the above factors into consideration, it is indicative that a part of the reason a person loses self-confidence is related to the underlying social stigma attached to tooth loss. Evidence points to social consequences which includes shying away from relationships or socializing with peers [13, 14]. This ultimately leads to patients who had dental trauma having less meaningful social interactions that can affect their overall well-being, as compared to others with no trauma that affects their esthetics.

Evidence [15] shows that essential functional activities that are compromised in children affected by dental trauma include: chewing, speaking, showing their teeth and brushing. Peers also engage in social judgment [16, 17] and tend to judge those with visible facial trauma more negatively than they judge others, with younger age groups being more negatively judgmental than older children. This can also be attributed to a greater degree of mental maturity in older children [18, 19]. Unfortunately, these negative social judgments can then have a lifetime of consequences, impacting career and even relationship success [16, 17].

Due to a lower self-esteem and poor confidence levels stemming from these traumatic events, affected individuals are then prone to neglect their self-care and may even start to lack in basic hygiene. This ultimately leads to poor social interactions and eventually impacts on financial status and income in later years. The lack of social interaction also impacts individuals negatively because this then impairs their ability to form close friendships or engage in romantic relationships later in life. Thus, the long term impacts of poorly managed dental trauma can significantly impact on individuals well-being and be pervasive in all areas of their lives [20].

4. Management guidelines for managing dental trauma amongst children and adolescents

Management guidelines for the holistic treatment of dental trauma amongst young individuals include the following:

4.1 Treatment of immediate pain and full history of complaint

As a first step, the oral health professional should immediately conduct all the necessary steps that entail selection of appropriate trauma treatment as needed. Pain elimination should be a high priority. The clinician should also simultaneously reassure the child and the parents/caregivers in order to alleviate their high levels of anxiety. This stage of treatment is also crucial for building rapport with the child and the parent/caregiver. The element of trust needs to be solidified early in this relationship between clinician and the affected child with parents/caregiver included.

Because there will be pain involved this first step is crucial because all individuals associate new experiences with past experiences and if the past experience was accompanied by pain, then future dental visits may be construed in the same light. Parents/caregivers may also be anxious about long term impacts on the child's esthetics as well as the added financial burden that this injury now presents with. Thus, by alleviating all these concerns, the oral health professional will help to allay long-term consequences that could significantly impact long-term treatment and care.

During this visit, a full medical, behavioral and social history of the patient should be detailed out in the patients file. All this information can be garnered from the parent who can then be distracted from their anxiety during this information session as well since they will be kept busy, even if for a short period of time. The importance of attending all follow-up visits must also be constantly reiterated with patients and if needed, a financial plan drawn up together with the patient in order to consider all factors that may impact upon long term follow-up visits.

4.2 Strategies to ease anxiety in affected individuals

The entire oral health team will need to work together to ensure that these young individuals are afforded a very low stress environment in order for treatment procedures to be meted out successfully. The following recommended treatment and behavioral strategies can be considered when managing these individuals who will be fearful and anxious due to the uncertainties surrounding the short and long-term consequences of their injuries:

4.2.1 Restoration of esthetics: after the initial clinical examination, radiographic examination and sensibility tests to determine condition of the pulp, recommended treatment strategies for dental traumatic injuries should be followed

According to Flores et al., for an uncomplicated crown fracture the following can be done: if any portion of the broken tooth is available, this can be bonded to the affected tooth. Emergency care involves covering of the exposed dentin with either permanent restoration material or a glass ionomer using a compatible bonding agent. The use of accepted dental restorative materials is recommended in order to restore esthetics to the highest level of suitability as possible [21].

According to Flores et al., for complicated crown fractures the following can be done: for teeth that are still developing, all attempts to preserve pulp vitality by a partial pulpotomy or pulp capping. This treatment procedure can also be used in children with completely formed teeth. Esthetically pleasing materials for such procedures include calcium hydroxide and Mineral Trioxide Aggregate (white). With patients more advanced in age, root canal treatment can be the treatment of choice and factors that also further determine this would include how much time has lapsed between the incident and treatment [21].

Behavioral strategies to ease anxiety in children during their clinical examination and treatment include the following:

4.2.2 Distraction

This technique involves talking to the child in a comforting manner throughout the treatment procedure in order to veer their thoughts away from what you are doing on them currently. All words and terminology used should meet the mental maturity of the individual at all times. Distraction may also include allowing the child to watch cartoons or music videos whilst you are working on them.

4.2.3 Tell-show-do

This technique involves you showing the child the instrument you will be using on them whilst showing them the instrument itself and then only using the instrument on him/her. It thus focuses on using a step-by-step technique to draw the individual into this specific experience. For example, if you are planning on using a probe to start off with, then show the individual the probe whilst you explain the functions of the probe and what you are going to do in the mouth with it. This technique was introduced by Addelston [22] more than half a century ago and has been shown to be highly effective [22].

4.2.4 Behavior shaping

For this technique, you introduce everything that you are doing in small steps and praise the child after each accomplishment. Example, sitting on chair follows with praise, then opening mouth wide follows with praise then allowing you to treat them is followed by praise or even a reward, like a sticker. Ensure that you are always using basic language and terminologies that the individual will easily understand.

4.2.5 Modeling

In the modeling technique, one would show the affected child video clips of other children having dental procedures being done on them. This will hopefully prompt the child to feel that they are also capable of being like the children in the video clips.

4.2.6 Right of choice

In order for the individual to feel a sense of involvement in the procedure, it is important to involve them in some aspects of decision-making around their treatment which are non-impactful. An example of this would be what flavor of topical anesthetic to use or even which glove to put on which of the clinician's hands [22, 23].

4.2.7 Non-verbal communication

Patients can be informed that they can communicate at any time during the treatment by lifting their hand up or if questioned, they can use a thumbs up for affirmative and thumbs down for negative. The clinician will always stop for the hand up signal or thumbs down signal. This will help in reassuring the patient that they are still able to communicate with the clinician during the procedure and may reduce feelings of powerlessness that young individuals may feel when being treated in a clinical environment.

4.2.8 Management of psychological impacts

Children who experience dental trauma often develop anxiety and fear due to pain associated with the traumatic injury itself. Experiencing pain during such an episode can have lifelong consequences on future and long-term dental treatment. Because research [8] strongly indicates a negative impact on oral health quality of life and levels of anxiety in children, dentists are advised [23] to manage patients whilst taking into consideration the following factors: (a) Removing or minimizing of predisposing factors (example, do not keep extraction forceps within sight or do not have pictures/artwork of individuals in dental chairs having extractions done) in order to create a safe and comfortable environment within the dental setting to avoid further negative experiences; (b) educating children and their caregivers on how to avoid situations leading to dental trauma (example, having seatbelts on at all times or using mouthguards during extreme sports); (c) encouraging use of and providing protective devices for children who are susceptible to dental traumatic injuries (example, mouthguards and head/face protective helmets for those children engaging frequently in high impact and/or contact sports); and (d) immediately treat any signs of traumatic dental injury. Since the occlusion is a predisposing factor for traumatic dental injuries, early orthodontic treatment for such children may be a factor worth considering as a long term preventive strategy. Subjective and objective evaluations of anxious, fearful and phobic patients who display negative psychological behavior in the dental setting are suggested in order to enhance the diagnosis for comfortable and successful patient management.

Psychophysiological patient responses can include the following:

- Muscle tightness
- Restlessness
- Unsteady hands
- Excess sweating
- Constant clearing of throat
- Strong startle response
- Frequent urination
- Holding things very tightly
- Pulsation in the temporal and carotid arteries
- Depth and speed of respiration

Subsequent behavioral and emotional responses can include the following:

- Inattentiveness
- Irritation
- Talking fast
- Hyperactivity
- Getting tongue-tangled
- Outbursts of emotions
- Sitting on the edge of the chair
- Pacing
- Rapidly thumbing through magazines
- Confusion
- Poor memory
- In a hurry
- Nervousness
- Leaning forward whilst sitting

- Excessive worrying
- Outbursts of emotions

Based on the dentist's experience and expertise, anxiety and phobias can be managed by psychotherapeutic interventions, pharmacologic interventions, or a combination of both.

According to Appukuttan [24], psychotherapeutic interventions can include the following [24]:

- Communication skills: a two-way communication strategy between dentist and patient where both parties are given an opportunity to converse freely. This must start at first visit as it also helps to build rapport and trust between both clinician, the patient and their caregivers/guradians/families.

- Relaxation techniques: deep breathing and muscle relaxation can be encouraged in patients because it is almost impossible to be psychologically upset whilst being simultaneously physically relaxed. It is further suggested that dentists acquire training in this technique and practice it with anxious or phobic patients prior to the commencement of treatment.

- Guided imagery: this technique can be performed by an adequately trained dentist or with the use of audio recordings. It involves teaching patients to create a mental image of a personally comforting experience that consciously navigates their attention toward complete body relaxation, thereby minimizing anxiety.

- Biofeedback: requires trained dentists or therapists to use specific instruments to monitor patients and to then use the information obtained to help patients practice and obtain self-regulation of their emotions.

- Acupuncture: a procedure whereby tiny needles are inserted in specific areas on the body to target healing of ailments, in this case anxiety. It is a procedure used widely but does require special training before it can be introduced into practice.

- Enhancing control: a procedure where patients get to feel like they have a sense of control over the procedure. This includes them giving the dentist a signal to pause treatment when they need a break (and dentist should adhere to this agreement) or giving patient a mirror to watch the procedure beign conducted on them.

- Positive reinforcement: this technique rewards desired behaviors and subsequently encourages the continuation of those behaviors. Such reinforcers include verbal praise, positive facial expressions and/or positive voice modulation.

- Cognitive behavioral therapy (CBT): this technique attempts to redefine the content of negative cognitions and thereby increase the patient's control over their own negative thoughts by redirecting their thoughts. This technique is a mixture of cognitive and behavioral approaches and includes learning to change negatively distorted thoughts and actions. Basically, new skills are learned to manage anxiety symptoms over s series of visits. However, dentists do need specialized training before this therapy can be instituted by them.

4.3 Multi-disciplinary team approach

Oral health professionals should have a comprehensive referral list on hand where patients can be referred and duly accommodated at the practice being referred to. At one of the initial dental visits, families should be comprehensively informed about all the possible consequences of traumatic dental injuries and who they could see if any issues arise post-treatment if the issue does not have a dental focus. The referral list should then be shared with all families of young individuals experiencing dental trauma—whether they ask to be referred to other healthcare professionals or not. This list should include amongst others: social workers, psychologists, trauma counselors, play therapists, pediatric specialists and maxillofacial surgeons who specialize in treating children. There should also be regular communication amongst these professionals as this is imperative to long-term treatment success for any of these professionals.

5. Conclusion

Traumatic dental injuries that are not effectively and holistically managed are significant in that they have been shown to impact on an individual's quality of life. In most societies, esthetics is held in high regard, specifically facial esthetics. Trauma to the outer and inner oral structures can leave an individual with dental anomalies or deformities. This can then cause body dysmorphic issues in that a person battles to accept their changed appearance leaving them stressed and anxious. The traumatic event itself can have lasting negative repercussions which when combined with a changed appearance, can cause long term psychological effects for the patient. These negative impacts can be negated by means of a comprehensive emergency care strategy that is accompanied by a comprehensive referral system and multidisciplinary team approach.

Conflict of interest

The author confirms that there are no conflicts of interest related to this piece of work.

Author details

Aneesa Moolla
Faculty of Health Sciences, Health Economics and Epidemiology Research Office, University of the Witwatersrand, Johannesburg, South Africa

*Address all correspondence to: aneesa.moolla@wits.ac.za

IntechOpen

© 2023 The Author(s). Licensee IntechOpen. This chapter is distributed under the terms of the Creative Commons Attribution License (http://creativecommons.org/licenses/by/3.0), which permits unrestricted use, distribution, and reproduction in any medium, provided the original work is properly cited.

References

[1] Andersson L. Epidemiology of traumatic dental injuries. Journal of Endodontia. 2013;**39**:S2-S5. DOI: 10.1016/j.joen.2012.11.021

[2] Lam R. Epidemiology and outcomes of traumatic dental injuries: A review of the literature. Australian Dental Journal. 2016;**61**:4-20. DOI: 10.1111/adj.12395

[3] Petti S, Glendor U, Andersson L. World traumatic dental injury prevalence and incidence, a meta-analysis-one billion living people have had traumatic dental injuries. Dental Traumatology. 2018;**34**:71-86. DOI: 10.1111/edt.12389

[4] Rodd H, Noble F. Psychosocial impacts relating to dental injuries in childhood: The bigger picture. Dentistry Journal. 2019;7(1):23. DOI: 10.3390/dj7010023

[5] Arhakis A, Athanasiadou E, Vlachou C. Social and psychological aspects of dental trauma, behavior management of young patients who have suffered dental trauma. The Open Dentistry Journal. 2017;**11**:41-47. DOI: 10.2174/1874210601711010041

[6] Kumar S, Kaur G, Kashyap N, Radhe A. Social and psychological impact of traumatic dental injuries in children and adolescents: A review of literature. Interventions in Pediatric Dentistry Open Access Journal. 2020;**11**:330-333. DOI: 10.32474/IPDOAJ.2020.04.000188

[7] Das P, Mishra L, Jena D, Govind S, Panda S, Lapinska B. Oral health-related quality of life in children and adolescents with a traumatic injury of permanent teeth and the impact on their families: A systematic review. International Journal of Environmental Research and Public Health. 2022;**19**:3087. DOI: 10.3390/ijerph19053087

[8] El-Kalla IH, Shalan HM, Bakr RA. Impact of dental trauma on quality of life amongst 11-14 years schoolchildren. Contemporary Clinical Dental. 2017;**8**(4):538-544. DOI: 10.4103/ccd42817

[9] Seehra J, Newton J, Dibiase A. Bullying in schoolchildren – its relationship to dental appearance and psychosocial implications: An update for GDPs. British Dental Journal. 2011;**210**(9):411-415. DOI: 10.1038/sj.bdj.2011.339

[10] Stallard P, Velleman R, Langsford J, Baldwin S. Coping and psychological distress in children involved in road traffic accidents. The British Journal of Clinical Psychology. 2001;**40**:197-208. DOI: 10.1348/014466501163643

[11] Odenbach J, Newton A, Gokiert R, Falconer C, Courchesne C, Campbell S, et al. Screening for post-traumatic stress disorder after injury in the pediatric emergency department—a systematic review protocol. Systematic Reviews. 2014;**3**(1):19-23. DOI: 10.1186/2046-4053-3-19

[12] Kaur P, Singh S, Mathur A. Impact of dental disorders and its influence on self-esteem levels amongst adolescents. Journal of Clinical and Diagnostic Research. 2017;**11**(4):ZC05-ZC08. DOI: 10.7860/JCDR/2017/23362.9515

[13] Locker D, Allen F. What do measures of 'oral health related quality of life' measure? Community Dentistry and Oral Epidemiology. 2007;**35**:401-411. DOI: 10.1111/j.1600-0528.2007.00418.x

[14] Allison PJ, Locker D, Feine JS. Quality of life: A dynamic construct. Social Science & Medicine. 1997;**45**(2):221-230. DOI: 10.1016/s0277-9536(96)00339-5

[15] Ramos-Jorge ML, Bosco VL, Peres MA, Nunes AC. The impact of treatment of dental trauma on the quality of life of adolescents – a case control study in southern Brazil. Dental Traumatology. 2007;**23**(2):114-119. DOI: 10.1111/j.1600-9657.2005.00409.x

[16] Karunakaran T, Gilbert D, Asimakopoulou K, Newton T, Newton JT. The influence of visible dental caries on social judgments and overall facial attractiveness amongst undergraduates. Journal of Dentistry. 2011;**39**:212-217. DOI: 10.1016/j.jdent.2010.12.006

[17] Stolier RM, Hehman E, Keller MD, Walker M, Freeman JB. The conceptual structure of face impressions. Proceedings of the National Academic Science USA. 2018;**115**:9210-9215. DOI: 10.1073/pnas.1807222115

[18] Awooda EM, Ali YA. Social judgments made by children (10-15 year old) in relation to visible incisors trauma: School-based cross-sectional study in Khartoum state, Sudan. Journal of International Society of Preventive & Community. 2015;**5**(5):423-431. DOI: 10.4103/2231-0762.165931

[19] Rodd HD, Barker C, Baker SR, Marshman Z, Robinson PG. Social judgments made by children in relation to visible incisor trauma. Dental Traumatology. 2010;**26**(1):2-8. DOI: 10.1111/j.1600-9657.2009.00849.x

[20] Wilson JP, Rule NO. Facial trustworthiness predicts extreme criminal-sentencing outcomes. Psychological Science. 2015;**26**:1325-1331. DOI: 10.1177/0956797615590992

[21] Flores MT, Andersson L, Andreasen JO, Bakland LK, Malmgren B, Barnett F, et al. Guidelines for the management of traumatic dental injuries. I. Fractures and luxations of permanent teeth. Dental Traumatology. Apr 2007;**23**(2):66-71. DOI: 10.1111/j.1600-9657.2007.00592.x

[22] Addelston HK. Child patient training. Fortnight review. Chicago Dental Society. 1959;**38**(7-9):27-29

[23] Kotsanos N. Pediatric Dentistry-Evidence Based Total Care. Thessaloniki: Fylatos Publishing; 2015. pp. 77-97. DOI: 10.2174/1874210601711010041

[24] Appukuttan DP. Strategies to manage patients with dental anxiety and dental phobia: Literature review. Clinical, Cosmetic and Investigational Dentistry. 2016;**8**:35-50. DOI: 10.2147/CCIDE.S63626

Section 2

Periodontal Disease and Cysts

Chapter 10

Trauma and the Periodontal Tissues: A Narrative Review

Santo Grace Umesh, Lakshmi Ramachandran, Janani Karthikeyan and Sindhuja M. Shankar

Abstract

The health of the periodontium including the soft tissues – gingiva and periodontal ligament; and the hard tissues – cementum and alveolar bone is of key importance in the overall homeostasis of the dentition. Injury to the periodontal tissues in any form such as microbial, physical, thermal, chemical, mechanical, occlusal and habitual injury affects the harmony of the periodontal attachment apparatus thereby altering the entire functioning of the dentition. The type of tissue damage when trauma is unintentional and iatrogenic tends to be acute and self-limiting. On the other hand, mechanical and occlusal forces could result in chronic damage. This book chapter provides a review on the various forms of non-microbial trauma to the periodontal tissues, their clinical manifestations and its management.

Keywords: periodontal trauma, gingival trauma, chemical injury, trauma from occlusion, iatrogenic trauma

1. Introduction

A traumatic dental injury represents acute transmission of energy to a tooth and its supporting structures, which results in fracture and/or displacement of the tooth and/ or separation or crushing of the supporting tissues (gingival, periodontal ligament, PDL and bone) [1, 2]. Dental injuries can be divided into different categories based on their genesis, anatomy, pathology, or treatment implications (**Figure 1**) [3, 4].

1.1 Injuries to the hard dental tissues: pulp, periodontal ligament, alveolar process and supporting tissues

1.1.1 Crown-root fracture

A fracture involving enamel, dentin and cementum. It may or may not expose the pulp.

1.1.2 Root fracture

A fracture involving dentin, cementum and the pulp. Root fractures can be further classified according to displacement of the coronal fragment.

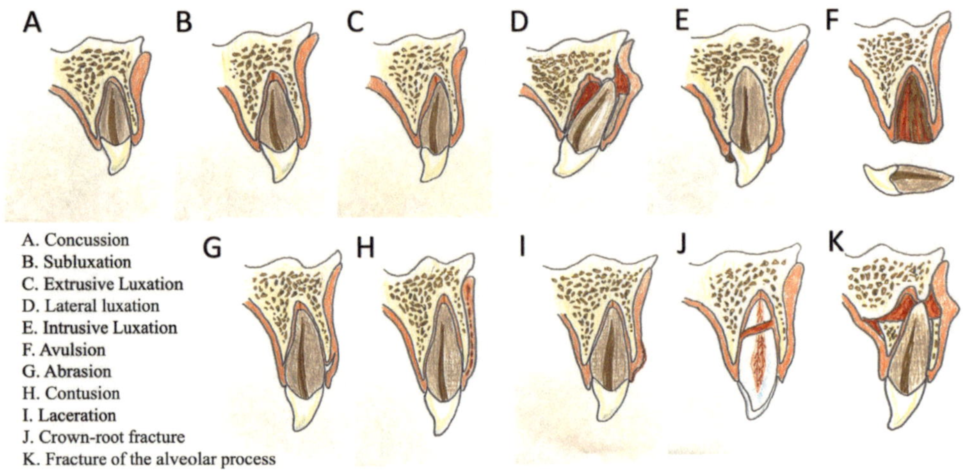

Figure 1.
Traumatic injuries to the periodontal tissues.

1.1.3 Fracture of the alveolar socket wall

A fracture of the alveolar process which involves the alveolar socket.

1.1.4 Fracture of the alveolar process

Fracture of the alveolar process that may or may not involve the alveolar socket.

1.1.5 Concussion

An injury to the tooth- supporting structures without abnormal loosening or displacement of the tooth, but with marked pain to percussion.

1.1.6 Subluxation (loosening)

An injury to the tooth-supporting structures resulting in increased mobility, but without displacement of the tooth.

1.1.7 Extrusive luxation (peripheral dislocation, partial avulsion)

Partial displacement of the tooth out of its socket.

1.1.8 Lateral luxation

Displacement of the tooth in a direction other than axially. Displacement is accompanied by comminution or fracture of either the labial or the palatal/lingual alveolar bone.

1.1.9 Intrusive luxation (central dislocation)

Displacement of the tooth into the alveolar bone. This injury is accompanied by comminution or fracture of the alveolar socket.

1.1.10 Avulsion (exarticulation)

The tooth is completely displaced out of its socket.

1.1.11 Abrasion

A superficial wound produced by rubbing or scraping of the skin or mucosa leaving a raw, bleeding surface.

1.1.12 Contusion

A bruise without a break in the skin or mucosa. Subcutaneous or submucosal haemorrhage in the tissue. A contusion may be isolated to the soft tissue but may also indicate an underlying bone fracture.

1.1.13 Laceration

A shallow or deep wound penetrating into the soft tissue, usually produced by a sharp object. May disrupt blood vessels, nerves, muscles and involve salivary glands. Most frequently seen in lips, oral mucosa and gingiva. More seldom the tongue is involved.

1.1.14 Soft tissue avulsion

Avulsion (loss of tissue) injuries are rare but seen with bite injuries or as a result of a very deep and extended abrasion.

2. Thermal traumatic injuries (TTI)

The use of overheated handpieces and ultrasonic scalers can iatrogenically result in thermal traumatic injuries to the gingiva. Thermal burns, however, have been listed as one of the potential side effects that could be brought on by using ultrasonic scalers [5]. TTI can also be brought on by consuming unusually hot/cold meals or drinks. However, persons with psychiatric illnesses have been documented to experience severe cases of intraoral and laryngopharyngeal burn brought on by hot foods or beverages [6]. Because the supporting periodontal tissue is unconstrained by space and has a larger blood supply than the pulp, heat-generating devices are more likely to cause a temperature increase in the periodontal ligament than the pulp [7].

3. Mechanical traumatic injuries (MTI)

Accidents, assaults, falls during play or sports, and convulsions can all lead to mechanical traumatic injuries (MTI) to the gingival tissue. It has also been noted that malocclusions such a deep bite or an enhanced overbite can harm the gingiva [8, 9]. Dental appliances that were manufactured incorrectly and defective dental restorations might cause iatrogenic mechanical stress [10, 11]. MTI can also occur when one bites or sucks on a fingernail or other hard, sharp object, improper flossing [12].

Gingivitis artefacta are the most frequently described self-inflicted MTI to the gingival tissue [13]. According to reports, gingivitis artefacta minor is more prevalent, whereas gingivitis artefacta major is more severe and spreads to the periodontium's deeper tissues. In gingivitis artefacta minor, there is typically a previous source of irritation, such as a habit of biting one's fingers or eating foods that are abrasive. As a result, the condition can be treated effectively by removing the irritant from its source. On the other hand, gingivitis artefacta major requires specialised treatment approaches because the condition may have an emotional and extraoral component [14].

Stewart and Kernohan [15] grouped gingival injuries resulting from self-inflicted physical trauma into three categories: Type A injuries are those that are added on top of pre-existing lesions (or irritations) where the patient continues to cause harm to the area, Type B injuries are those that are caused by habits like fingernail biting or finger sucking, and Type C injuries are those with unknown and/or complex etiologies that are typically brought on by emotional disturbances [15]. Oral piercing is another MTI to the oral soft tissues that is self-inflicted [16]. The prevalence of oral and peri-oral piercings among young adults ranged from 0.8 percent to 12 percent, according to a comprehensive review [17].

Oral and peri-oral tissues are perforated in order to place jewellery on various facial features, including the tongue, lips, cheek, and labial frenum. However, complications could develop after surgery [17–20]. In addition to increased plaque and calculus production, gingival inflammation may also be one of the main post-operative periodontal problems [17, 20]. Chronic bad oral hygiene, particularly in people who smoke a lot, can lead to secondary post-operative periodontal problems. Additionally, when the jewellery material is porous, there may be a change in the bacterial population and a rise in the pathogenic potential of the periodontopathogens bacteria leading to mucogingival defects and abscesses of the supporting tissues [17, 20].

While the only reasons for getting an oral piercing may be a trend, group identification, attractiveness, other types of self-inflicted MTI to the gingival tissue may be caused by potentially dangerous oral behaviour [16, 21]. Neuroses, occupational habits, and other habits were used to categorise these oral behaviour [22]. Neuroses include biting the lips, cheeks, pencils, pens, and fingernails. Occupational habits include holding nails in the mouth by upholsterers, carpenters and biting thread by tailors. Miscellaneous habits include smoking pipes or cigarettes, thumb sucking, mouth breathing, and using the wrong toothbrushing technique [22].

3.1 Clinical presentations and management of trauma to the gingiva

The numerous factors already mentioned lead to a wide range of potential clinical manifestations. Depending on the unique characteristics of each instance, the history elicited will vary from case to case. Patients who engage in self-harming behaviour may have a history of continuous gingival irritation, which leads to picking or scratching of the gingiva, as well as a history that may point to an emotional disorder or psychological imbalance [13, 14, 23]. A history may also indicate long-standing behaviour like compulsive toothbrushing, digit sucking, or biting on potentially harmful things, as well as interaction with other potentially harmful mechanical, chemical, or thermal objects.

When examined, there may be significant ulcerative lesions affecting the lips, tongue, and gingival oral mucosa in addition to intense burns, scorching, and bleeding [13]. The ulcer may occasionally appear as coagulative necrosis coated in slough.

In factitious injuries, bite marks on the lips and nail marks on the gingiva can both be seen [14]. Usually, there is gingival recession, which can be severe and widespread, affecting numerous teeth. Depending on the affected location, mouth opening may be restricted and chewing may be challenging. It's possible that there is not any laboratory or radiologic proof of an underlying systemic illness.

Complete re-epithelialization of the gingival tissue, complete or considerable root covering, and an expansion of the zone of keratinized gingiva are the treatment's primary objectives [24]. Additionally, it's crucial to stop a recurrence by getting rid of any identified causal factors. Therefore, the first step in treatment is to cure any improper oral hygiene habits and get rid of any dangerous substances. To eliminate the accumulated plaque, gentle mechanical oral hygiene techniques are implemented; if necessary, this may be done with topical or local anaesthetic medications. In the beginning, regular brushing in the other areas may be continued while chemical plaque management is advised as the only oral hygiene measure in the affected area. Two times a day, chlorhexidine mouthwash may be recommended. Warm saline mouth wash and Betadine has also been found helpful [25, 26].

Supportive symptomatic care is provided to preserve the patient's overall health, and this includes the recommendation of a non-spicy, soft food, as well as multivitamins and topical analgesics such triamcinolone acetate and benzocaine to ease discomfort [26]. Topical steroid triamcinolone should be administered in conjunction with carboxymethyl cellulose in cases of significant tissue injury [25]. To eliminate the infection, antibiotic treatment could be required. Factitious situations may necessitate professional psychiatric care, which may involve the use of antidepressants and/or antianxiety medications [14]. A significant loss of gingival tissue may need the use of a free gingival graft to repair the damage [12].

3.2 Trauma to periodontal ligaments

The soft complex connective tissue that serves as an interface between the cementum covering the roots and the inner wall of the alveolar bone is vascular, highly cellular, and specialised [27, 28]. The periodontal ligaments may become overextended and inflamed in circumstances where there are too many bilateral opposing vector stresses. The term "sprained tooth syndrome" is sometimes used to describe this (STS.). This can happen when someone unintentionally bites down on a hard object, when a tooth is improperly or excessively filled, when teeth are drifting, or in cases of sinusitis or allergies. The aberrant outward lateral pressure from the tongue to the teeth that results in temporary orthodontic pressure and outer movement outward and abnormal tooth mobility has been linked to STS in cases of upper respiratory tract infection.

Every effort must be made to avoid iatrogenic forms of trauma to the periodontal ligament because its attempts at healing may have unpredictable outcomes. Periodontal ligament may heal favourably without resorption or with repair related surface resorption and it can also heal unfavourably with osseous replacement resorption (ankylosis) or with inflammatory resorption [29].

Treatment for sprained teeth focuses mostly on reversing the opposing vector forces that caused the strain. A broken tooth, on the other hand, can wait a few days to see whether it heals by itself. Rest is necessary for the treatment of a sprained tooth because using the injured teeth for chewing and speaking causes further discomfort [23].

Radiographic evaluation, tooth realignment, surgical or orthodontic extrusion of the afflicted tooth, splinting, occlusal correction, antimicrobial therapy, endodontic treatment, and follow-up are all necessary for the management of invasive luxation [30]. All of the aforementioned procedures are likewise necessary for lateral and extrusive luxation, with the exception of tooth extrusion. While concussion simply needs a radiographic evaluation and follow-up to monitor the tooth over time, subluxation only needs a radiographic evaluation, splinting, and follow-up [30]. Only if there is no contamination and the tooth was transported and stored in a manner that ensured the health of the periodontal ligaments could an avulsed tooth be successfully reimplanted. After reimplantation, the tooth will be immobilised, and endodontic procedure may be initiated later [31].

It has been established that higher temperatures have detrimental effects on the periodontal ligament [32]. Clinical signs of protein denaturation in periodontal ligaments, disruption of the blood supply to the periodontal ligament, and tooth ankylosis may result from thermal injury to periodontal disorders [32, 33]. Thermal injuries are mostly managed by prevention. Using enough cooling water for tooth preparation or when dry cutting is required, applying gentle pressure, and limiting the bur-contact duration to less than 20 seconds at a time are just a few of the clinical recommendations that have been made to help prevent thermal injuries during dental treatment [17].

4. Chemical burns

4.1 Classification

Chemical burns majorly occur by the action of irritants on the mucosal tissues (**Table 1**). Mucosal damage caused by chemical burns could be

1. Iatrogenic as in irrigation performing endodontic procedures

2. Inappropriate application of chemicals and non-therapeutic agents by the patients.

4.1.1 Alendronate

It is a constituent of the diphosphonate family and has been used to treat osteoporosis caused on by glucocorticoids as well as a number of other bone disorders. Alendronate may have side effects, such as esophagitis on the mucosa of the upper

Dental materials	Medications	Nontherapeutic agents	Drugs
• Arsenic [34] • Calcium hydroxide [35, 36] • Cavity varnish [37] • Chromic acid [38] • Dentine-bonding agent [39] • Ferric sulfate [40] • Formocresol [41] • Iodine [42] • Paraformaldehyde [42] • Eugenol [43, 44]	Alendronate [45, 46] Aspirin [47, 48] Chlorpromazine [49] Promazine [49] Tetracycline hydrochloride [50–52]	• Arrack [53] • Battery acid [49] • Denture cleansers [54, 55] • Garlic [56] • Gasoline [57] • H_2O_2 [58, 59] • Minard's Liniment [60] • Mouthwashes [61–64] • NaOCl [65, 66]	Amphetamine [67] Cocaine [68–72] MDMA [72]

Table 1.
Aetiology for chemical burns of the oral mucosa.

aerodigestive tract is the most typical one. Patients must be instructed to take the drug with a glass of water, not to chew or suck the tablet, and to stand up straight for around 30 minutes in order to avoid this side effect [45].

4.1.2 Aspirin

Acetylsalicylic acid, popularly known as aspirin, is a frequently prescribed drug for the treatment of pain, fever, and inflammation. Aspirin and its derivatives, commonly prescribed for alleviating oral and tooth pain, are responsible for the majority of chemical burn incidences when they are sucked, administered as a gel, mouthwash, powder, or as a tablet near to a sore tooth in an effort to relieve pain [73]. When aspirin is applied to the mucosa for a long time, it exerts a caustic impact. A cell-mediated response might result in an aphthous-like ulceration of the oral mucosal layer due to the acidic nature of acetylsalicylic acid (pH 3.5–5.0) [47]. Further, aspirin's organic and inorganic components adhere to the oral cavity epithelium, causing denaturation and coagulative necrosis [48].

4.1.3 Calcium hydroxide

Calcium hydroxide ($Ca(OH)_2$) is frequently used in the field of endodontics due to its notable characteristics of mineralisation induction and promotion, antimicrobial capabilities, and necrotic material disintegration. Its adverse effects include cellular damage, epithelial damage, necrosis of bone, and cytotoxicity.

4.1.4 Cocaine (benzoylmethylecgonine) ($C_{17}H_{21}NO_4$)

It is an alkaloid obtained from *Erythroxylum coca* leaves. Europe has the second-highest prevalence of cocaine use, with about 910,000 persons taking it. Cocaine's nonionized form diffuses across the lipid membranes of neurons. It transforms back into the active cationic form in the axoplasm, binds to the sodium channels, and stops the action potential from forming, producing a reversible anaesthetic effect [72].

4.1.5 Denture cleansers

Patients clean their dentures with a variety of homemade and store-bought cleaners. Potassium monopersulfate, sodium perborate, sodium carbonate, surfactant, sodium bicarbonate, citric acid, and an additive are ingredients in immersion-type denture cleaners sold as tablets or powders. The perborate breaks down into an alkaline peroxide solution when the tablet or powder is dissolved in water, and it continues to break down to release oxygen. Debris is mechanically loosened by this process. The newly formed oxygen may interact with substances required for cell metabolism, interact with cell structures, or accelerate metabolism at the expense of cell growth [54].

4.1.6 Eugenol

Eugenol has a scorching flavour, a strong carnation aroma and is a pale yellow liquid. It has been included in a number of products, including dental cement, endodontic sealants, impression pastes, and dressings for dry sockets. Unprocessed eugenol is combined with zinc oxide to create zinc oxide-eugenol, which demonstrates a combination of physical and therapeutic qualities and can be used as a foundation material, root canal filler, and temporary restorative material. The tissue reaction caused by eugenol's byproducts might range from mild local allergic reactions to the uncommon catastrophic anaphylactic reactions [43, 44].

4.1.7 Formocresol

Ever since Buckley introduced formocresol to dentistry in 1904, it has been frequently utilised in paediatric dentistry. In pulpotomy, formocresol is employed as a medication because of its ability to repair tissue when exposed to pulp. In the field, there has been a lot of concern stated and debated regarding the safety of using formocresol. There have been reports of widespread necrosis of soft tissues in the oral cavity due to improper formocresol use.

4.1.8 Garlic burn

Allium sativum, also known as garlic, is regarded as a valuable herbal remedy and has been used for ages to treat a variety of illnesses. Additionally, studies have indicated that garlic has fibrinolytic, antihypertensive, and lipid-lowering properties. It has antiviral, antifungal, and antibacterial effects. Garlic's most frequent adverse reactions are nausea, diarrhoea, heartburn, and digestive distress. Rhinitis, asthma, anaphylaxis, contact dermatitis, and pemphigus are manifestations of garlic allergy. In 1987, Parish et al. reported the first instance of garlic burn. Garlic's precise ingredients that cause skin lesions are still a mystery. Allicin, diallyl disulfide, and allyl propyl disulfide are presumed to be the causes of chemical burn [56].

4.1.9 Hydrogen peroxide

The method by which H_2O_2 exerts its antimicrobial effects is owing to the release of nascent oxygen, which is harmful to anaerobes. The action of H O on bacterial cell wall debridement is the other antibacterial property mechanism [58]. H2O2 is used in mouthrinses (1–3%) and as a bleaching agent (3–5%) among other applications. Oral use of solutions containing 3 percent H2O2 may result in nausea, minor mucosal irritability, and burns to the mouth, throat, oesophagus, and stomach. Ingestion of greater concentrations (>10 percent) can have more hazardous side effects, like burns to the gut mucosa and mucous membranes [59]. It is because it can directly react with proteins to create conjugates and reactive haptens that it triggers localised hypersensitivity reactions to oral mucosa, known as "contact stomatitis," and to the dermis, known as "contact dermatitis," in lower doses [43, 44].

4.1.10 Sodium hypochlorite

NaOCl is a transparent, straw-coloured solution with 5% accessible chlorine in it. It creates chloramines upon ionisation, those are providing the antibacterial properties. The drawback of NaOCl is that if it is used outside of a root canal, it can lead to soft-tissue irritation and necrosis [40]. It reacts with the oral mucosa's proteins and lipids, which could cause subsequent infections [42]. NaOCl should be used as an irrigant in the root canal at a concentration of between 0.5 percent and 5.2 percent. Localised or widespread tissue necrosis has resulted from NaOCl's extension into the periradicular tissue. In the epidermis and subcutaneous tissues, a significant acute inflammatory response causes rapid intraoral and extraoral tissue swelling. It causes acute sinusitis if it spreads into the maxillary sinus [65].

4.2 Clinical features

The degree of tissue damage, the causative agent's destructive qualities, and the method of application all affect how chemical burns look clinically [56]. Clinical lesions can range in severity from mild to severe depending on the substance used, pH level, chemical agent concentration, quantity used, method and length of tissue contact, depth of tissue penetration, and mechanism of action. Chemical burns on the mucosa manifest as diffuse erosive lesions that can range in severity from conventional desquamation to full mucosal detachment with penetration into the submucosa [50]. Chemical exposure causes changes in the vascularity, colour, texture, and consistency of the tissues. The general chemical burn appears as a shallow, wrinkled lesion that ranges in colour from white to yellow.

The characteristics of coagulative necrosis are seen through histopathological analysis [56]. Salivary gland duct involvement may result in temporary obstructive salivary glanditis, but subsequent ductal opening scarring may result in chronic obstruction. Excision of the duct or gland may be necessary in cases of chronic sialadenitis [41]. Chemical burns frequently have a localised distribution and are not always restricted to the anatomic distribution of the masticatory mucosa [74].

4.2.1 Alendronate

Clinically, it may present as ulcers located on the palate, tongue, and lower lip. The ulcers cause intense pain [45].

4.2.2 Aspirin

It causes a localised white scurf with a reddened and thickened border [47, 73], while chromic acid produces a characteristic yellow lesion with a flat border [74].

4.2.3 Calcium hydroxide

Patients present with a swollen lip and mucosa, no history of pain and an extensive necrotic zone on gingiva with perforation [37].

4.2.4 Cocaine

Lesions develop at the site of application. A white slough, which could easily be removed, showing underlying ulceration and erythema seen on the gingiva. Patients may report painful, retracted gingiva [72].

4.2.5 Denture cleansers

Denture cleansers on chewing and swishing it around the mouth show burning sensation, swelling of the floor of the mouth and the salivary glands, inflammation of the soft palate and tongue. The orifices of the submandibular glands can also present with red and ulcerated with sloughing of the mucosa. There have been several reports of upper digestive tract injury associated with the accidental ingestion of denture cleansers. Furthermore, it can depict as diffuse erosive lesions ranging from simple desquamation to complete obliteration of the oral mucosa with extension past the basement membrane into the submucosa. On ingestion, it also presented with perioral, glossal, and laryngeal edema and respiratory stridor leading to death. On autopsy, it showed extensive hemorrhagic bronchopneumonia and widespread gastrointestinal ulceration [54].

4.2.6 Eugenol

Eugenol burns usually presents with burning sensation and pain over the exposed area. Patient also complains of itching sensation. Intraoral examination may reveal allergic reaction “contact stomatitis” over the gingiva and adjacent mucosa [43].

4.2.7 Formocresol

Formocresol burns usually presents with pain and swelling on the exposed area. Extensive ulcerative lesion extending along exposed surface will appear like coagulative necrosis covered by slough. Patient also presents with symptoms of restricted mouth opening and reduced food intake [41].

4.2.8 Garlic

Garlic burns are clinically manifested as an area of slough and mucosal ulceration extending along the area of placement. The lesion may be painful on palpation [56].

4.2.9 Hydrogen peroxide

H_2O_2 burns present as extensive areas of ulceration and erythema involving the alveolar mucosa and the marginal and attached gingival regions. Focal areas of ulceration and sloughing with necrosis of the surface layers of the epithelium may be seen [59].

4.2.10 Sodium hypochlorite

NaOCl burns manifest clinically as soft-tissue inflammation and necrosis if it is expressed outside the confines of root canal. The swelling may be edematous, hemorrhagic, or both and may extend beyond the region that might be expected with an acute infection of the affected tooth. The sudden onset of pain is a hallmark of tissue damage and may occur immediately or be delayed for several minutes or hours. Associated bruising and ecchymosis of adjacent tissues may occur due to bleeding into interstitial spaces [65].

4.2.11 Tetracycline hydrochloride

Tetracycline hydrochloride burns are manifested as loosely adherent yellowish white slough on gingiva. It may show erythematous margins, and patients complain of severe pain [38].

4.3 Treatment

A correct clinical history must be obtained in order to diagnose a chemical burn because the patient may not be aware of the relevance of these potentially harmful chemicals [41]. Early patient screening and prompt implementation of therapeutic measures will guarantee a speedy recovery and potentially stop additional mucosal damage [74].

The reason might be entirely eliminated by just getting rid of the agent permanently. Multiple irrigations with sterile water or betadine. If needed, analgesics, corticosteroids and benzocaine applied topically. Dietary supplements in the form of multivitamins would accelerate the recovery. When necessary, medications to stop secondary infections. Encourage the patient to follow a soft, chilled diet devoid of spices for a week. After a week, recall.

5. Occlusal trauma

The role of occlusion and how it interacts with the periodontium has been extensively researched. Occlusal trauma, also known as traumatism or trauma from occlusion(TFO), is an injury that causes tissue alterations inside the attachment apparatus as a result of occlusal force. Clinicians' knowledge of the impacts of damaging occlusal forces and the periodontium's adaptive, reparative, and destructive responses is mostly based on retrospective observations of human postmortem specimens and laboratory animal investigations. Unfortunately, there is a scarcity of scientific information from well-controlled prospective trials in people, making it difficult to comprehend this intricate host interaction [75].

5.1 Definitions

- Trauma from occlusion was defined by Stillman [76] as "a condition where injury results to the supporting structures of the teeth by the act of bringing the jaws into a closed position."

- According to Carranza (AAP, 1986) [77], when occlusal forces exceed the adaptive capacity of the tissues, tissue injury results, the resultant injury is termed trauma from occlusion.

- WHO in 1978 defined trauma from occlusion as "damage in the periodontium caused by stress on the teeth produced directly or indirectly by teeth of the opposing jaw."

- In the "Glossary of Periodontic Terms" (AAP 1986); occlusal trauma was defined as "An injury to the attachment apparatus as a result of excessive occlusal force".

5.2 Glickman's concept

Glickman asserted that a plaque-associated gingivitis can be altered by abnormal occlusal forces [28]. That suggests that the Periodontal apparatus is gradually being affected by these forces. The response of a traumatised tooth with subgingival plaque is different when compared to tissues around a tooth without deliterious forces. He suggested that there exists two distinct zones (**Figure 2**).

Zone of irritation: The interdental gingival papillae and marginal gingiva make up the zone of irritation, which is restricted by the gingival fibres. In this area, local irritations cause inflammation. The most harmful effects are epithelium ulceration, suppuration, and gingival connective tissue degeneration and necrosis. Even (horizontal) bone loss is could occur [78].

Zone of co-destruction: This contains the alveolar bone, the root cementum, and the periodontal ligament. Transseptal collagen fibre bundles (interdental and dentoalveolar) demarcate it coronally. The formation of an angular bony defect may result from the progression of inflammation from the zone of irritation directly into the periodontal ligament [79].

5.3 Adaptive capacity of the periodontium to occlusal forces

Adaptive capacity varies from person to person and from time to time within the same person. The size, direction, duration, and frequency of occlusal forces on the periodontium all determine their effect (**Figure 3**).

When occlusal stresses are raised in amplitude, the periodontium responds with

1. The periodontal ligament space is being widened.

2. The quantity and width of PDL fibres significantly increased.

3. An increase in the alveolar bone density [76].

The reorientation of stress and strains inside the periodontium is caused by changing the direction of occlusal pressures. The main fibres are positioned along the long

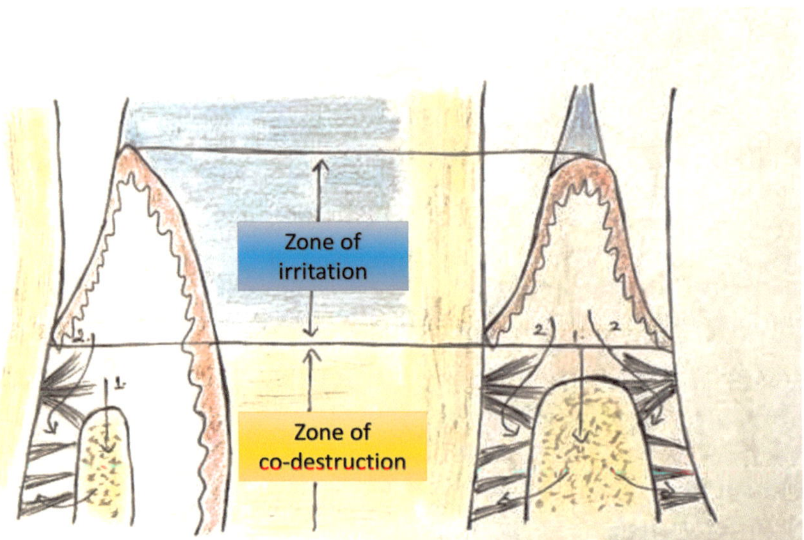

Figure 2.
Spread of inflammation in TFO-Glickman Concept-zone of irritation, zone of co-destruction [28].

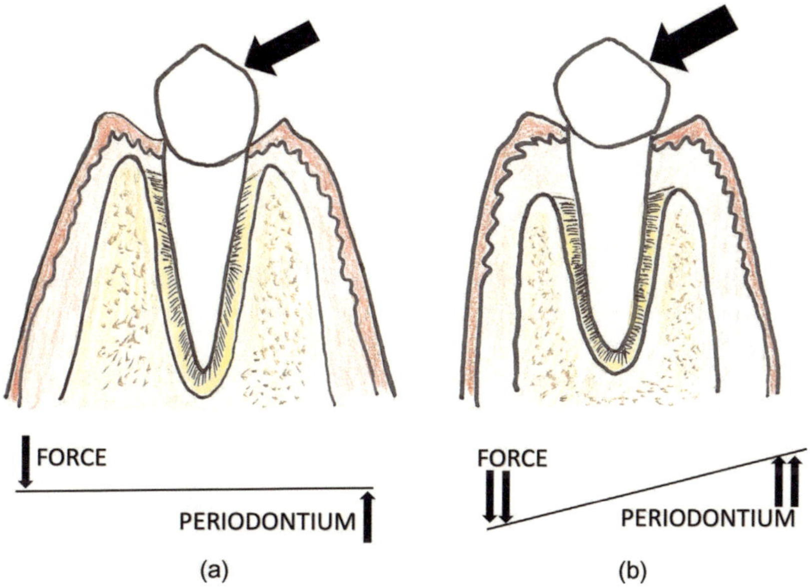

Figure 3.
Response to occlusal forces (a) normal periodontium can withstand normal occlusal forces, and (b) excessive occlusal forces causes damage to the periodontium [28].

axis of the tooth to best tolerate occlusal stresses. The periodontium is more prone to be injured by lateral (horizontal) and torque (rotational) forces.

5.4 Trauma caused by occlusion

5.4.1 Acute vs chronic TFO

5.4.1.1 Acute TFO

Acute TFO is a type of TFO that occurs suddenly. It is usually caused by

1. Biting down on a hard object causes an abrupt occlusal impact.

2. Prosthetic appliances that interfere with or change the direction of occlusal force are known as restorations [80].

Characteristics: Tooth pain, percussion sensitivity, and increased tooth movement.
Consequence: If the force is removed by a shift in the position of the tooth or by wearing away or correcting the restoration, the injury heals and the symptoms disappear if not, injury may worsen, leading to necrosis and the creation of a periodontal abscess.In some instances, it may persist as a symptomless chronic illness or end up in formation of cemental tears.

5.4.1.2 Chronic

It's more common and has a higher clinical impact. Rather than developing as a result of acute TFO, it develops as a result of gradual alterations in occlusion caused by tooth attrition combined with parafunctional habits like as bruxism and clenching [81].

Characteristics: Increasing mobility is one of the clinical characteristics.

5.4.2 Primary vs secondary TFO

5.4.2.1 Primary TFO

Occlusion trauma is the key etiologic cause in periodontal deterioration, and occlusion trauma is the only local modification to which a tooth is susceptible. Insertion of a “high filling” insertion of a prosthetic replacement that places excessive forces on the abutment and antagonist teeth drifting movement or extension of teeth into spaces created by unreplaced missing teeth drifting movement or extension of teeth into functionally unacceptable positions drifting movement or extension of teeth into spaces created by unreplaced missing teeth.

The amount of connective tissue attachment is not altered by original trauma, and pocket development is not initiated. This is likely because the supracrestal gingival fibres are unaffected, preventing the junctional epithelium from migrating apically [81].

5.4.2.2 Secondary TFO

Occurs when bone loss caused by marginal inflammation impairs the tissues’ adaptive capacity to bear occlusal stresses. This changes the leverage on the remaining tissues by reducing the periodontal attachment area. The periodontium becomes more prone to injury, and occlusal forces that were previously tolerated become traumatic [82].

5.5 Tissue response to increased occlusal forces

5.5.1 Effect on periodontal ligament

5.5.1.1 Stage I: injury

Excessive occlusal forces result in tissue destruction. The periodontium is modified to buffer the impact of the offending force if it is chronic. The ligament widens at the expense of the bone, resulting in angular bone defects and loose teeth without periodontal pockets. The fulcrum or axis of rotation, which in single-rooted teeth is located in the junction of the middle third and the apical third of the clinical root, rotates under the stresses of occlusion. On opposite sides of the fulcrum, pressure and tension are created. These various lesions may coexist in the same region if jiggling pressures are applied.

Slightly too much pressure induces alveolar bone resorption, resulting in a widening of the periodontal ligament space. Blood vessels become more numerous and smaller in places with increased pressure.

Excessive tension promotes elongation of the PDL fibres and alveolar bone opposition. The size of blood vessels expands in locations of high strain.

Greater pressure caused a gradation of alterations in the periodontal ligament, beginning with the compression of the fibres, resulting in areas of hyalization. Following insult to the fibroblasts and other connective tissue cells, portions of the ligament undergo necrosis.

Within 30 minutes, blood vessels appear to be constricted and stagnant with erythrocytes, which begin to fragment at the end of 3 hours.

Disintegration of the blood vessel walls and discharge of the contents into the surrounding tissue occurs between 1 and 7 days.

Resorption of alveolar bone and root surface also occurs.

Severe strain causes periodontal ligament expansion, thrombosis, bleeding, ripping of the periodontal ligament, and alveolar bone resorption.

Necrosis of the periodontal ligament and bone occurs when there is enough pressure to drive the tooth against the bone. Undermining resorption occurs when bone is resorbed from viable periodontal ligament close to necrotic areas and from marrow gaps.

The furcations are the parts of the periodontium that are most vulnerable to harm from high occlusal stresses. When the periodontium is injured, there is a temporary decrease in mitotic activity and fibroblast proliferation, as well as in the creation of collages and bone. After the forces have dissipated, these restore to normal levels.(6).

5.5.1.2 Stage 2

Repair TFO induces greater reparative activity in the typical periodontium, which is always occurring. In order to heal the injured periodontium, the damaged tissues are eliminated and new connective tissue cells and fibres, bone, and cementum are created. The body seeks to reinforce the thinned bony trabeculae with new bone when bone is damaged by high occlusal forces. This attempt to compensate for missing bone is known as buttressing bone growth, and it is a key part of the TFO recovery process. Within the jaw, buttressing bone production occurs when endosteal cells deposit new bone, which repairs the bony trabeculae and minimises the size of the marrow gaps. On the bone, buttressing bone development can also occur [77].

5.5.1.3 Stage3: periodontal adaptive remodelling

If the repair process is unable to keep up with the occlusion's damage, the periodontium is reformed in an attempt to establish a structured relationship in which forces are no longer harmful to the tissues. This causes a thicker periodontal ligament with a funnel-shaped crest, as well as angular flaws in the bone and no pocket formation. The teeth that are implicated grow loose. There has also been evidence of increased vascularization [83].

Apart from occlusal forces, the forces such as orthodontic forces, jiggling forces etc. also play a role in remodelling (**Figures 4–7**).

5.5.2 Pathologic tooth destruction

Each tooth is expected to have a force threshold at which an occlusal traumatic lesion in the attachment apparatus occurs. This threshold force may be extremely strong, but it may be greater than a tooth's resistance to wear. Wear on the occlusal and incisal surfaces. As a result of the trauma, cartilage-like material might form in the periodontal ligament spare. It has also been demonstrated that erythrocytes can form crystals [84].

5.5.3 Soft-tissue effects

Because occlusal forces only affect the attachment apparatus of the periodontium, they have no effect on the supracrestal soft tissues of the periodontium. Excessive

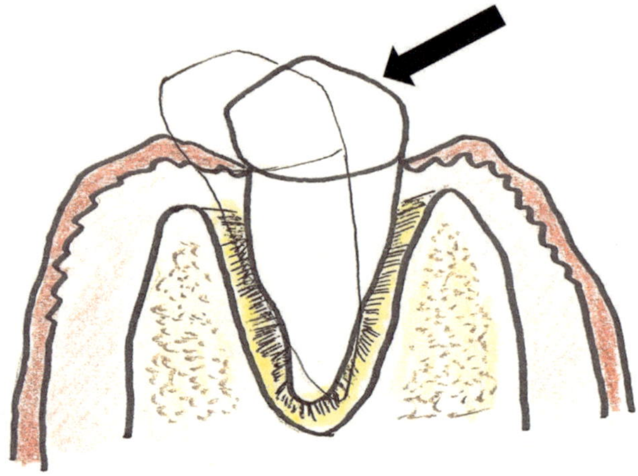

Figure 4.
Physiological response, intra-socket adaptation of the tooth to the normal occlusal forces [28].

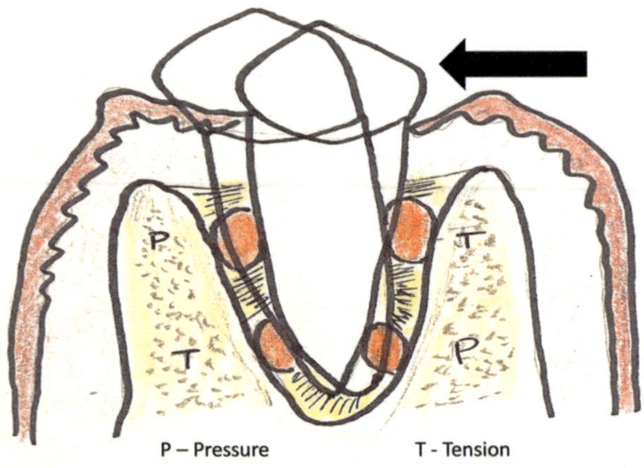

Figure 5.
Response to orthodontic forces—results in areas of pressure and tension [28].

force on a tooth does not harm the attachment of gingival soft tissues coronal to the bone (the C.T. attachment and JE). Pocketing and recession are marginal disease entities (occlusal trauma is not a marginal illness) that are initiated at the gingival margin by plaque-related pathosis [84]. As a result of the trauma, cartilage-like material might form in the periodontal ligament spare. It has also been demonstrated that erythrocytes can form crystals.

5.6 Clinical and radiographic

5.6.1 Signs

Increased tooth mobility is the most prevalent clinical symptom of periodontal damage. Destruction of PDL fibres increases mobility in the early stages.

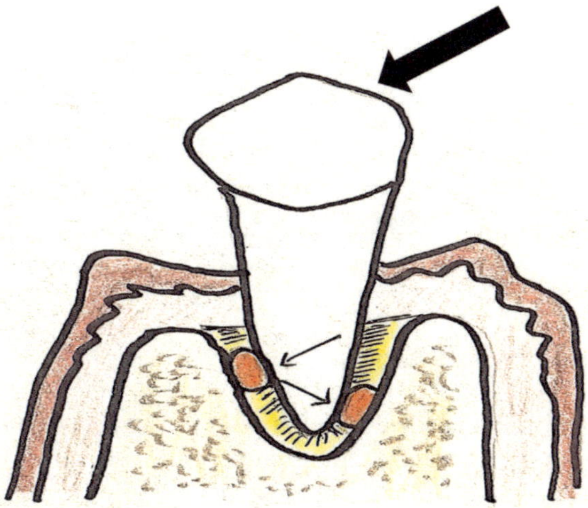

Figure 6.
Response to excessive occlusal forces by a compromised periodontium results in tooth mobility [28].

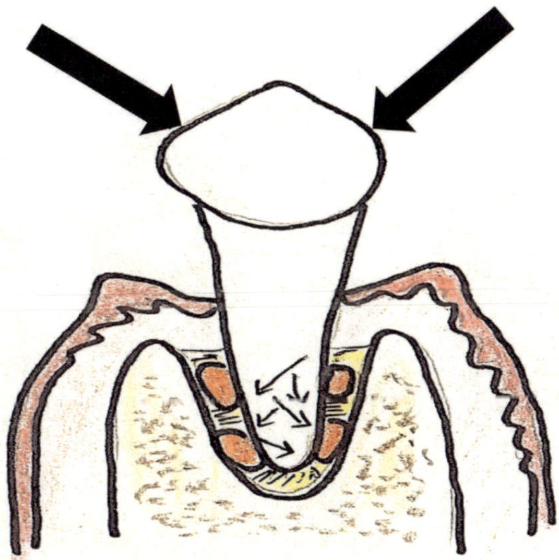

Figure 7.
Periodontal response to jiggling forces results in multiple areas of pressure and tension causing extensive tissue damage [28].

Accommodation of PDL to force widening of PDL to promote mobility is not pathologic in the ultimate stage. It becomes pathogenic when it gets worse over time [85].

5.6.2 Radiographic features

The following radiographic features of TFO may be seen:

1. Wider periodontal space, often accompanied with thickening of the lamina dura along the lateral face of the root, in the apical region, and at bifurcation points.

These changes may be due to thickening and strengthening of the periodontal ligament and alveolar bone as a positive reaction to increasing occlusal stresses, and so are not necessarily detrimental.

2. Interdental septum damage that is "vertical" rather than "horizontal."

3. Alveolar bone radiolucence and condensation.

4. Resorption of the roots.

5.7 Traumatic lesions can be reversed

Occlusion-related trauma is reversible. When the artificially induced force is removed from experimental animals, the tissues begin to heal. TFO, on the other hand, does not always fix itself (by going away or intruding), hence it is not always transitory or of minor clinical relevance. For repair to take place, the injurious force must be alleviated. Periodontal injury persists or worsens in people if the teeth are unable to escape or adapt to severe occlusal force. Inflammation may make this reversibility more difficult [86].

Occlusal trauma cannot be identified without a block section biopsy since TFO is characterised and diagnosed based on histologic abnormalities in the periodontal supporting system. Because this is manifestly unfeasible in periodontics therapy, the doctor must rely on clinical symptoms of possible occlusal trauma. These are some of the indicators:

1. Fremitus

2. Flexibility (progressive)

3. Occlusal inconsistencies

4. Additional signs such as wear facets.

5. Migration of teeth

6. Broken tooth/teeth

7. Sensitivity to heat

The method in which the teeth make contact can also be used to assess the occlusal relationship of the teeth. This is accomplished by gradually retruding the patient's jaw (retruded occlusion/centric relation) and softly closing the patient's mouth, until the first tooth-to-tooth contact is made After that, the patient is asked to close their mouth to a comfortable intercuspated position (central occlusion/habitual occlusion). The centric relation to centric occlusion slide (or CR/CO shift) is the distance the patient moves from the retruded position to the greatest intercuspation. It is possible to capture both the initial contact point and the approximate amount of slide. Tooth interactions are also documented in eccentric jaw positions (i.e. lateral and protrusive jaw positions). Contacts are frequently noticed and may also be documented with a thin inked silk ribbon or Mylar film to record tooth contact during an examination.

5.8 Occlusal therapy

After nonsurgical treatment is completed, occlusal treatment is frequently carried out. When the periodontal supporting structures become inflamed, the teeth's mobility often increases. The periodontal ligament may be inflamed, resulting in more movement. When inflammation is under control, teeth are less dynamic, resulting in a more stable occlusal association after occlusal therapy. To make the patient more comfortable, occlusal treatment may be recommended as the first stage of periodontal therapy in these circumstances [87]. If occlusal therapy is started before inflammation is controlled, it will almost certainly be essential to do additional occlusal treatment once the inflammation has been controlled. Prior to starting treatment, the patient should be advised about this.

There are two primary techniques to occlusal therapy.

(1) Using a bite device (bite guard) and/or (2) Altering the occlusal connections between the teeth to adjust the occlusion.

Orthodontic therapy or selective occlusal surface grinding can permanently alter the relationship between teeth.

Coronoplasty/Selective grinding- Selective grinding is a process that involves modifying the occlusal surfaces of teeth to improve the overall contact pattern. Tooth structure is eliminated selectively until the reshaped teeth make contact in a way that achieves the treatment goals [88].

The following are some of the goals of coronoplasty that have been met as a consequence of occlusal adjustment:

1. Afferent impulse pattern and intensity change.
2. Excessive tooth movement is reduced.
3. To provide occlusal stabilisation, multiple simultaneous contacts are dispersed across the occlusal scheme.
4. A beneficial adjustment in chewing or swallowing habits.
5. Mandibular movement patterns in multiple directions.
6. Occlusal stresses on implants are verticalized.

The occlusion is generally modified once gingival inflammation and periodontal pockets have been removed in treatment planning for the following reasons:

1. Evidence of aetiology and healing features suggests that coronoplasty effects are incomplete unless inflammation is addressed initially.
2. When the inflammation is gone, the teeth frequently shift back to their original place. As a result, if the occlusion is modified before the inflammation has subsided, it may need to be corrected again once gingival health has been restored.

This treatment sequence is altered if the following conditions are met:

a. In infrabony pockets, where excessive occlusal stresses are vital in deciding the pattern of osseous defects, the occlusion is altered to give best conditions for development of bony flaws.

b. Bacterial plaque is often thought to be the cause of periodontal disease. It's possible that a localised mechanism interacts with bacterial plaque when high occlusal stresses are applied. It's also possible that high occlusal forces produce an environment in which bacterial plaque's harmful effects are amplified, or that there's a whole new process at work that has not been discovered yet. Treatment of the occlusion to reduce occlusal interferences, in combination with other modalities of periodontal treatment, may, however, have a positive impact on the progression and treatment of periodontal deterioration. Excessive occlusal forces is a risk factor that can be reduced using current clinical tools, as can any risk factors that can be reduced using current clinical tools.

6. Food impaction

Food impaction is the forceful wedging of food into the tooth supporting tissues by occlusal force. It may occur interdentally or in the buccal and palatal surfaces. It is perceived to be the most common cause of gingival and periodontal inflammation. If left unidentified it could alter the pathogenesis and leads to adverse therapeutic outcomes [89]. Food is typically prevented from being forced into the mouth by the integrity and placement of the proximal contact, the contour of the marginal ridge and developing grooves, and the contour of the lingual and facial surfaces (**Figure 8**).

6.1 Types of food impaction

6.1.1 Vertical impaction

A. Open contacts

B. Irregular marginal ridge

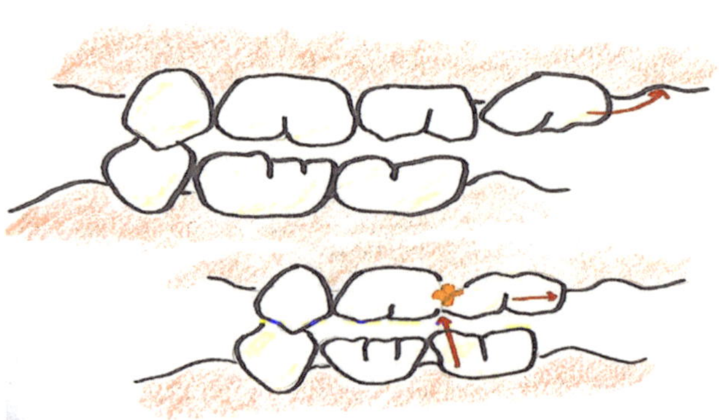

Figure 8.
Food impaction—wedging of food into the deeper tissues by plunger cusp [89].

C. Plunger cusp: Cusp that tend to forcibly wedge food interproximal region of opposing teeth.

6.1.2 Horizontal/lateral food impaction

Periodontal disease/gingival recession results frequently in enlargement of gingival tissues in the interdental embrasure area which is subjected to forces from the lips, cheek and tongue resulting in food lodgment in the proximal areas.

6.2 Management

6.2.1 Periodontal treatment

Curettage, interproximal brushing, flossing, and scaling.

6.2.2 Occlusal adjustment

Plunger cusp—Go around these angular plunger cusp peaks. The palatal cusp of maxillary teeth, the buccal cusp of mandibular teeth, and occasionally the palatal incline of the maxillary buccal cusp and the buccal incline of the lingual cusp are the functional cusps that make up these plunger teeth. Additional advantages could result from reviewing the study cast to assess the relationship between the lingual cusps. Equalise the marginal ridges' occlusal heights.

7. Iatrogenic injury

In 1912, Black recognised the strong connection between iatrogenic causes and periodontal degeneration [90]. It has been well established for many years that dental restorations and periodontal health are related. The position of the restoration in relation to the gingival margin, the presence of overhangs, the presence of marginal leakage, the roughness of the surfaces, and the type of restorative material are a few examples of the various aspects of the periodontal-restorative interaction that have received attention in numerous studies [91]. The most consistent way that dental restorations can harm marginal health is by increasing plaque formation, but overhanging metal restorations have also been linked to changes in the subgingival microbiota, including an increase in potential periodontal pathogenic microflora [92].

The areas of restorative dentistry and periodontics that overlap are the marginal periodontium. In contrast, special attention should be paid to how the periodontium reacts to the irritants caused by negligent procedures, which might start or exacerbate gingival inflammation already present. If the illness is not identified and treated in its early stages, loss of periodontal support and subsequent tooth loss may follow. Particularly when they are subgingivally positioned, dental restorations or appliances are usually linked to the development of gingival inflammation. This may be true for orthodontic bands, crowns placed onlays, fillings, and subgingivally. By being positioned deep inside the sulcus or within the junctional epithelium, restorations may have an impact on the biologic width. With apical migration of the junctional epithelium and re-establishment of the attachment apparatus at a higher apical level, this may encourage inflammation and loss of clinical attachment.

7.1 Margins of restorations

The following characteristics of dental restorations and detachable partial dentures are important for maintaining periodontal health:

1. Where the gingival margin should be placed for the restoration

2. The distance between the restoration's edge and the unprepared tooth

3. The design of restorations

4. The occlusion

5. The restoration's components

6. The practical restoration process

7. The removable partial denture's design

When positioning the restorative margins, especially in the aesthetic zone where the major treatment objective is to cover the junction of the margin with the tooth, the biologic width information should be used. The placement of the restoration margin depends greatly on:

1. Aesthetics.

2. The need for extra restorative retention.

3. The level of oral hygiene.

4. The person's vulnerability to root caries.

5. The marginal gingiva's susceptibility to irritants.

6. The marginal gingival's morphological features.

7. The severity of gingival recession.

8. Significant cervical abrasion.

9. Dental restorations with overhanging margins.

Overhanging dental restoration margins increase the severity of periodontal disease by changing the gingival sulcus' ecological balance to one that favours the growth of disease-associated organisms (mostly gram-negative anaerobic species) at the expense of healthy organisms (primarily gram-positive facultative species) [93] and by preventing the patient's access to remove accumulated plaque.

7.2 Placing the matrix/rubber dam

After cavity preparation, a correctly planned and contoured matrix needs to be implanted so that it may be accurately adjusted to the margins without harming the biologic width. For class II restorations, extra interdental wedge placements are necessary for a well-contoured restoration, but they must be done carefully. To repeat proper form and avoid intracrevicular overhangs, the matrix should be stiff and well-contoured (**Figure 9**).

7.3 Hypersensitivity to dental materials

Nonprecious alloys used in dental restorations have been linked to inflammatory gingival reactions, according to reports [94]. Although the frequency of these events is debatable [95], the reactions have typically been to alloys containing nickel. Rarely do precious alloys cause hypersensitivity reactions, and these alloys offer a simple fix for the issues with nonprecious alloys.

7.4 Marginal fit

Marginal fit has unmistakably been linked to the periodontium's inflammatory response. According to research, the degree of gingival inflammation might rise in direct proportion to the degree of marginal opening [96]. Significantly open marins (more than a few tenths of a millimetre) are capable of hosting huge numbers of bacteria and may be the cause of the observed inflammatory response. However, the periodontium is significantly more affected by the quality of the marginal finish and the location of the margin in relation to the attachment than by the distinction between a 20-m fit and a 100-m fit [97].

7.5 Crown contour

The preservation of periodontal health has been said to depend heavily on restoration contours [98]. Access for hygiene is made possible by proper contour, which also

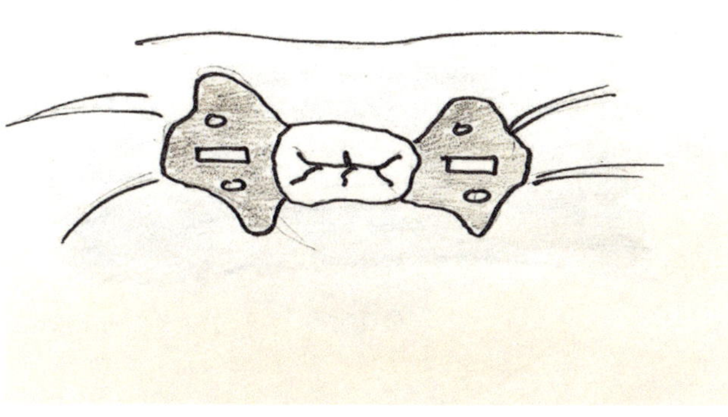

Figure 9.
Improper rubber dam placement can cause injury to the periodontal tissues.

has the capabilities to create the ideal gingival form and has a pleasant visible tooth contour in places that matter aesthetically.

Studies on both humans and animals conclusively show a link between gingival inflammation and over-contouring, whereas under-contouring has no negative effects on periodontal health [99]. Inadequate tooth preparation by the dentist is the most frequent cause of over-contoured restorations, which compels the technician to create a bulky restoration to make place for the restorative material. A flatter contour is always acceptable in parts of the mouth where aesthetic concerns are not important.

8. Discussion

There is a potential risk that the periodontium's soft tissues will sustain accidental, intentional, or fictitious trauma, which can have a negative impact on periodontal health. Also, studies on animals and humans have suggested a connection between periodontal disease progression and occlusal trauma/occlusal differences [100]. However, all researchers came to the consensus that high occlusal forces do not cause plaque-induced periodontal disease or loss of periodontal attachment, and more recent research confirms this [101]. The treatment strategy for traumatic dental injuries differs depending on the amount of damage to the teeth and supporting tissues. It should be remembered that the treatment strategy must be properly developed in this situation. By doing so, additional traumas that might exacerbate the prognosis—which is not always favourable—would be avoided. Because it is impossible to determine the exact extent of damage to the tooth and supporting structures, follow-up after any form of trauma is crucial [102].

9. Conclusion

In order to maintain the general homeostasis of the dentition, the periodontium, which includes the cementum and alveolar bone as well as the soft tissues gingiva and periodontal ligament, must be in good health. The harmony of the periodontal attachment system is affected by injury to the periodontal tissues in any form, including microbiological, physical, thermal, chemical, mechanical, occlusal, and habitual injury, which changes how the dentition functions as a whole. Prior to receiving any other dental treatment, the periodontium must first be restored which comprehends that gingival irritants are eliminated, functional and occlusal interferences are fixed, morphologic and pathologic gingival problems are treated, and bone abnormalities of the supporting periodontium are corrected.

Author details

Santo Grace Umesh*, Lakshmi Ramachandran, Janani Karthikeyan
and Sindhuja M. Shankar
SRM Dental College, Ramapuram, Chennai, Tamil Nadu, India

*Address all correspondence to: grace.santo@gmail.com

IntechOpen

© 2022 The Author(s). Licensee IntechOpen. This chapter is distributed under the terms of the Creative Commons Attribution License (http://creativecommons.org/licenses/by/3.0), which permits unrestricted use, distribution, and reproduction in any medium, provided the original work is properly cited.

References

[1] Gottrup F, Andreasen JO. Wound Healing Subsequent to Injury. Textbook and Color Atlas of Traumatic Injuries to the Teeth. 4th ed. Oxford: Blackwell; 2007. pp. 1-61

[2] Andreasen JO, Andreasen FM, Andersson L, editors. Textbook and Color Atlas of Traumatic Injuries to the Teeth. John Wiley & Sons; 2018

[3] Andreasen JO, Andreasen FM. Classification, etiology and epidemiology. Textbook and Color Atlas of Traumatic Injuries to the Teeth. 1994; **3**:151-179

[4] Glendor U, Marcenes W, Andreasen JO. Classification, epidemiology and etiology. Textbook and Color Atlas of Traumatic Injuries to the Teeth. 2007;**4**: 217-254

[5] Thennukonda RA, Natarajan BR. Adverse events associated with ultrasonic scalers: A manufacturer and user facility device experience database analysis. Indian Journal of Dental Research. 2015;**26**(6):598

[6] Iyama K, Ueki T, Yamano S, Tajima G, Inokuma T, Hirao T, et al. An adult case of laryngopharyngeal burn by drinking hot water. Acute Medicine & Surgery. 2017;**4**(2):198-201

[7] Kwon SJ, Park YJ, Jun SH, Ahn JS, Lee IB, Cho BH, et al. Thermal irritation of teeth during dental treatment procedures. Restorative Dentistry & Endodontics. 2013;**38**(3):105-112

[8] Ustun K, Sari Z, Orucoglu H, Duran I, Hakki SS. Severe gingival recession caused by traumatic occlusion and mucogingival stress: A case report. European Journal of Dentistry. 2008;**2** (02):127-133

[9] Gupta ND, Maheshwari S, Prabhat KC, Goyal L. A critical review of the management of deep overbite complicated by periodontal diseases. European Journal of General Dentistry. 2012;**1**(01):2-5

[10] Meeran NA. Iatrogenic possibilities of orthodontic treatment and modalities of prevention. Journal of Orthodontic Science. 2013;**2**(3):73

[11] Safa'a AA, Fadel EI. Hazards of prosthodontic devices and materials. Tanta Dental Journal. 2017;**14**(1):7

[12] Dilsiz A, Aydin T. Self-inflicted gingival injury due to habitual fingernail scratching: A case report with a 1-year follow up. European Journal of Dentistry. 2009;**3**(02):150-154

[13] Chalkoo AH, Peerzada GY, Makroo NN. Case report of gingivitis artefacta (self-injurious behavior). Journal of Indian Academy of Oral Medicine and Radiology. 2016;**28**(3):317

[14] Mazumdar U, Mazumdar B, Rajkumar IR. Gingivitis artefacta–self injurious behaviour in adult patients of depression report of 2 cases. Journal of Orofacial Research. 2011;**1**(1):45-48

[15] Stewart DJ, Kernohan DC. Self-inflicted gingival injuries. Gingivitis artefacta, factitial gingivitis. The Dental Practitioner and Dental Record. 1972;**22** (11):418-426

[16] Khalia N, Vemanaradhya GG, Mehta DS. Oral piercing: Style statement or a state of disharmony? International Journal of Oral Health Sciences. 2013;**3**(2):84

[17] Hennequin-Hoenderdos NL, Slot DE, Van der Weijden GA. The

prevalence of oral and peri-oral piercings in young adults: A systematic review. International Journal of Dental Hygiene. 2012;**10**(3):223-228

[18] Bone A, Ncube F, Nichols T, Noah ND. Body piercing in England: A survey of piercing at sites other than earlobe. BMJ. 2008;**336**(7658):1426-1428

[19] Hickey BM, Schoch EA, Bigeard L, Musset AM. Complications following oral piercing. A study among 201 young adults in Strasbourg, France. Community Dental Health. 2010;**27**(1): 35-40

[20] Gill JB, Karp JM, Kopycka-Kedzierawski DT. Oral piercing injuries treated in United States emergency departments, 2002–2008. Pediatric Dentistry. 2012;**34**(1):56-60

[21] Mishra P, Gupta M, Shrivastava K, Singh N, Singh P. Oral tattoos:"beauty lies in the eyes of the beholder". Advances in Human Biology. 2015;**5**(2): 17-21

[22] Bathla S. Periodontics Revisited. India: JP Medical Ltd; 2011

[23] Odai ED, Ehizele AO. Trauma to the soft tissues of the periodontium: A review. Nigerian Journal of Dental and Maxillofacial Traumatology. 2019;**2**(1& 2):7-14

[24] Griffin TJ, Cheung WS, Zavras AI, Damoulis PD. Postoperative complications following gingival augmentation procedures. Journal of Periodontology. 2006;**77**(12):2070-2079

[25] Girish MS, Anandakrishna L, Chandra P, Nandlal B, Srilatha KT. Iatrogenic injury of oral mucosa due to chemicals: A case report of formocresol injury and review. IOSR Journal of Dental and Medical Sciences. 2015;**14**:1-5

[26] Gonçalves PS, Mendez DA, Santos PS, Damante JH, Rios D, Cruvinel T. The diagnosis and treatment of multiple factitious oral ulcers in a 6-year-old boy. Case Reports in Dentistry. 2017;**2017**

[27] Mcculloch CA, Lekic P, Mckee MD. Role of physical forces in regulating the form and function of the periodontal ligament. Periodontology 2000. 2000;**24** (1):56-72

[28] Lindhe J, Lang NP, Karring T. Clinical Periodontology and Implant Dentistry. 5th ed. Pan America, Mexico: Wiley-Blackwell; 2012. pp. 3-49

[29] Goswami M, Chaitra TR, Chaudhary S, Manuja N, Sinha A. Strategies for periodontal ligament cell viability: An overview. Journal of Conservative Dentistry: JCD. 2011;**14**(3):215

[30] Pedrini D, Panzarini SR, Poi WR, Sundefeld ML, Tiveron AR. Dentists' level of knowledge of the treatment plans for periodontal ligament injuries after dentoalveolar trauma. Brazilian Oral Research. 2011;**25**:307-313

[31] Trope M. Clinical management of the avulsed tooth. Dental Clinics of North America. 1995;**39**(1):93-112

[32] Kocak FZ, Talari AC, Yar M, Rehman IU. In-situ forming pH and thermosensitive injectable hydrogels to stimulate angiogenesis: Potential candidates for fast bone regeneration applications. International Journal of Molecular Sciences. 2020;**21**(5):1633

[33] Gluskin AH, Ruddle CJ, Zinman EJ. Thermal injury through intraradicular heat transfer using ultrasonic devices: Precautions and practical preventive strategies. The Journal of the American Dental Association. 2005;**136**(9):1286-1293

[34] Maron FS. Mucosal burn resulting from chewable aspirin: Report of case. Journal of the American Dental Association (1939). 1989;**119**(2):279-280

[35] Santos-Pinto L, Campos JA, Giro EM, Cordeiro R. Iatrogenic chemical burns caused by chemical agents used in dental pulp therapy. Burns: Journal of the International Society for Burn Injuries. 2004;**30**(6):614-615

[36] De Bruyne MA, De Moor RJ, Raes FM. Necrosis of the gingiva caused by calcium hydroxide: A case report. International Endodontic Journal. 2000; **33**(1):67-71

[37] Murrin JR, Abrams H, Barkmeier WW. Chemical burn of oral tissue caused by dental cavity varnish. Report of a case. Illinois Dental Journal. 1978;**47** (10):580-581

[38] Dayakar MM, Pai PG, Sooranagi RP, Vijayan V, Waheed A. Chemical burns of gingiva and its management. SRM Journal of Research in Dental Sciences. 2018;**9**(4):174

[39] Harris JH. Soft-tissue burns from a dentin bonding agent. General Dentistry. 1991;**39**(5):350-351

[40] Loe H. Reaction of marginal periodontal tissues to restorativie procedures. International Dental Journal. 1968;**18**:759-778

[41] Ozcelik O, Haytac MC, Akkaya M. Iatrogenic trauma to oral tissues. Journal of Periodontology. Oct 2005;**76**(10): 1793-1797

[42] Pindborg JJ. Atlas of Diseases of the Oral Mucosa. Copenhegan: Munksgaard; 1980

[43] Deshpande A, Verma S, Macwan C. Allergic reaction associated with the use of eugenol containing dental cement in a young child. Austin Journal of Dental. 2014;**1**(2):1-3

[44] Sarrami N, Pemberton MN, Thornhill MH, Theaker ED. Adverse reactions associated with the use of eugenol in dentistry. British Dental Journal. 2002;**193**(5):257-259

[45] Gonzalez-Moles MA, Bagan-Sebastian JV. Alendronate-related oral mucosa ulcerations. Journal of Oral Pathology & Medicine. 2000;**29**(10): 514-518

[46] Krasagakis K, Krüger-Krasagakis S, Ioannidou D, Tosca A. Chronic erosive and ulcerative oral lesions caused by incorrect administration of alendronate. Journal of the American Academy of Dermatology. 2004;**50**(4): 651-652

[47] Dellinger TM, Livingston HM. Aspirin burn of the oral cavity. Annals of Pharmacotherapy. 1998;**32**(10):1107

[48] Ramalingam K, Abdalla KA. Traumatic chemical oral ulceration—Aspirin burn—A case report from Libya. CIBTech Journal of Surgery. 2016;**5**(2): 2319-3875

[49] Neville BW, Damm DD, Allen CM, Bouquot JE. Oral and Maxillofacial Pathology. 2nd ed. Philadelphia, PA: Saunders; 2002. pp. 337-369

[50] Dayakar MM, Pai PG, Madhavan SS. "Tetracycline hydrochloride chemical burn" as self-inflicted mucogingival injury: A rare case report. Journal of Indian Society of Periodontology. 2012; **16**(2):282

[51] Sánchez AR, Rogers RS III, Sheridan PJ. Tetracycline and other tetracycline-derivative staining of the teeth and oral

cavity. International Journal of Dermatology. 2004;**43**(10):709-715

[52] Kapoor A, Malhotra R, Grover V, Grover D. Systemic antibiotic therapy in periodontics. Dental Research Journal. 2012;**9**(5):505

[53] Baruchin AM, Lustig JP, Nahlieli O, Neder A. Burns of the oral mucosa: Report of 6 cases. Journal of Cranio-Maxillofacial Surgery. 1991;**19**(2):94-96

[54] Murdoch-Kinch CA, Mallatt ME, Miles DA. Oral mucosal injury caused by denture cleanser tablets: A case report. Oral Surgery, Oral Medicine, Oral Pathology, Oral Radiology, and Endodontics. 1995;**80**(6):756-758

[55] Bundgaard T. Chemical burns in the oral cavity and esophagus after accidental intake of a Steradent denture-cleansing tablet. Tandlaegebladet. 1985; **89**(19):711-713

[56] Bagga S, Thomas BS, Bhat KM. Garlic burn as self-inflicted mucosal injury—A case report and review of the literature. Quintessence International. 2008;**39**(6)

[57] Isenberg SR, Hier LA, Chauvin PJ. Chemical burns of the oral mucosa: Report of a case. Journal (Canadian Dental Association). 1996;**62**(3):262-264

[58] Putt MS, Proskin HM. Custom tray application of peroxide gel as an adjunct to scaling and root planing in the treatment of periodontitis: Results of a randomized controlled trial after six months. The Journal of Clinical Dentistry. 2013;**24**(3):100-107

[59] Shetty K. Hydrogen peroxide burn of the oral mucosa. The Annals of Pharmacotherapy. 2006;**40**(2)

[60] Moghadam BK, Gier R, Thurlow T. Extensive oral mucosal ulcerations caused by misuse of a commercial mouthwash. Cutis. 1999;**64**(2):131-134

[61] Bernstein ML. Oral mucosal white lesions associated with excessive use of Listerine mouthwash: Report of two cases. Oral Surgery, Oral Medicine, Oral Pathology. 1978;**46**(6):781-785

[62] Flötra L, Gjermo PE, Rölla G, Waerhaug J. Side effects of chlorhexidine mouth washes. European Journal of Oral Sciences. 1971;**79**(2):119-125

[63] Gagari E, Kabani S. Adverse effects of mouthwash use. A review. Oral Surgery, Oral Medicine, Oral Pathology, Oral Radiology, and Endodontics. 1995; **80**(4):432-439

[64] Kowitz GM, Lucatorto FM, Cherrick HM. Effects of mouthwashes on the oral soft tissues. Journal of Oral Medicine. 1976;**31**(2):47-50

[65] Singhal A, Vinaya V, Ahuja T, Longani P. Sodium hypochlorite: Complications and management. Journal of Dental Sciences and Oral Rehabiltation. 2013;**4**(1):7-10

[66] Mathew ST. Risks and management of sodium hypochlorite in endodontics. Journal of Oral Hygiene & Health. 2015;**3** (3):1-5

[67] Parry J, Porter S, Scully C, Flint S, Parry MG. Mucosal lesions due to oral cocaine use. British Dental Journal. 1996; **180**(12):462-464

[68] Gandara-Rey JM, Diniz-Freitas M, Gandara-Vila P, Blanco-Carrion A, Garcia-Garcia A. Lesions of the oral mucosa in cocaine users who apply the drug topically. Medicina Oral: Organo Oficial de la Sociedad Espanola de Medicina Oral y de la Academia Iberoamericana de Patologia y Medicina Bucal. 2002;**7**(2):103-107

[69] Blanksma CJ, Brand HS. Cocaine abuse: Orofacial manifestations and implications for dental treatment. International Dental Journal. 2005;**55**(6): 365-369

[70] Kapila YL, Kashani H. Cocaine-associated rapid gingival recession and dental erosion. A case report. Journal of Periodontology. 1997;**68**(5):485-488

[71] Brazier WJ, Dhariwal DK, Patton DW, Bishop K. Ecstasy related periodontitis and mucosal ulceration–a case report. British Dental Journal. 2003; **194**(4):197-199

[72] Brand HS, Gonggrijp S, Blanksma CJ. Cocaine and oral health. British Dental Journal. 2008;**204**(7):365-369

[73] Gilvetti C, Porter SR, Fedele S. Traumatic chemical oral ulceration: A case report and review of the literature. British Dental Journal. 2010;**208**(7): 297-300

[74] Touyz LZ, Hille JJ. A fruit—Mouthwash chemical burn: Report of a case. Oral Surgery, Oral Medicine, Oral Pathology. 1984;**58**(3):290-292

[75] Kar KM. Beobachtungen uber Pyorrhea alveolaris. Osterreichisch-Ungarische Vierteljahresschrift fur Zahnhelkunde. 1901;**17**:279

[76] Stillman PR. Early clinical evidence of disease in the gingiva and pericementum. Journal of Dental Research. Dec 1921;**3**(3):25-31

[77] Pihlstrom BL, Anderson KA, Aeppli D, Schaffer EM. Association between signs of trauma from occlusion and periodontitis. Journal of Peridontology. 1986;**57**:1-6

[78] Glickman I, Smulow J. The combined effects of inflammation and trauma from occlusion in periodontics. International Dental Journal. 1969;**19**: 393

[79] Glickman I, Sumlow JB. Effect of excessive occlusal forces upon the pathway of gingival inflammation in human. Journal of Periodontology. 1965; **36**:141-147

[80] Stillman PR. What is traumatic occlusion and how can it be diagnosed and corrected. Journal of the American Dental Association (1939). 1925;**12**:1330-1338

[81] American Academy of Periodontology. Glossary of Periodontal Terms. 2001. Available from: https://www.perio.org

[82] Reinhardt RA, Pao YC, Krejci RF. Periodontal ligament stressesin the initiation of occlusal traumatism. Journal of Periodontal Research. 1984;**19**:238-246

[83] Jin LJ, Cao CF. Clinical diagnosis of trauma from occlusion and its relation with severity of periodontitis. Journal of Clinical Periodontology. 1992;**19**:92-97

[84] Piotrowski BT, Gillette WB, Hancock EB. Examining the prevalence and characteristics of abfraction-like cervical lesions in a population of U.S. veterans. Journal of the American Dental Association (1939). 2001;**132**:1694-1701

[85] Lee WC, Eakle WS. Possible role of tensile stress in the etiology of cervical erosive lesions of teeth. Journal of Prosthetic Dentistry. 1984;**52**:374-380

[86] Nakatsu S, Yoshinaga Y, Kuramoto A, et al. Occlusal trauma accelerates attachment loss at the onset of experimental periodontitis in rats. Journal of Periodontal Research. 2014; **49**:314-322

[87] McCauley LK, Nohutcu RM. Mediators of periodontal osseous destruction and remodeling: Principles and implications for diagnosis and therapy. Journal of Periodontology. 2002;**73**:1377-1391

[88] Fleszar TJ, Knowles JW, Morrison EC, Burgett FG, Nissle RR, Ramfjord SP. Tooth mobility and periodontal therapy. Journal of Clinical Periodontology. 1980; **7**:495-505

[89] Khairnar M. Classification of food impaction-revisited and its management. Indian Journal of Dental Advancements. 2013;**5**(1):1113-1119

[90] Black A. Preventive treatment of periodontal diseases. NW Dental Journal. 1912;**10**:60-73

[91] Waerhaug J. Effect of rough surfaces upon gingival tissue. Journal of Dental Research. 1956;**35**:323-325

[92] Lang NP, Kiel RA, Anderhalden K. Clinical and microbiological effects of subgingival restorations with overhanging or clinically perfect margins. Journal of Clinical Periodontology. 1983;**10**:563-578

[93] Icon A. Amalgam restorations and periodontal disease. British Dental Journal. 1976;**140**:377

[94] Pierce LH, Goodkind RJ. A status report of possible risks in base metal alloys and their components. The Journal of Prosthetic Dentistry. 1989;**62**:234

[95] Pelton L. Nickel sensibility in the general population. Contact Dermatitis. 1979;**5**:2-7

[96] Felton DA, Be K, Bayne SC, et al. Effect of *in vivo* crown margin discrepancies on periodontal health. The Journal of Prosthetic Dentistry. 1991;**65**:357

[97] Marcum JS. The effect of crown margin depth upon gingival tissue. The Journal of Prosthetic Dentistry. 1967;**17**: 479

[98] Hochman N, Yaffe A, Ehrlich J. Crown contour variation in gingival health. The Compendium of Continuing Education in Dentistry. 1983;**4**:360

[99] Parkinson CF. Excessive crown contours facilitate endemic plaque niches. The Journal of Prosthetic Dentistry. 1976;**35**:424

[100] Reinhardt RA, Pao YC, Krejci RF. Periodontal ligament stresses in the initiation of occlusal traumatism. Journal of Periodontal Research. 1984;**19**: 238-246

[101] Flores MT, Andersson L, Andreasen JO, Bakland LK, Malmgren B, Barnett F, et al. Guideline for the management of traumatic dental injuries. I. Fractures and luxations of permanent teeth. Dental Traumatology. 2007;**23**(2):66-71

[102] Andreasen JO, Andreasen FM. Textbook and Color Atlas of Traumatic Injuries to the Teeth. Copenhagen: Munksgaard; 1994

Chapter 11

Perspective Chapter: Antioxidants as an Adjuncts to Periodontal Therapy

Sura Dakhil Jassim and Ali Abbas Abdulkareem

Some dreams cannot be actualized but without a doubt part of them can breathe the wonder of life ultimately

Abstract

It has been established that periodontal diseases are related with the hyperactivity of neutrophils. Reactive oxygen species are produced mainly by neutrophils. In order to maintain the balance with reactive oxygen species, the need for antioxidants is increasing. As for supplements to the conventional periodontal therapy, different antioxidants have been applied in an attempt to provide new possibilities in the periodontal treatment. This chapter focused on recent studies that used different antioxidants as adjuncts to conventional periodontal treatments.

Keywords: antioxidant, periodontal diseases, periodontal treatments, reactive oxygen species, neutrophils

1. Introduction

The most important immune response against periodontal pathogens attacks includes an increase in the numbers of neutrophils seen in gingival crevicular fluid (90%), junctional epithelium (50%), and connective tissue.

In order to control bacterial invasion, neutrophils have numerous mechanisms, which include extracellular and intracellular, non-oxidative, and oxidative killing mechanisms [1]. When macrophages and neutrophils are stimulated, they generate a "respiratory burst", which is characterized by a rise in the consumption of oxygen, Hexose-Monophosphate shunt activation, and generation of Reactive Oxygen Species (ROS) and Free Radicals (FR). There is significant overproduction of FR and reactive species at sites of chronic inflammation, including periodontal diseases. **Figure 1** shows the mechanisms of increased ROS production in periodontal disease.

Free radical may be defined as a molecular or atomic group capable of free existence with one or more unpaired electrons in its composition [3]. At low concentrations, these FRs are involved in performing a variety of cell signaling functions but at elevated concentrations, they react with certain cellular components such as proteins, DNA, and lipids, exerting oxidative stress in the periodontal ligament, gingival tissues, and alveolar bone associated with tissue damage.

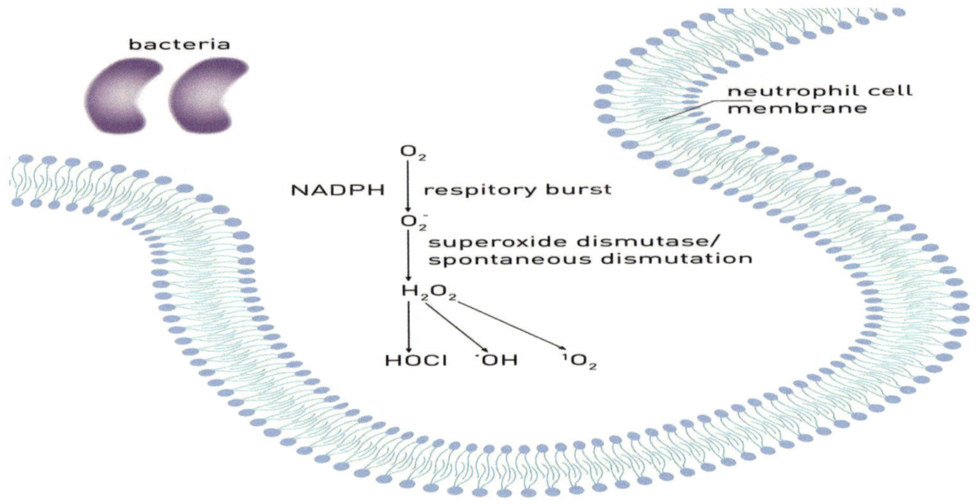

Figure 1.
Reactive oxygen species production in periodontal disease. Nicotinamide adenine dinucleotide phosphate (NADPH)-oxidase, hydroxyl radical (•OH), hypochlorous acid (HOCl) and singlet oxygen (1O2) [2].

Antioxidants define as the agents that scavenge ROS or FR; therefore, they prevent damage associated with them. Based on their mode of function, antioxidants can be categorized into two groups [4]. The first one includes preventive antioxidants which involve enzymatic antioxidants such as catalase (CAT), superoxide dismutase (SOD), DNA repair enzymes, glutathione reductase, and, glutathione peroxidase (GPx) as well as some metal ion sequestrators such as albumin. The second group involves chain-breaking antioxidants or scavenging antioxidants such as carotenoids (including retinol-vitamin A), ascorbic acid (vitamin C), a-tocopherol (vitamin E), polyphenols (flavonoids), reduced glutathione, and uric acid, **Table 1** shows types of antioxidants.

Many studies have tried to detect the uses of antioxidants in the management of periodontitis because antioxidants are associated with a strong defense function against ROS. It has been concluded that enhanced clinical periodontal parameters, lower levels of systemic and local ROS as well as higher activities of systemic and local antioxidants in comparison with usual periodontal treatment resulted from periodontal treatments that are supplemented with antioxidants like lycopene, vitamin C, and vitamin E [5–7].

Muniz et al. performed a review and they examined the effects of the supplemental application of vitamin C, lycopene, vitamin E, capsules with fruits/vegetables/berry and dietary changes on periodontal treatment [8]. It established that only the

Preventive antioxidants	Scavenging antioxidants
Catalase	Carotenoids
Superoxide dismutase	Ascorbic acid
DNA repair enzymes	Tocopherol
Glutathione reductase	Polyphenols
Glutathione peroxidase	Reduced glutathione
Metal ion sequestrators	Uric acid

Table 1.
Types of antioxidants.

use of vitamin E and lycopene is related with improved clinical periodontal parameters [8]. These results are associated with a beneficial effect not only on periodontal status but also on systemic oxidative status.

2. Methodology

For the assessment of the association between antioxidant and periodontal diseases all available studies that we could find were included. PubMed, Scopus, and Google Scholar were searched to select appropriate papers. The following combinations of search terms were used: "periodontal disease" OR "periodontitis" OR "periodontal therapies" OR "antioxidants" OR "periodontitis AND antioxidants" OR "periodontal disease AND antioxidants" OR "periodontal therapies AND antioxidant".

Only studies written in the English language were accepted, while pilot studies and case reports were not accepted for this chapter. All reference lists of the selected studies were screened for additional papers.

3. Lycopene

Lycopene is one of the most efficient antioxidants which provides prevention against various chronic disorders, and it was found in a wide range of foods [9]. It has been classified into the class of components known as carotenoids, which are the red, yellow, and orange pigments produced by plants [10].

Lycopene is considered as the most competent biological antioxidant agent because it has the exceptional characteristic of binding to chemical groups that react with oxygen [11].

Di Mascio et al. showed that lycopene is the most effective biological carotenoid singlet oxygen quencher [12].

It has been concluded by Chandra et al. [13] and Arora et al. [5] that systemic lycopene and oral prophylaxis showed a statistically significant drop in Gingival index, compared to the placebo oral prophylaxis group. Patients were followed up in both studies for 2 weeks in gingivitis patients and 2 months in chronic periodontitis patients respectively.

Kaur et al. evaluated the influences of systemically administered extracts of piperine, curcumin, and lycopene as an adjunct to conventional periodontal treatment in patients with moderate gingivitis. They recognized a reduction in gingival index, plaque index, and bleeding scores with statistically significant differences between the control and the test groups at the 21st day period [14].

4. Vitamin C

For a long period of time, the importance of ascorbic acid (vitamin C) for periodontal health was known. In the eighteenth century, sailors often suffered from scurvy, the disease of vitamin C deficiency, associated with loosening of the teeth and bleeding of the gums. James Lind in 1747 performed his classic experiments aboard the ship "the Salisbury"; he cured scurvy with lemons and oranges in this experiment [15].

Vitamin C is considered as an important dietary nutrient that is essential as a cofactor needed by numerous enzymes. As well as vitamin C is considered as an electron donor and this characteristic accounts for every identified function of vitamin C. In addition, vitamin C is a strong water-soluble antioxidant in humans by its electron donor property. It has been suggested by many lines of studies that vitamin C is a potent antioxidant in vitro [16]. Although records from clinically controlled trials have not confirmed that elevated consumption of ascorbic acid only will assist in the protection against chronic pathological conditions, however, the verification that vitamin C is considered as an essential antioxidant in several body tissues is persuasive [17].

Even though the precise function of ascorbic acid insufficiency in periodontitis is not well recognized, ascorbic acid is considered as a candidate for handling periodontal diseases for a long period of time [18]. It has been identified that supplemental ascorbic acid is necessary for tissue regeneration and infectious diseases, however, low ascorbic acid intake does not cause periodontitis [19].

Collagen fibers, which are present in different forms of the periodontal ligament, connective tissues, and bone, depending on vitamin C for synthesis as well as other intercellular substances depend on it [20]. In addition, vitamin C has immune-regulatory role in affecting the vulnerability of the body to infectious diseases [21].

Sulaiman and Shehadeh [22], found that the supplemental dose of ascorbic acid did not provide additional improvements in comparison to non-surgical periodontal therapy alone. They attributed their finding to the possibility that vitamin C is considered as a poor antioxidant in vivo and its antioxidant activity could have no physiologic function, or its function could be inconsiderable. As well as they supposed that the antioxidant functions of ascorbic acid occur only at particular locations and may be particular to definite reactions [22].

Shimabukuro et al. [23] used dentifrice containing L ascorbic acid 2-phosphate magnesium salt, they found that gingival redness and gingival index significantly decreased in the test group in comparison with the control group [23].

Rajaram et al. evaluate the effects of a diet rich in antioxidants, vitamin C, and fiber on clinical outcomes in patients with gingival inflammation for 1 month. They concluded that gingival inflammation is significantly reduced with a diet rich in antioxidants, vitamin C, and fibers [24]. However, interventional studies, evaluating vitamin C alone, are necessary for proper evaluation of the nutritional impact on periodontal status.

5. Vitamin E

Vitamin E is a well-known antioxidant that prevents the production of ROS formed from fat oxidation [25]. Vitamin E gained its antioxidant effects by its incorporation into cellular membranes, where it inhibits the peroxidation of lipids [26, 27].

Rattanasuan et al. [28] studied the adjunctive use of vitamin E supplementation (vitamin E soft gel 200 mg/day) to the conventional periodontal therapy and they found that antioxidant defense, as well as periodontal healing, were improved [28].

6. Melatonin

It has been reported by several studies that melatonin is considered as an active component with antioxidant properties [29]. It is secreted mainly by Pinealocytes; it is a derivative of tryptophan (indoleamine) [30]. Regulation of the sleep cycle is the main function of melatonin. In addition, studies showed that melatonin is involved in energy metabolism and homeostasis [31].

Melatonin has the ability to activate brown adipose tissue and consequently increase energy expenditure. Furthermore, another research pointed out its immunomodulatory, anti-inflammatory, and antioxidant properties [32]. Melatonin can enhance the expression of antioxidant enzymes (CAT, GPx, and SOD) as well as scavenges free radicals [33].

Javid et al. investigated the anti-inflammatory and antioxidant properties of melatonin in patients with periodontal disease and type 2 diabetes mellitus (T2DM) who experience non-surgical periodontal therapy, they found that the adjunctive effects of melatonin and nonsurgical periodontal therapy may improve antioxidant and inflammatory parameters in T2DM patients with periodontal disease [34].

7. Green tea

Green tea is associated with active ingredients, which include polyphenols. The majority of them are catechins (flavan-3-ols). Furthermore, entire green tea has other antioxidants in the structure of vitamins, such as tocopherols, ascorbate and carotenoids [35].

The mechanism of action of polyphenols as antioxidants is summarized via the stimulation of antioxidant enzymes for example superoxide dismutase and glutathione S-transferase.

In a study performed by Kushiyama and co-workers, they showed that when green tea is taken regularly, it has a protective outcome. Green tea may even decrease the development of existing periodontitis [36].

Generally, green tea catechins have anti-bacterial properties besides their antioxidant properties by their actions on pathological periodontal bacteria such as *Prevotella intermedia* and *Porphyromonas gingivalis.* Inhibition of cysteine proteases of *P. gingivalis* is considered as the mechanism of action [37, 38].

Kudva et al. [39] and Chava and Vedula [40] used green tea as a supplementary to nonsurgical periodontal therapy and they follow the patients for a period of 21 days and 4 weeks respectively, and they found declines in probing pocket depth parameters in test groups with statistically significant differences in comparison to control groups [39, 40].

8. Discussion

This chapter evaluated the efficacy of antioxidants as an adjunct to scaling and root planing. It has been concluded that systemic lycopene and oral prophylaxis showed a statistically significant drops in clinical periodontal parameters [5, 13, 14].

Although vitamin C has a strong effect on gingival parameters and gingival health conditions, some studies showed that there is no benefit from using vitamin C as an adjunct to periodontal therapy this maybe due to the weak antioxidant capacity of vitamin C in vivo [22].

Adjunctive use of both vitamin E and melatonin in the conventional periodontal therapy results in an improvement in antioxidant defense and periodontal healing [28, 34].

Green tea not only decreases the development of existing periodontitis but also when used as supplementary to nonsurgical periodontal therapy, it resulted in a drop in periodontal parameters.

Although antioxidants have a wide range of beneficial effects for overall health, numerous studies have raised doubt about possible side effects. It has been shown that antioxidants may have a harmful effect in the development of lung cancer [41]. The antioxidants reduced the expression of p53, a key tumor suppressor protein. However, further studies are required to improve a procarcinogenic role of antioxidants.

9. Conclusion

Uses of antioxidants as an adjunct to periodontal treatment is not a new concept. Nearly all of the evaluated studies showed that there was an improvement in clinical periodontal parameters when using antioxidants as an adjunct to periodontal treatment.

Author details

Sura Dakhil Jassim[1*] and Ali Abbas Abdulkareem[2]

1 Department of Periodontology, College of Dentistry, University of Babylon, Iraq

2 Department of Periodontology, College of Dentistry, University of Baghdad, Iraq

*Address all correspondence to: suradak85@yahoo.com

IntechOpen

© 2022 The Author(s). Licensee IntechOpen. This chapter is distributed under the terms of the Creative Commons Attribution License (http://creativecommons.org/licenses/by/3.0), which permits unrestricted use, distribution, and reproduction in any medium, provided the original work is properly cited.

References

[1] Dennison DK, Van Dyke TE. The acute inflammatory response and the role of phagocytic cells in periodontal health and disease. Periodontology 2000. 2000;**1997**(14):54-78

[2] Wang et al. Oxidative stress and antioxidant system in periodontitis. Frontiers in Physiology. 2017;**8**:910

[3] Halliwell B. Tell me about free radicals, doctor: A review. Journal of the Royal Society of Medicine. 1989;**82**:747-752

[4] Chapple IL, Matthews JB. The role of reactive oxygen and antioxidant species in periodontal tissue destruction. Periodontology 2000. 2007;**43**:160-232

[5] Arora N, Avula H, Avula JK. The adjunctive use of systemic antioxidant therapy (lycopene) in nonsurgical treatment of chronic periodontitis: A short-term evaluation. Quintessence International. 2013;**44**:395-405

[6] Singh N, Chander Narula S, Kumar Sharma R, Tewari S, Kumar Sehgal P. Vitamin E supplementation, superoxide dismutase status, and outcome of scaling and root planing in patients with chronic periodontitis: A randomized clinical trial. Journal of Periodontology. 2014;**85**:242-249

[7] Sree SL, Sethupathy S. Evaluation of the efficacy of taurine as an antioxidant in the management of patients with chronic periodontitis. Dental Research Journal. 2014;**11**:228-233

[8] Muniz FW, Nogueira SB, Mendes FL, Rosing CK, Moreira MM, de Andrade GM, et al. The impact of antioxidant agents complimentary to periodontal therapy on oxidative stress and periodontal outcomes: A systematic review. Archives of Oral Biology. 2015;**60**:1203-1214

[9] Mathur A, Mathur L, Manohar B, Mathur H, Shankarapillai R, Shetty N, et al. Antioxidant therapy as monotherapy or as an adjunct to treatment of periodontal diseases. Journal of Indian Society of Periodontology. 2013;**17**:21-24

[10] Belludi SA, Verma S, Banthia R, Bhusari P, Parwani S, Kedia S, et al. Effect of lycopene in the treatment of periodontal disease: A clinical study. The Journal of Contemporary Dental Practice. 2013;**14**:1054-1059

[11] Rao AV, Agarwal S. Role of antioxidant lycopene in cancer and heart disease. Journal of the American College of Nutrition. 2000;**19**:563-569

[12] Di Mascio P, Kaiser S, Sies H. Lycopene as the most efficient biological carotenoid singlet oxygen quencher. Archives of Biochemistry and Biophysics. 1989;**274**:532-538

[13] Chandra RV, Prabhuji ML, Roopa DA, Ravirajan S, Kishore HC. Efficacy of lycopene in the treatment of gingivitis: A randomised, placebo-controlled clinical trial. Oral Health & Preventive Dentistry. 2007;**5**:327-336

[14] Kaur S, Sharma R, Sarangal V, Kaur N, Prashar P. Evaluation of anti-inflammatory effects of systemically administered curcumin, lycopene and piperine as an adjunct to scaling and root planing: A clinical study. Ayu. 2017;**38**:117-121

[15] Sutton G. Putrid gums and 'dead men's cloaths': James Lind aboard the

Salisbury. Journal of the Royal Society of Medicine. 2003;**96**:605-608

[16] Padayatty SJ, Katz A, Wang Y, et al. Vitamin C as an antioxidant: Evaluation of its role in disease prevention. Journal of the American College of Nutrition. 2003;**22**:18-35

[17] Jacob RA, Sotoudeh G. Vitamin C function and status in chronic disease. Nutrition in Clinical Care. 2002;**5**: 66-74

[18] Nishida M, Grossi SG, Dunford RG, Ho AW, Trevisan M, Genco RJ. Dietary vitamin C and the risk for periodontal disease. Journal of Periodontology. 2000;**71**:1215-1223

[19] Rubin MB. Vitamins and wound healing. Plastic Surgical Nursing. 1984;**4**:16-19

[20] Geesin JC, Darr D, Kaufman R, Murad S, Pinnell SR. Ascorbic acid specifically increases type I and type III procollagen messenger RNA levels in human skin fibroblast. The Journal of Investigative Dermatology. 1988;**90**:420-424

[21] Field CJ, Johnson IR, Schley PD. Nutrients and their role in host resistance to infection. Journal of Leukocyte Biology. 2002;**71**:16-32

[22] Sulaiman, Shehadeh. Assessment of total antioxidant capacity and the use of vitamin C in the treatment of non-smokers with chronic periodontitis. Journal of Periodontology. 2010;**81**(11):1547-1554

[23] Shimabukuro Y, Nakayama Y, Ogata Y, et al. Effects of an ascorbic acid-derivative dentifrice in patients with gingivitis: A double-masked, randomized, controlled clinical trial. Journal of Periodontology. 2015;**86**:27-35

[24] Rajaram SS, Nisha S, Ali NM, Shashikumar P, Karmakar S, Pandey V. Influence of a low-carbohydrate and rich in Omega-3 fatty acids, ascorbic acid, antioxidants, and fiber diet on clinical outcomes in patients with chronic gingivitis: A randomized controlled trial. Journal of International Society of Preventive and Community Dentistry. 2021;**11**:58-67

[25] Traber MG, Atkinson J. Vitamin E, antioxidant and nothing more. Free Radical Biology & Medicine. 2007;**43**(1):4-15

[26] Packer L, Weber SU, Rimbach G. Molecular aspects of α-tocotrienol antioxidant action and cell signalling. The Journal of Nutrition. 2001;**131**(2):369S-373S

[27] Roy S, Lado BH, Khanna S, Sen CK. Vitamin E sensitive genes in the developing rat fetal brain: A high-density oligonucleotide microarray analysis. FEBS Letters. 2002;**530**(1): 17-23

[28] Rattanasuwan K, Rassameemasmaung S, Sangalungkarn V, Komoltri C. Clinical effect of locally delivered gel containing green tea extract as an adjunct to non-surgical periodontal treatment. Odontology. 2016;**104**(1):89-97

[29] Reiter RJ, Tan DX. Melatonin: An antioxidant in edible plants. Annals of the New York Academy of Sciences. 2002;**957**(1):341-344

[30] Reiter RJ, Tan DX, Galano A. Melatonin: Exceeding expectations. Physiology. 2014;**29**(5):325-333

[31] Hardeland R, Madrid JA, Tan DX, Reiter RJ. Melatonin, the circadian multioscillator system and health: The need for detailed analyses of peripheral

melatonin signaling. Journal of Pineal Research. 2012;**52**(2):139-166

[32] Reiter RJ, Mayo JC, Tan DX, Sainz RM, Alatorre-Jimenez M, Qin LJ. Melatonin as an antioxidant: Under promises but over delivers. Journal of Pineal Research. 2016;**61**(3):253-278

[33] Rodriguez C, Mayo JC, Sainz RM, et al. Regulation of antioxidant enzymes: A significant role for melatonin. Journal of Pineal Research. 2004;**36**(1):1-9

[34] Javid Z et al. Antioxidant and anti-inflammatory properties of melatonin in patients with type 2 diabetes mellitus with periodontal disease under non-surgical periodontal therapy: A double-blind, placebo-controlled trial. Diabetes, Metabolic Syndrome and Obesity: Targets and Therapy. 2020;**13**:753-761

[35] Narotzki B, Reznick AZ, Aizenbud D, Levy Y. Green tea: A promising natural product in oral health. Archives of Oral Biology. 2012;**57**(5):429-435

[36] Kushiyama M, Shimazaki Y, Murakami M, Yamashita Y. Relationship between intake of green tea and periodontal disease. Journal of Periodontology. 2009;**80**(3):372-377

[37] Okamoto M, Sugimoto A, Leung KP, Nakayama K, Kamaguchi A, Maeda N. Inhibitory effect of green tea catechins on cysteine proteinases in *Porphyromonas gingivalis*. Oral Microbiology and Immunology. 2004;**19**(2):118-120

[38] Okamoto M, Leung KP, Ansai T, Sugimoto A, Maeda N. Inhibitory effects of green tea catechins on protein tyrosine phosphatase in Prevotella intermedia. Oral Microbiology and Immunology. 2003;**18**(3):192-195

[39] Kudva P, Tabasum ST, Shekhawat NK. Effect of green tea catechin, a local drug delivery system as an adjunct to scaling and root planing in chronic periodontitis patients: A clinicomicrobiological study. Journal of Indian Society of Periodontology. 2011;**15**(1):39-45

[40] Chava VK, Vedula BD. Thermo-reversible green tea catechin gel for local application in chronic periodontitis: A 4-week clinical trial. Journal of Periodontology. 2013;**84**(9):1290-1296

[41] Sayin VI, Ibrahim MX, Larsson E, Nilsson JA, Lindahl P, Bergo MO. Antioxidants accelerate lung cancer progression in mice. Science Translational Medicine. 2014;**6**:221

Chapter 12

Management of Periodontal Emergency during COVID-19 Pandemic

Desy Fidyawati, Adrianus Wicaksono, Veronica Septnina Primasari and Suci Amalia

Abstract

The novel coronavirus disease (COVID-19) caused by the SARS-CoV-2 virus presents with nonspecific symptoms such as fever, dry cough, shortness of breath, weakness, headache, and diarrhea. The primary mode of transmission of SARS-CoV-2 is through direct or indirect inoculation of the mucous membranes (eyes, nose, or mouth) with infectious respiratory droplets or fomites. Periodontal tissue can serve as a barrier to the SARS-CoV-2 virus in infected individuals. There are similarities between COVID-19 and periodontal disease, based on pro-inflammatory cytokines released by the body. A periodontal emergency arises when an acute condition involving the periodontium causes pain, forcing the patient to seek urgent care; therefore, most periodontal treatment can be considered as dangerous work compared to other dental procedures regarding the aspect of bioaerosol generation procedure. Transmission can occur through direct doctor-patient contact, as well as contamination from instruments or surfaces in the dentist's practice room, and it is recommended to use PPE, to avoid aerosol splashes that occur during the work procedure, where aerosol granules and droplets can last 30 minutes after the treatment procedure is performed. The use of teledentistry is very important in periodontal care, in communication with patients regarding chief compliant, risk factor control, and oral hygiene instruction.

Keywords: COVID-19, periodontal disease, dental management, periodontal emergency, periodontal treatment

1. Introduction

Coronavirus disease 2019 (COVID-19) was first reported in Hubei Province of China at the end of December 2019. Later, in March 2020, after observing the nature of the virus and its course, the World Health Organization (WHO) announced it as a pandemic [1]. SARS-CoV-2 is mainly transmitted *via* direct contact with respiratory droplets, through cough, sneeze, and droplet inhalation, or *via* indirect contact of oral, nasal, and mucous membranes with contaminated fomites or saliva, which may be of particular interest for dental settings, that invariably carries the risk of

SARS-CoV-2 transmission, especially considering the interpersonal proximity, the exposure to blood and saliva, the handling of sharp instruments, and the variety of aerosol-generating dental procedures [2, 3]. Therefore, dental patients are very vulnerable and at risk of transmission of the SARS-CoV-2 virus infection, where this virus can be transmitted through direct contact through the mouth and nose in the form of droplets and aerosols containing the virus, originating from infected individuals or through indirect contact with contaminated dental instruments or contaminated teeth [4]. Not only patients but also clinicians who treat patients are also at risk of transmission caused by direct contact with patients who are not wearing masks, as well as aerosols and droplets produced from the mouth of the patient [5]. So, caution is needed for clinicians and patients in carrying out dental actions and treatments.

2. COVID-19 and periodontal disease

Severe acute respiratory syndrome coronavirus 2 (SARS-CoV-2) is a new type of novel coronavirus that causes COVID-19 [6]. The target of SARS-CoV-2 infection is cells in the respiratory tract, where Protein S in SARS-CoV-2 will bind to (angiotensin-converting enzyme 2 (ACE2) as the receptor [7]. ACE2 is found in pulmonary epithelial cells, myocardial cells, gastrointestinal system, proximal cells of renal tubules, arterial smooth muscle cells, and oral epithelial cells, where the expression of ACE2 will increase in patients with certain conditions, such as, in elderly individuals, obesity, kidney disease, and lung disease that results in individuals with the condition being more susceptible to the transmission of COVID-19 [8–10]. The SARS-CoV-2 virus will replicate, and the virus that has entered the body will be presented by *antigens-presenting cells* (APCs) and will induce T cells and B cells as humoral and cellular immune responses [11].

Periodontal disease is an inflammatory disease of dental support tissue that is commonly found in individuals over the age of 30 years and is often found in the elderly population. Severe periodontitis, now known as stage III and IV periodontitis, is the 6th rank disease commonly suffered by adults, affecting 11% of the adult population globally Several studies have shown a link between COVID-19 and periodontal disease, and this is due to the similarity of pro-inflammatory cytokines released by the body. Periodontal disease is a multifactorial disease caused by the involvement of microorganisms and a host response characterized by the production of pro-inflammatory cytokines [12, 13]. Pathogenesis of periodontal begins from the expansion of the subgingival plaque into the gingival sulcus, where microorganisms residing in the subgingival plaque can cause changes in the coronal attachment of the epithelium on the surface of the tooth, and this is due to the presence of an immune response to pathogenic bacteria and endotoxins through the activity of neutrophils, macrophages, and lymphocytes. Host factors also influence the development of periodontal disease, where an inadequate host response in destroying bacteria can damage periodontal tissue [14]. Pathophysiology periodontitis stimulates the occurrence of cytokine responses. Research conducted by Wu et al. (2020) on COVID-19 shows that there is an unfavorable relationship that can cause cytokine storms, where certain elements have similarities with cytokine profiles commonly encountered in periodontitis. Individuals infected with the COVID-19 virus that was accompanied by aggravation so that they had to be treated in the ICU showed an increase in IL-2, IL-7, IL-10, macrophage, monocytes, and TNF alpha. Th17 cells were also found in individuals suffering from SARS-Co V and MERS-CoV [15]. Th17 cells are found in cytokine storms, {Formatting Citation} pulmonary edema, and damaging tissues that may result in lung infections caused by the SARS-CoV-2 virus [16]. An increase in IL-17 was also found in individuals experiencing inflammatory gingivitis and periodontitis [17]. Gupta et al. (2021) found the accumulation of the corona virus in gingival crevicular fluid (GCF) in asymptomatic or mildly symptomatic COVID-19 patients, where the condition is in line with the hypothesis in a study conducted by Badran et al. (2020) where periodontal can serve as a reservoir for the SAR-CoV-2 virus in infected individuals [18, 19].

3. Dental management during COVID-19

Dental care during the pandemic should not be delayed, especially in emergency cases, dental care during the pandemic should be linked to patient risk assessment, patient triage, and infection prevention measures for clinicians or health professionals and nosocomial transmission in dental clinics (**Figure 1**) [20].

Treatment in the field of dentistry can generally be categorized as an emergency, urgent, nonurgent, and advise/self-care (**Figure 2**). In principle, emergency care in the field of dentistry is associated with acute pain that is urgent for treatment, as well as life-threatening possibilities, including uncontrolled bleeding, significant infections, bending, and orofacial trauma that has the potential to block the airway. Meanwhile, urgent (essential) treatment is the treatment of severe or uncontrolled symptoms that require patients to see a dentist. Nonurgent care or categorized as daily care is a routine treatment carried out by individuals, while advise/self-care treatment is dental care that can be done through telemedicine, related to it the instruction and prescribing of either analgesic or antimicrobial (**Figure 3**) [21].

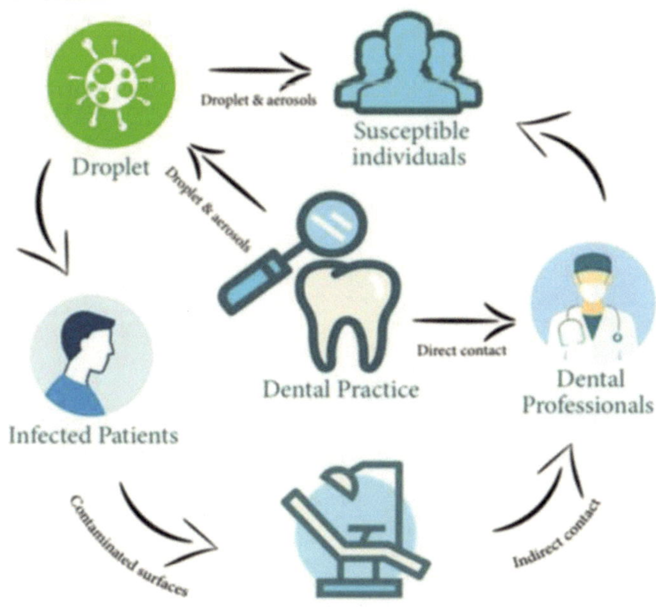

Figure 1.
Illustration of COVID-19 transmission in dental clinic.

Orofacial problem	Recommended management: Advice and self help	Urgent care	Emergency care
Acute apical abscess Acute periodontal abscess Perio-endo lesions	-Recommend analgesics(*) -Prescribe antibiotics(**) if there is concern about swelling or if there is sign and symptoms of systemic infection -Advice patient to call again after 2 days if the symptoms not resolve	In case of spreading infection without airway obstruction refer to designated dental clinic in the local area for extraction or drainage	If spreading infection with airway obstruction refer to medical emergency
Acute pericoronitis	-Recommend analgesics(*) -Recommend chlorhexidine(***)/ saltwater mouthwash -Prescribe antibiotics(**) if there is concern about swelling or if there is sign and symptoms of systemic infection -Advice patient to call again after 2 days if the symptoms not resolved	In case of spreading infection without airway obstruction refer to designated dental clinic in the local area for possible extraction	If spreading infection with airway obstruction refer to medical emergency
Irreversible pulpitis	-Recommend analgesics(*) -Advice for cold water rinse -Advice patient to call again if the symptoms get worse	If pain is severe and uncontrollable, preventing sleep refer for designated dental clinic for possible initial endodontic therapy or extraction	
Reversible pulpitis Dentine hypersensitivity	-Recommend analgesics(*) if needed -Avoid stimuli (cold, hot and acidic drinks or food) -Apply desensitizing toothpaste regularly to the sensitive area with finger. -Advice the patient to call back if symptoms get worse	-Recommend analgesics -Advice for cold water rinse -Advice patient to call again if the symptoms get worse	
Suture removal	-Advice to keep good oral hygiene -Mouth wash with salt water -Dissolvable sutures can stay longer than 2 weeks	If unabsorbable suture was used refer to the designated dental center for suture removal	

Orofacial problem	Recommended management: Advice and self help	Urgent care	Emergency care
Dry socket	-Recommend analgesics(*) -Advice for warm saltwater mouthwash -In case of signs of spread of infection or immunocompromised patient prescribe antibiotics(**)	If pain is severe and uncontrollable, preventing sleep refer for designated dental clinic for dressing	
Oral ulcer	If less than 3 weeks: -Advice for chlorhexidine mouthwash(***) (> 7 years old) -Recommend analgesics(*) (topical-systemic) -If due to denture, advice to keep the denture out where possible -In case of herpetic gingivostomatitis or herpes zoster, if the symptoms are severe or immunocompromised, prescribe anti-viral agents(****)	If more than 3 weeks: refer to local dental care	If the patient is severely dehydrated, refer to emergency medical care
Post extraction hemorrhage Uncontrolled bleeding in the orofacial region	-Advice the patient not to spit -Advice to place a rolled piece of gauze or cotton over the socket or injured area and press firmly for 20 minutes -Avoid drinking hot drinks or smoking for 24 hrs.	If the bleeding fails to stop but is not brisk and persistent refer to designated urgent dental care Centre for management	If the bleeding fails to stop and is brisk and persistent, or the patient is taking anticoagulant medication refer to medical emergency care
Fracture/loose tooth fragments or restorations (Tooth-Crown-Bridge)	For sensitive tooth -Recommend analgesics(*) -Advice to call again if the symptoms are worsened	Refer to the designated dental clinic if the symptoms are worse or temporary restoration is lost or broken or causing gingival inflammation for temporary restoration or cementation	For inhaled tooth, crown or bridge refer immediately to the medical emergency care
Dento-alveolar trauma Including : (Avulsed, displaced or fractured tooth)	-If patient didn't need emergency care advice to: -Clean the affected area gently with mild antiseptic and remove any foreign object if it is present -Apply ice pack to the soft tissue and swelling -Recommend analgesics(*) if needed - If tooth is knocked out <u>Therapeutic protocol of Avulsed tooth in primary and permanent teeth could be followed</u>	Refer to the designated dental care in case of: -Large wound laceration - Permanent tooth fracture involving the pulp, moved out of its place or knocked out	If bleeding is severe and will not stop in 15-30 min, and/or significant facial trauma and/or loss of consciousness and/or tooth inhaled refer immediately to the medical emergency care

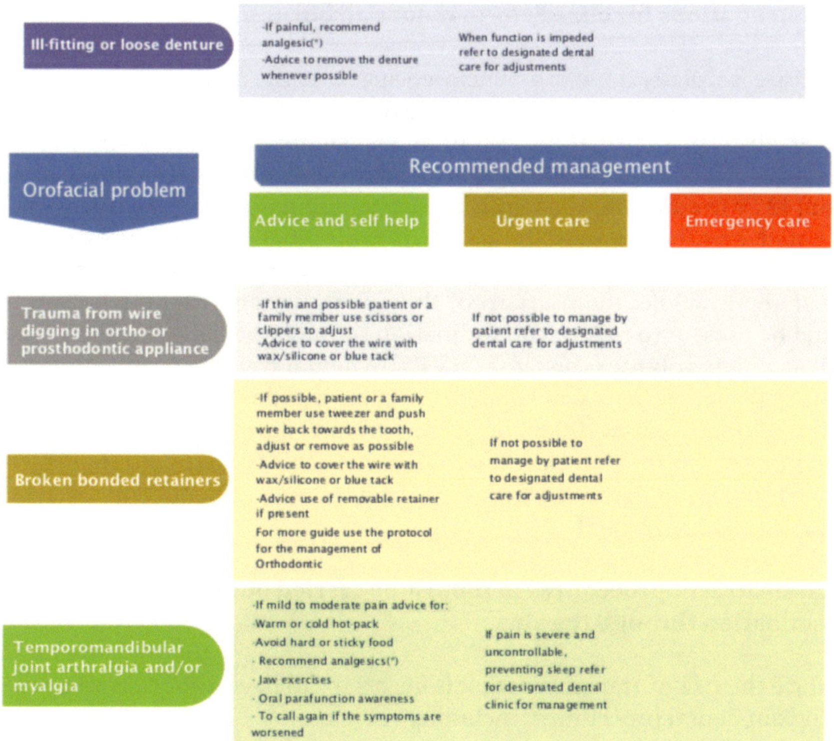

Figure 2.
Dental care management that occurs during COVID-19.

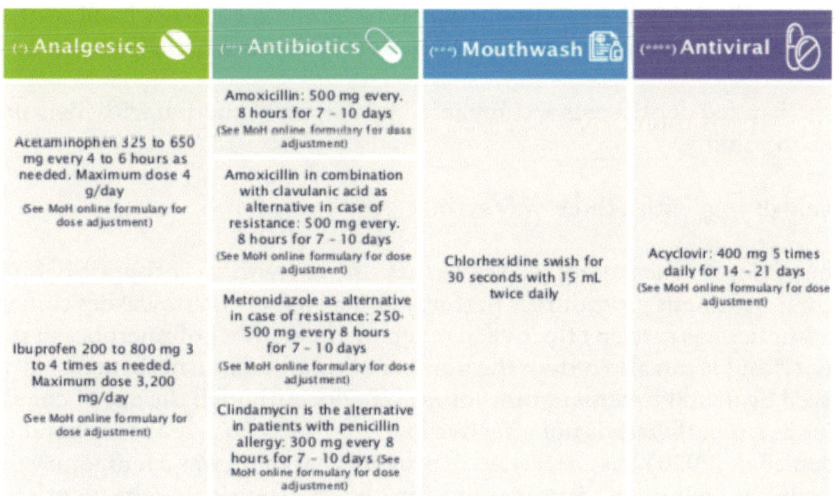

Figure 3.
Medical dosage recommendations.

Note: Patients with substantial swellings can progress to life-threatening emergencies, which can increase risks in the setting of reduced health care availability. For that patient, extraction of the causative pathogenic teeth should be prioritized over the restorative rescue. Close follow-up by telephone is recommended [21].

3.1 Recommendations for clinicians to reduce airborne viral contamination

Dental care is usually done in an enclosed space, so the dentist needs to equip himself with some protection, such as masks, gloves, goggles, head coverings, and gowns that reduce saliva splashes that may occur during dental procedures. Aerosol granules or droplets can stay in the air for 30 minutes after the dental treatment procedure is carried out [22]. In addition, the regulation of air circulation in the clinic room is also must be noted, and the common thing to do is to eliminate airborne transmission in the clinic room is to equip the room with the use of a good quality air filter and the presence of an ultraviolet room as part of the air ventilation system [23]. Another tool that should be present to reduce contamination through the air is extraoral suction or known as a high-volume evacuator (HVE), in dental treatment procedures, and a good extra oral suction has a wide opening or mouth and is connected to a drain that reduces the volume of air to 100 cubics of per minute. Several previous studies have suggested that the use of HVE can reduce airborne virus contamination by up to 90%, if the clinic room is not equipped with HVE, and it is recommended to use air vents to facilitate air exchange [24, 25].

3.2 Dental treatment procedures that must be carried out to eliminate viral contamination through the air

To reduce the risk of transmission, it is necessary to have a good strategy in terms of carrying out dental procedures, including [26].

1. The use of rubber dam

The use of a rubber dam is needed for dental treatment procedures that require isolation of the work area, and if it is not possible to isolate the work area such as curettage or other periodontal measures, it is recommended to use hand instruments instead of ultrasonic tools, to reduce the chances of aerosols being generated.

1. Four-handed dentistry is accompanied by the use of suction with high-pressure sucking ability.

2. Avoid drying with a three-way syringe

3. The advice for the patient is to rinse their mouth with an antiseptic before the dental treatment procedure is performed. The use of mouthwashes containing antiseptics has proven effective in reducing the number of microbes in the oral cavity, and it can also reduce the number of microorganisms in aerosols produced by dental treatment procedures [27–29]. Although the use of chlorhexidine as a mouthwash is not effective in killing SAR-CoV-2, a study conducted by Yoon et al. (2020) has succeeded in proving that there was a temporary reduction in the amount of virus in saliva for 2 hours after rinsing the mouth with chlorhexidine [30–32]. According to Mady et al. (2020), the use of povidone iodine as a mouthwash before dental treatment can reduce the SARS-CoV-2 virus and also MERS-CoV in 15 seconds with a dilution ratio of 1:30 [33]. While, the use of hydrogen peroxide as a mouthwash is recommended for reducing the SARS-CoV-2 virus still needs further study [34].

Protection type	Hand hygiene	Waterproof apron	Cap	Surgical mask	N95/ PFF2 masks	Glasses or face protector	Gloves	Appropriate shoes
Dental staff								
Administrative/receptionist				✔		✔		
Screening patients	✔	✔	✔		✔	✔	✔	
Anamnesis	✔	✔	✔		✔	✔	✔	
Radiology services	✔	✔	✔		✔	✔	✔	
Dental assistance without generating aerosol	✔	✔	✔		✔	✔	✔	
Dental assistance with aerosol generation	✔	✔	✔		✔	✔	✔	
Asymptomatic individuals	✔	✔	✔		✔	✔	✔	
Outpatient care	✔	✔	✔		✔	✔	✔	✔
Ward	✔	✔	✔		✔	✔	✔	✔
Individuals with COVID-19	✔	✔	✔		✔	✔	✔	
Intensive care unit	✔	✔	✔		✔	✔	✔	✔

Figure 4.
Recommended PPE during COVID-19.

3.3 PPE (personal protective equipment)

For professional dentists, the risk of transmission can be prevented by the use of PPE. The recommended use of PPE (**Figure 4**) includes head coverings, gowns, gloves, face shields, masks, footwear covers, or other equipment that aims to protect against injury or contamination bacteria derived from aerosols or droplets produced during dental treatment procedures [26]. The recommended use of masks is N95/PFF2 because it provides good protection and is recommended internationally; in addition, if needed due to inadequate amount of availability, N95/PFF2 masks can be disinfected first before reuse [26, 35, 36].

4. Periodontal management during COVID-19

4.1 Prevention of droplet transmission before treatment measures

Dentists who perform periodontal treatment are at risk of being contaminated with the COVID-19 virus through droplets or aerosols generated during the periodontal treatment procedure, through the use of ultrasonic scalers, rotary instruments, and water syringes and air polishers that potentially increase the risk of transmission through cross-transmission between dentists and patients [37–39]. All dental health care facilities are required to implement triage protocols including detailed medical record data, which contains specific questions that can identify individuals suspected of COVID-19. All patients seeking treatment should be considered potentially infectious. All patient screening actions must be carried out in strict health protocols, and operators should be equipped with PPE during the patient screening process [37, 40]. When the screening process is carried out, the dental professional should ask questions related to patient complaints that lead to emergency care and conduct an assessment to determine whether or not emergency care is necessary [39, 41, 42]. To reduce the occurrence of transmission through direct contact, screening can be done via telemedicine or tele-triage, which can be done via the internet or telephone, and if the patient states to have had contact with an infected individual with COVID-19 recently or is known to have the symptoms of COVID-19, the patient can be prescribed if needed [39, 43].

4.2 Prevention of droplet transmission during treatment measures

Some preventive measures that can be carried out before periodontal treatment include cleaning the surface of the dental unit with material containing 0.5% sodium hypochlorite for 1 minute and sterilizing non-disposable tools [44]. Using an extraoral suction, air purifier and exhaust fan are still being evaluated for effectiveness for dental clinics, if there are patients who are suspected of having COVID-19, and it is recommended that their dental treatment should be carried out in a negative pressure room to reduce the spread of the virus through droplets and aerosols [45]. However, the use of negative pressure rooms has issues because it requires quite expensive costs [38, 45]. After the initial examination, the periodontist is advised to take periodontal treatment measures that are not emergency in nature unless there is pain that is a complaint. The effectiveness of the use of ultrasonic scalers is basically the same as that of manual scalers except that on ultrasonic scalers, and it is more risky in aerosol dispersing, which allows to stick to the corners of the eyes and nose operator [46]. However, if the patient complains of pain leading to emergency measures, it is advisable to perform a scaling procedure manual rather than scaling by using an ultrasonic scaler. The use of mouthwashes containing povidoneiodine 0.2% or 0.5–1% of hydrogen peroxide is recommended before the periodontal treatment procedure to reduce the accumulation of virus in the saliva and also as an infection control for operators [37]. Patients should not do self-medication independently, and if necessary, it is recommended to consult through telemedicine in advance for planning pain-related treatments complained by patients [40]. Dental care and periodontal is a treatment that requires close physical contact, so it would be better if the treatment was made as short as possible, or the treatment procedure was carried out in the area that became complaints only, and the patient's recall time for maintenance is made a bit long, at least 2 weeks to see the possibility of COVID-19 symptoms in patients [5, 47]. Periodontal disease is a disease with biofilm plaque as the primary etiology, so plaque control is very important, and the use of mouthwashes as an ingredient in dentrifices gives good results especially when combined with scaling treatment. The administration of antibiotics in the treatment of periodontitis is not recommended, since it allows the occurrence of resistance, except in certain cases such as aggressive periodontitis and recurrent periodontitis, which requires evaluation of certain specific bacteria [48]. For periodontal surgical therapy, in the current pandemic situation, it is rather difficult to do, given the necessity of a strict control schedule, so for cases of intra bony defects that require regenerative therapy, and it is advisable to do conservative therapy, such as the use of enamel matrix derivative, for control that can be done via telemedicine/teledentistry as already described above to get good results after regenerative or conservative therapy. It is necessary to motivate the maintenance of good oral hygiene so that good results are obtained well. On the contrary, mucogingival surgery is advised not to be performed or done limitedly during the COVID-19 pandemic [5, 48]. Complex periodontal cases that require cooperation between disciplines as one of the ways to control the inflammation of periodontitis and also rehabilitate the mastication function [49] must be carefully analyzed to obtain the right diagnosis and treatment plan which is accurate, avoid excessive maintenance, and minimize surgical procedures [50]. Teledentistry plays a very important role in periodontal care (**Figure 5**) among others to regulate patient schedule based on complaint priority, pre-check triage monitoring, diagnosis determination based on staging, grading, and also communication with patients regarding risk factor control and oral hygiene instruction [5].

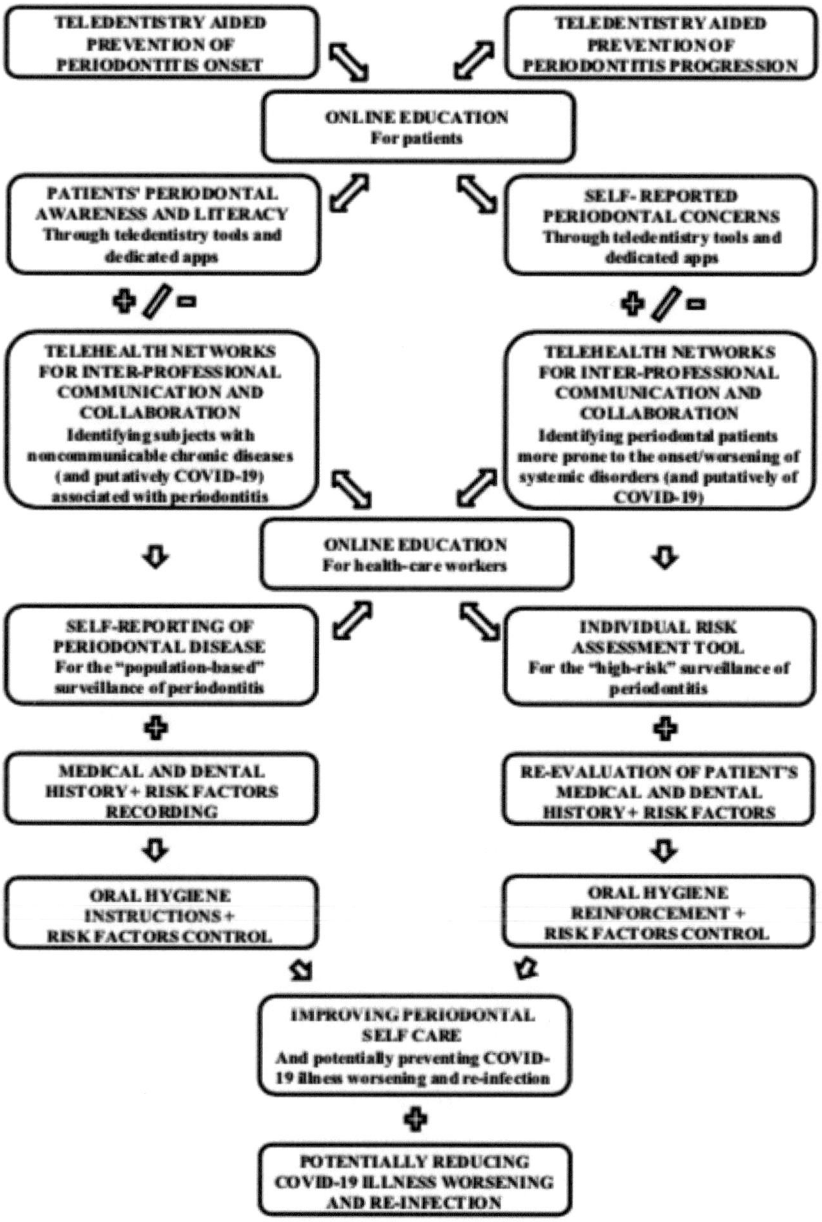

Figure 5.
Periodontal care flowchart during COVID-19 pandemic.

5. Periodontal emergency management during COVID-19

Cases of periodontal emergence arise when an acute condition that causes pain in the periodontal tissue forces the patient to seek treatment on the spot. Time management is key to avoiding more severe periodontal tissue damage as well as its effect psychically and functionally on patients [51]. Cases related to periodontal emergencies are basically limited, including acute abscesses involving periodontal tissue or

Emergency	Urgent	Elective
Gingivitis with conditions of stage III gingival index according to Loe and Sillness (1963)	Gingivitis with conditions of stage III gingival index according to Loe and Sillness (1963)	Gingivitis with conditions of stage III gingival index according to Loe and Sillness (1963)
Periodontitis—All stages according to Tonetti's classification	Mucogingival tissues-related complaints other than esthetic issues	Routine follow-up visits
Replacement of missing teeth (immediate implant)	Peri-implant mucositis	Depigmentation
Peri-implantitis and related mucogingival conditions	Trauma caused due to occlusal discrepancies	Frenectomy
Necrotizing periodontitis and stomatitis	Necrotizing gingivitis	Vestibular deepening
Abscesses	Prosthesis-related issues	Hopeless teeth extraction
Endo-perio lesions	Replacement of missing teeth (delayed implant)	Esthetic-related issues
Pericoronitis		

Table 1.
Periodontal condition based on treatment needs.

endo-perio lesions, necrotizing ulcerative gingivitis and periodontitis caused by stress during the pandemic, dentin hypersensitivity, and lesions oral effects on the quality of life such as ulcers, viral and fungal infections, and cases requiring biopsy [52]. During the pandemic, pharmacological treatment is the best and safest option [37]. According to group disease conditions through the periodontal disease classification approach and the latest conditions 2017, it is actually very unfortunate that there is no grouping of cases periodontal as an emergency, urgent, or elective (**Table 1**) because the disease can initially be recognized as urgent which can then become an emergence if ignored, which then can trigger irreversible damage, and it should all be done in parallel with the periodontal treatment procedure, minimizing the production of aerosols produced during the treatment periodontal [47, 49].

5.1 Necrotizing periodontitis

Clinical and etiology: Necrotizing periodontitis is also known as an inflammatory disease of severe dental support tissue (**Figure 6**), associated with the presence of biofilm plaques, which are grouped into acute necrotizing ulcerative gingivitis (ANUG) and necrotizing ulcerative periodontitis (NUP) [51]. ANUG, the necrotic

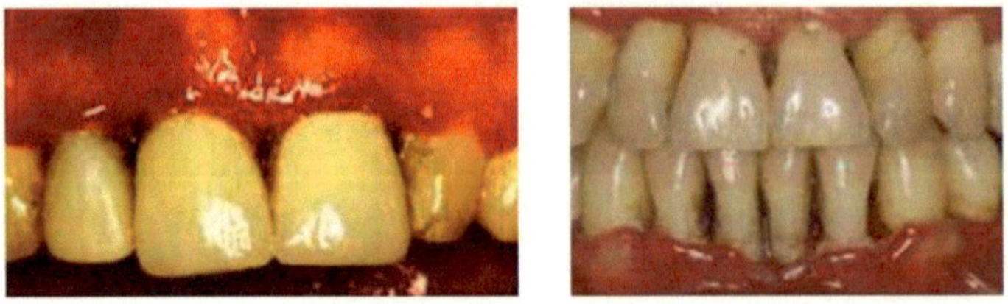

Figure 6.
(left) NUG and (right) NUP.

state of tissue, only involves the gingival with a clinical picture of the presence of ulcers and necrotic tissue in the attached gingival, while in NUP there has been damage to periodontal tissue and alveolar bone which results in loss of attachment. Periodontal necrotizing is characterized by the presence of pseudo-membranes. The pain felt by the patient is generally based on the expansion and severity of the lesion area, sometimes accompanied by halitosis. In NUP, there is an interdental crater. This inflammation generally hits the anterior region of the lower jaw. ANUG or NUP is often associated with HIV/AIDS disease or immunosuppressant disease. The etiology of the disease is associated with infection of organisms and is often associated with Spirochaeta and fusiform bacteria, with compromised immunology predisposing factors [53].

Emergency treatment: For the elimination of plaque deposits and calculus through superficial debridement, it is recommended to use an ultrasonic scaler instead of a hand instrument to minimize pressure on the ulcerated soft rareness, during the pandemic currently, and the use of ultrasonic scalers should be done briefly and quickly, combined with hand instruments. Debridements should be performed daily in the acute phase for 2–4 days. Patients are advised to brush their teeth on a limited basis to avoid pain and disruption of the healing process. Patients are also recommended to rinse their mouth with chlorhexidine 0.2% as much as 2x a day or with 3% hydrogen peroxide diluted with warm water 1: 1 and also with other mouthwashes that function as oxygen-releasing agents, which have an antibacterial effect through the release of oxygen [54]. If it does not also improve, then the patient can be given a systemic antibiotic with metronidazole content (400 mg 3x1 a day) as a drug of choice for cases of periodontitis necrotizing [55].

5.2 Abscesses

5.2.1 Gingival abscesses

Clinically and etiology: Gingival abscesses are generally purulent and localized on the marginal or interdental gingival. A common cause of a gingival abscess is the "trapping" of a foreign body inside a healthy gingival in the sub-gingival region. Foreign objects include fish bones or nail pieces from individuals with a bad habit of biting nails (**Figure** 7) [51, 56].

Emergency treatment: Preparation of incision and irrigation with saline solution to reduce symptoms. Short-term treatment is recommended through the use of chlorhexidine mouthwash (0.2%) or warm saline solution, especially for areas where brushing is not possible [51].

KEY FEATURES OF THE GINGIVAL, PERIODONTAL, PERI-CORONAL AND PERI-ENDO ABSCESS

	Gingival abscess	Periodontal abscess	Peri-coronal abscess	Perio-endo abscess
Symptoms	Painful, especially to touch	Painful, tooth may feel more mobile and 'high' in occlusion	Painful to touch, extraoral swelling, difficulty opening fully, radiating pain to the ear	Painful, tooth tender to bite on and may feel more mobile
Site	Marginal gingiva/ interdental papilla	Attached gingiva/mucosa	Partially erupted/ impacted tooth	Attached gingiva/mucosa usually close to the root apex
Peridontal	Periodontally healthy	Deep pocket depths	False pocketing possible around partially erupted tooth but adjacent teeth with no increased probing pocket depths	Deep pocket depths
Sensibility testing	Positive	Positive	Positive	Negative

Figure 7.
Periodontal abscess features.

5.2.2 Periodontal abscess

Clinically and etiology: Periodontal abscesses are defined as the accumulation in the periodontal pocket produced by the destruction of collagen fibers accompanied by bone damage [51, 57]. The most prominent clinical sign is the presence of enlargement in the gingival along the length of the lateral root of the tooth, which is characterized by redness, diffuse, and soft consistency. There is a deep periodontal pocket accompanied by bleeding during probing (**Figure 7**) [51]. The presence of suppurations that come out through fistulas or walls of periodontal pockets spontaneously or through suppression is also accompanied by the presence of tooth shakes and pain during percussion. Generally, patients complain that their teeth feel rather high. Periodontal abscesses generally come from further periodontitis, derived from pockets, bifurcation abnormalities, or vertical defects [58].

Emergency treatment: Treatment in the case of periodontal abscess is found in the pre-elimination phase, including the management of acute conditions, and drainage, either through a pocket or an external incision. Sometimes, an occlusal adjustment is needed to eliminate the symptom. The administration of antibiotics is necessary if there are indications of infection (fever or lymphadenopathy). If the tooth is no longer maintainable, then the most likely treatment is the removal [51].

5.2.3 Pericoronitis or pericoronal abscess

Clinically and etiology: Pericoronitis is an inflammation of the soft tissue surrounding the crown of a partially erupted tooth. Pericoronal abscesses are generally localized accumulations on the gingival flaps that envelop the crown of a tooth that has not been perfectly erupted [57]. The clinical picture of a periodontal abscess lesion is the gingival redness, softness, suppurative, and pain when touched aching. There is a bending at the angle of the mandible, trismus pain that radiates to the ear area, accompanied by fever and bending lymphadenopathy. The etiology of pericoronitis is the accumulation of plaque on the operculum that covers part of the molar 3 mandibles that are partial eruption and can also be caused by trauma from the opponent's teeth (**Figure 7**) [51].

Emergency treatment: The operculum area should be cleaned with an irrigation solution slowly, to remove debris, if needed, that can be done under anesthesia. The operculum removal and occlusal adjustment should be performed to eliminate trauma to the 3-mandibular molar tooth. Antibiotic administration is carried out if there is an indication of infection [51].

5.2.4 Peri-endo abscess

Clinically and etiology: It is a combination of periodontal/endodontic lesions, localized, covering areas that have infection originating from periodontal/pulp tissue. It is the result of "communication" between the periodontal tissue and the pulp. The clinical picture is characterized by the presence of periodontal pockets surrounding non-vital teeth, and soft lesions of the gingival, accompanied by the formation of exudate and fistulas. Teeth that have a peri-endo abscess will hurt when there is percussion and shake, and sometimes there is a vertical fracture of the root (crack). The etiology of this lesion is the presence of an infection that begins with inflammation of the pulp which then extends to the periodontal ligament, or it can also be preceded by inflammation of the periodontal tissue through the formation of a pocket that extends to the musty from the tooth and then radiates to the pulp through the accessory canal (**Figure 7**) [51, 55].

Emergency treatment: For the drainage through periodontal canal debridement or root canal treatment, incision can be done if the abscess appears to be fluctuating. If necessary, occlusal adjustments should be done. The administration of antibiotics is recommended for the comfort of the patient and if there is an indication of the expansion of infection [51].

6. Discussion

Several studies have shown a link between COVID-19 and periodontal disease, and this is due to the similarity of pro-inflammatory cytokines released by the body [13]. The pathogenesis of periodontal disease begins with the expansion of the subgingival plaque into the gingival sulcus, where microorganisms in the subgingival plaque can cause changes in the coronal attachment of the epithelium on the tooth surface, and this is due to the immune response to pathogenic bacteria and endotoxins through the activity of neutrophils, macrophages, and lymphocytes [14]. Research conducted by Wu et al. (2020) on COVID-19 shows that there is an unfavorable relationship that can lead to cytokine storms, where certain elements have similarities with cytokine profiles commonly encountered in periodontitis [15]. Treatment in dentistry can generally be categorized as an emergency, urgent, nonurgent, and advise/self-care [21]. Dental and periodontal care are treatments that require close physical contact, so it would be better if the treatment was made as short as possible or done as a complaint only, and the patient's recall time for maintenance was made rather long, at least 2 weeks to see the possible symptoms of COVID-19 in the patient [5, 47]. Cases of periodontal emergence arise when an acute condition that causes pain in the periodontal tissue forces the patient to seek treatment on the spot. Time management is the key to avoiding more severe periodontal tissue damage and its effect psychically and functionally on patients [51]. Cases related to periodontal emergencies are essentially limited, including acute abscesses involving periodontal tissue or endo-perio lesions, necrotizing ulcerative gingivitis and periodontitis resulting from stress during the pandemic, hypersensitivity to dentin, and oral lesions that affect the quality of life such as ulcers, viral and fungal infections, and also cases requiring biopsy. During the pandemic, pharmacological treatment is the best and safest option [37, 52]. During the treatment, if direct contact is required, dentists recommended to use PPE to avoid aerosol splashes that occur during the work procedure, where aerosol granules and droplets can last 30 minutes after the treatment procedure is performed [21, 26]. The use of teledentistry is very important in periodontal care, including organizing patient schedules based on complaint priority, pre-checking triage monitoring, diagnosing determination based on staging, grading, and also communicating with patients regarding risk factor control and oral hygiene instruction [5].

7. Conclusion

Periodontitis is an inflammatory disease of periodontal tissue that is multifactorial; in some cases, it can be aggravated by the presence of systemic abnormalities so that individuals with certain systemic disorders become more at risk, which allows the use of telehealth to be one of the ways of communicating between patients and professionals of various disciplines. Control of routine maintenance of periodontal tissue, monitoring of periodontal tissue health, and control of risk factors aim to reduce the progression of periodontal disease and reduce the risk of tooth loss, which during this pandemic is difficult to do, so far teledentistry is quite reliable for monitoring the health of periodontal tissue, motivating, and provision of periodontal health maintenance instructions. Increased motivation related to the prevention of periodontal tissue abnormalities can be done through teledentistry and other applications by increasing individual motivation and awareness related to periodontal tissue maintenance, especially for individuals with risk factors for systemic disorders who have a more severe risk of transmission of COVID-19.

Acknowledgements

The authors would like to express their gratitude to everyone who facilitated and enabled us to carry out this successfully.

Conflict of interest

There were no conflicts of interest as declared by the authors.

Author details

Desy Fidyawati[1,2]*, Adrianus Wicaksono[1], Veronica Septnina Primasari[1] and Suci Amalia[1]

1 Department of Periodontology, University of Prof. Dr. Moestopo (B), Jakarta, Indonesia

2 Faculty of Dentistry, Doctoral's Candidate, University of Indonesia, Jakarta, Indonesia

*Address all correspondence to: desyfidyawati@dsn.moestopo.ac.id

IntechOpen

© 2022 The Author(s). Licensee IntechOpen. This chapter is distributed under the terms of the Creative Commons Attribution License (http://creativecommons.org/licenses/by/3.0), which permits unrestricted use, distribution, and reproduction in any medium, provided the original work is properly cited.

References

[1] Organization WH. WHO Director-General's Opening Remarks at the Media Briefing on COVID-19-11. WHO; 2020

[2] Aldahlawi SA, Afifi IK. COVID-19 in dental practice: Transmission risk, infection control challenge, and clinical implications. The Open Dentistry Journal. 2020;**14**(1):348-354. DOI: 10.2174/1874210602014010348

[3] Ren Y, Rasubala L, Malmstrom H, Eliav E. Dental care and oral health under the clouds of COVID-19. JDR Clinical and Translational Research. 2020;**5**(3):202-210

[4] Diegritz C, Manhart J, Bücher K, et al. A detailed report on the measures taken in the Department of Conservative Dentistry and Periodontology in Munich at the beginning of the COVID-19 outbreak. Clinical Oral Investigations. 2020;**24**(8):2931-2941. DOI: 10.1007/s00784-020-03440-z

[5] Di Spirito F, Iacono VJ, Alfredo I, Alessandra A, Sbordone L, Lanza A. Evidence-based recommendations on periodontal practice and the Management of Periodontal Patients during and after the COVID-19 era: Challenging infectious diseases spread by airborne transmission. The Open Dentistry Journal. 2021;**15**(1):325-336. DOI: 10.2174/1874210602115010325

[6] Siddharthan S, Naing NN, Arfah NW. Periodontal disease and COVID 19. Journal of Pharmaceutical Research International. 2020;**3**:88-91

[7] Zhang H, Penninger JM, Li Y, Zhong N, Slutsky USA. Angiotensin-converting enzyme 2 (ACE2) as a SARS-CoV-2 receptor: Molecular mechanisms and potential therapeutic target. Intensive Care Medicine. 2020;**46**(4):586-590. DOI: 10.1007/s00134-020-05985-9

[8] Zou X, Chen K, Zou J, Han P, Hao J, Han Z. Single-cell RNA-seq data analysis on the receptor ACE2 expression reveals the potential risk of different human organs vulnerable to 2019-nCoV infection. Frontiers in Medicine. 2020;**14**(2):185-192. DOI: 10.1007/s11684-020-0754-0

[9] Xu H, Zhong L, Deng J, et al. High expression of ACE2 receptor of 2019-nCoV on the epithelial cells of oral mucosa. International Journal of Oral Science. 2020;**12**(1):1-5. DOI: 10.1038/s41368-020-0074-x

[10] Cai W, Marouf N, Said KN, Tamimi F. Nature of the interplay between periodontal diseases and COVID-19. Frontier in Dental Medicine. 2021;**2**(December):1-9. DOI: 10.3389/fdmed.2021.735126

[11] Li X, Geng M, Peng Y, Meng L, Lu S. Molecular immune pathogenesis and diagnosis of COVID-19. Journal of Pharmaceutical Analysis. 2020;**10**(2):102-108

[12] Vos T, Barber RM, Bell B, et al. Global, regional, and national incidence, prevalence, and years lived with disability for 301 acute and chronic diseases and injuries in 188 countries, 1990-2013: A systematic analysis for the global burden of disease study 2013. Lancet. 2015;**386**(9995):743-800. DOI: 10.1016/S0140-6736(15)60692-4

[13] Do JH, Takei HH, Carranza FA. Periodontal examination and diagnosis. In: Carranza. Elsevier; 2019. pp. 378-396

[14] Luis Muñoz-Carrillo J, Elizabeth Hernández-Reyes V, Eduardo García-Huerta O, et al. Pathogenesis of periodontal disease. In: Periodontal Disease – Diagnostic and Adjunctive Non-Surgical Considerations. London, UK: IntechOpen; 2020. pp. 1-14. DOI: 10.5772/intechopen.86548

[15] Wu D, Yang XO. TH17 responses in cytokine storm of COVID-19: An emerging target of JAK2 inhibitor Fedratinib. Journal of Microbiology, Immunology, and Infection. 2020;**53**(3):368-370. DOI: 10.1016/j.jmii.2020.03.005

[16] Sahni V, Gupta S. COVID-19 & periodontitis: The cytokine connection. Medical Hypotheses. 2020;**144**:1-3. DOI: 10.1016/j.mehy.2020.109908

[17] Graves D. Cytokines that promote periodontal tissue destruction. Journal of Periodontology. 2008;**79**(8s):1585-1591. DOI: 10.1902/jop.2008.080183

[18] Gupta S, Mohindra R, Chauhan PK, et al. SARS-CoV-2 detection in gingival crevicular fluid. Journal of Dental Research. 2021;**100**(2):187-193. DOI: 10.1177/0022034520970536

[19] Badran Z, Gaudin A, Struillou X, Amador G, Soueidan A. Periodontal pockets: A potential reservoir for SARS-CoV-2? Medical Hypotheses. 2020;**143**: 4-5. DOI: 10.1016/j.mehy.2020.109907

[20] Baba Y, Takahashi K, Kato Y. The management of periodontitis patients should not be postponed during the COVID-19 era. Journal of Dental Oral Health.

[21] Saudi Arabia Ministry of Health. Dental Emergency. 2020

[22] van Doremalen N, Bushmaker T, Morris DH, et al. Aerosol and surface stability of HCoV-19 (SARS-CoV-2) compared to SARS-CoV-1. medRxiv The Present Server for Health Sciences. 2020

[23] Harrel SK, Molinari J. Aerosols and splatter in dentistry: A brief review of the literature and infection control implications. Journal of the American Dental Association (1939). 2004;**135**(4):429-437. DOI: 10.14219/jada.archive.2004.0207

[24] Dahlke WO, Cottam MR, Herring MC, Leavitt JM, Ditmyer MM, Walker RS. Evaluation of the spatter-reduction effectiveness of two dry-field isolation techniques. Journal of the American Dental Association. 2012;**143**(11):1199-1204. DOI: 10.14219/jada.archive.2012.0064

[25] Holloman JL, Mauriello SM, Pimenta L, Arnold RR. Comparison of suction device with saliva ejector for aerosol and spatter reduction during ultrasonic scaling. Journal of the American Dental Association (1939). 2015;**146**(1):27-33. DOI: 10.1016/j.adaj.2014.10.001

[26] Souza AF, de Arruda JAA, Costa FPD, et al. Safety protocols for dental care during the Covid-19 pandemic: The experience of a Brazilian hospital service. Brazilian Oral Research. 2021;**35**:1-13. DOI: 10.1590/1807-3107bor-2021.vol35.0070

[27] Marui VC, Souto MLS, Rovai ES, Romito GA, Chambrone L, Pannuti CM. Efficacy of preprocedural mouthrinses in the reduction of microorganisms in aerosol: A systematic review. Journal of the American Dental Association (1939). 2019;**150**(12):1015-1026. DOI: 10.1016/j.adaj.2019.06.024

[28] Feres M, Figueiredo LC, Faveri M, Stewart B, De Vizio W. The effectiveness of a preprocedural mouthrinse

containing cetylpyridiniuir chloride in reducing bacteria in the dental office. Journal of the American Dental Association. 2010;**141**(4):415-422. DOI: 10.14219/jada.archive.2010.0193

[29] Retamal-Valdes B, Soares GM, Stewart B, et al. Effectiveness of a pre-procedural mouthwash in reducing bacteria in dental aerosols: Randomized clinical trial. Brazilian Oral Research. 2017;**31**:1-10. DOI: 10.1590/1807-3107BOR-2017.vol31.0021

[30] Association AD. American Dental Association (ADA) Interim Guidance for Minimizing Risk of COVID-19 Transmission. 2020. Available from: https://www.ada.org/en/publication

[31] Ministério da Saúde (BR). Secretaria de Vigilância Em Saúde. Técnica GVIMS/GGTES/ANVISA Memorandum No 04/2020. Orientações Para Serviços de Saúde: Medidas de Prevenção e Controle Que Devem Ser Adotadas Durante a Assistência Aos Casos Suspeitos Ou Co. 2020

[32] Yoon JG, Yoon J, Song JY, et al. Clinical significance of a high SARS-CoV-2 viral load in the saliva. Journal of Korean Medical Science. 2020;**35**(20):1-6. DOI: 10.3346/JKMS.2020.35.E195

[33] Mady LJ, Kubik MW, Baddour K, Snyderman CH, Rowan NR. Consideration of povidone-iodine as a public health intervention for COVID-19: Utilization as "Personal Protective Equipment" for frontline providers exposed in high-risk head and neck and skull base oncology care. Oral Oncology. 2020;**105**:1-2. DOI: 10.1016/j.oraloncology.2020.104724

[34] Cavalcante-Leão BL, de Araujo CM, Basso IB, et al. Is there scientific evidence of the mouthwashes effectiveness in reducing viral load in Covid-19? A systematic review. Journal of Clinical and Experimental Dentistry. 2021;**13**(2):179-189. DOI: 10.4317/JCED.57406

[35] Bartoszko JJ, Farooqi MAM, Alhazzani W, Loeb M. Medical masks vs N95 respirators for preventing COVID-19 in healthcare workers: A systematic review and meta-analysis of randomized trials. Influenza and Other Respiratory Viruses. 2020;**14**(4):365-373. DOI: 10.1111/irv.12745

[36] Derraik JGB, Anderson WA, Connelly EA, Anderson YC. Rapid review of SARS-CoV-1 and SARS-CoV-2 viability, susceptibility to treatment, and the disinfection and reuse of ppe, particularly filtering facepiece respirators. International Journal of Environmental Research and Public Health. 2020;**17**(17):1-31. DOI: 10.3390/ijerph17176117

[37] Kurt B, Ilhan B, Sevki B, Kurt A, Orhan K. Periodontal management during COVID-19 pandemic: Mini review. Balkan Journal of Dental Medicine. 2021;**25**(3):135-138. DOI: 10.2478/bjdm-2021-0021

[38] Proffitt E. What will be the new normal for the dental industry? British Dental Journal. 2020;**228**(9):678-680. DOI: 10.1038/s41415-020-1583-x

[39] Ather A, Patel B, Ruparel NB, Diogenes A, Hargreaves KM. Reply to "coronavirus disease 19 (COVID-19): Implications for clinical dental care". Journal of Endodontia. 2020;**46**(9):1342. DOI: 10.1016/j.joen.2020.08.005

[40] Lo GR. The severe acute respiratory syndrome coronavirus-2 (Sars cov-2) in dentistry. Management of biological risk in dental practice. International Journal of Environmental Research and Public Health. 2020;**17**(9):1-12. DOI: 10.3390/ijerph17093067

[41] Solina K. ADA Develops Guidance on Dental Emergency, Nonemergency Care. 2020. Available from: https://www.ada.org/en/publications/ada-news/2020-archive/march/ada-develops-guidance-on-dental-emergency-nonemergency-care

[42] Abramovitz I, Palmon A, Levy D, et al. Dental care during the coronavirus disease 2019 (COVID-19) outbreak: Operatory considerations and clinical aspects. Quintessence International. 2020;**51**(5): 418-429. DOI: 10.3290/j.qi.a44392

[43] de Almeida GR et al. Remote diagnosis of traumatic dental injuries using digital photographs captured via a mobile phone. Dental Traumatology. 2017;**33**(5):350-357. DOI: 10.1111/edt.12347

[44] WHO. Cleaning and Disinfection of Environmental Surfaces in the Context of COVID-19. 2020. Available from: https://www.who.int/publications-detail/cleaning-and-disinfection-of-environmental-surfaces-inthe-context-of- covid-19

[45] Halepas S, Ferneini EM. A pinch of prevention is worth a pound of cure: Proactive dentistry in the wake of COVID-19. Journal of Oral and Maxillofacial Surgery. 2020;**78**(6):860-861. DOI: 10.1016/j.joms.2020.03.036

[46] Nejatidanesh F, Khosravi Z, Goroohi H, Badrian H, Savabi O. Risk of contamination of different areas of dentist's face during dental practices. International Journal of Preventive Medicine. 2013;**4**(5):611-615

[47] Jafer MA, Hazazi MA, Mashi MH, et al. COVID-19 and periodontitis: A reality to live with. The Journal of Contemporary Dental Practice. 2020;**21**(12):1398-1403. DOI: 10.5005/jp-journals-10024-2961

[48] Graziani F, Karapetsa D, Alonso B, Herrera D. Nonsurgical and surgical treatment of periodontitis: How many options for one disease? Periodontology 2000. 2000;**75**:152-188. DOI: 10.1111/prd.12201

[49] Tonetti MS, Greenwell H, Kornman KS. Staging and grading of periodontitis: Framework and proposal of a new classification and case definition. Journal of Clinical Periodontology. 2018;**45**(January):S149-S161. DOI: 10.1111/jcpe.12945

[50] Ramaglia L, Di Spirito F, Sirignano M, La Rocca M, Esposito U, Sbordone L. A 5-year longitudinal cohort study on crown to implant ratio effect on marginal bone level in single implants. Clinical Implant Dentistry and Related Research. 2019;**21**(5):916-922. DOI: 10.1111/cid.12757

[51] Wadia R. The idea of M. periodontal emergencies in general practice. Dental Journal. 2017;**6**(2):46-51. DOI: 10.1308/205016817821281774

[52] Jamal M, Shah M, Almarzooqi SH, et al. Overview of transnational recommendations for COVID-19 transmission control in dental care settings. Oral Diseases. 2021;**27**(S3):655-664. DOI: 10.1111/odi.13431

[53] Holmstrup P, Westergaard J. Necrotising periodontal disease. In: Lindhe J, Lang NP, Karring T, editors. Clinical Periodontology and Implant Dentistry. 5th ed. Oxford: Wiley-Blackwell; 2008. pp. 459-474

[54] Wennström J, Lindhe J. Effect of hydrogen peroxide on developing plaque and gingivitis in man. Journal of Clinical Periodontology. 1979;**6**(2):115-130. DOI: 10.1111/j.1600-051X.1979.tb02190.x

[55] Loesche WJ, Syed SA, Laughon BE, Stoll J. The bacteriology of acute necrotizing ulcerative gingivitis. Journal of Periodontology. 1982;**53**(4):223-230. DOI: 10.1902/jop.1982.53.4.223

[56] Sousa D, Pintodn D, Araujo R, Rego RO, Moreira-Neto J. Gingival abscess due to an unusual nail-biting habit: A case report. The Journal of Contemporary Dental Practice. 2010;**11**(2):85-91. DOI: 10.5005/jcdp-11-2-85

[57] Oak Brook I. International workshop for a classification of periodontal diseases and conditions. Annals of Periodontology. 1999;**4**(1):112-141

[58] Herrera D, Roldan S, Gonzalez I. The periodontal abscess (I). Clinical and microbiological findings. Journal of Clinical Periodontology. 2000;**27**:387-394

Chapter 13

Perspective Chapter: Salivary Duct Cyst

Saurabh R. Nagar, Gabriela Fernandes, Shivani Bansal, Rajiv S. Desai and Diya Jayanth Kamdar

Abstract

Salivary duct cysts (SDCs) are true cysts caused by obstruction of salivary ducts and are rare in minor salivary glands. Intraoral SDCs and mucoceles represent clinically salivary gland neoplasms, making diagnosis difficult and subject to errors in treatment. It is important for Oral and Maxillofacial Surgeons to include SDC in the differential diagnosis of swelling affecting buccal mucosa.

Keywords: salivary duct cyst, minor salivary glands, oral pathology, oral surgery, maxillofacial surgery

1. Introduction

The two major groups of oral cysts are divided based on odontogenesis: odontogenic cysts (OCs) and non-odontogenic cysts (non-OCs). The odontogenic cysts are distinguished by specific odontogenic markers. They have histological similarities with odontogenic structures and anatomical considerations, whereas the non-odontogenic group includes cysts that originate from specific areas or organs of the oral cavity such as naso-palatine duct/mid-palatine cysts, nasolabial cysts, and salivary cysts. There are some cysts that are included in this group, that are ubiquitous in the body such as aneurysmal bone cysts, lympho-epithelial cysts, and dermoid cysts [1].

Odontogenic cysts develop from the tooth-producing tissues and on the other hand, they originate from the remnants of dental lamina epithelium entrapped within the gingival named epithelial rests of "Serres," or the epithelial remains of the "Malassez." These cellular remnants have limited growth potential and they fall within the concept of the post-functional state of the dental lamina. The two types of dental cysts are generated by the two types of embryological residues. Periodontal cysts originate from the remnants of Serres and the orthokeratocysts, which are a more aggressive type of cyst with a neoplastic variant. The inflammatory radicular cyst originates from the residues of the Malassez. For this particular type of cyst, an infectious and/or inflammatory stimulus acting on a genetic predisposition has been proposed as the first pathogenic event causing the proliferation of cellular odontogenic remnants.

Cytokeratins are ideal markers for differential diagnosis of these cysts, being involved in physiological odontogenesis epithelium-specific markers of differentiation

IntechOpen

and have been proposed as ideal markers for differential diagnosis of these cysts, being involved in physiological odontogenesis, thoroughly cytokeratins 5 and 14 are present in the basal cell layer of keratinized and non-keratinized epithelia along with a depletion in the layers above. Cytokeratins 1 and 10 are particular with respect to the spinous layer; cytokeratin 19 is specific with regard to the basal stratum layer of the non-kertinized epithelia; cytokeratins 13 as well as 4 are particular to the supra-basal cells of the tongue epithelium; there is the presence of K2p in the supra-basal epithelial cells of the hard palate and gingiva. In the course of odontogenesis, the cytokeratins form a unique expression; in the early bell stage, cytokeratin 14 is present in the "stellatum reticulum"

Cyst of oral bone tissue and periodontal	Soft tissue non-odontogenic cysts
Odontogenic cyst • Inflammatory origin Radicular necrotic cyst Collateral inflammatory cyst 1. Paradental cyst 2. Juvenile paradental cyst • Development origin Dentigerous cyst 1. Follicular cyst 2. Germinal cyst 3. Eruptive cyst • Parodontal cyst (Periodontal tissue) • Gingival cyst of infants 1. Newborn gingival cysts 2. Dental lamina cysts 3. Bohn's nodules Non Odontogenic cysts • Nasopalatine duct/midline palatine cyst • Mid-palatal raphe non-odontogenic cysts of infants (Epstein's Pearls)	Salivary cysts and salivary duct cysts Cysts of lymphatic tissue origin • Cystic hygromayour name • Lymphoepithelial cysts
Cysts of globulo-maxillary area	Dermoid and epidermoid congenital cysts
Cysts with malignant variant • Orthokeratinized odontogenic cyst • Calcifying odontogenic cyst Glandular cysts 1. Glandular odontogenic cyst 2. Sialo-odontogenic cyst	Nasolabial cysts
Cysts of maxillary sinus	Thyroglossal duct cyst
Pseudocysts of the bone in relation to the oral cavity • Solitary bone pseudo cyst • Aneurysmal bone cyst	

Table 1.
Cysts of the oral cavity.

along with cytokeratin 7; CK19 is expressed along with these cytokeratins in the cells of the enamel epithelium; although cytokeratin 14 is present during the early bell stages which are ultimately substituted by cytokeratin 19 in differential ameloblasts; cytokeratins 7 and 13 are present in the "rests of Serres." The structure of cytokeratins and their expression within the cells are based on the conditions of the environment and changes that occur in the functioning of the cell. Hence, an altered expression when detected becomes extremely helpful for the differential diagnosis of multiple diseases like cysts and tumors. Therefore, cytokeratins 5 and 6 are found in every single layer of the odontogenic cysts, cytokeratin 13 is present among the supra-basal cell layer of odontogenic cysts, while cytokeratin 20 is not present in any of the odontogenic cysts.

In this chapter, we suggest a simplified classification with regard to the cysts of the oral cavity. We plan to divide the various types of cysts into two main groups: (1) cyst of the osseous and periodontal tissue and (2) soft tissue origin non-odontogenic cyst. After which, these groups are further divided into subgroups depending on their relationship with the anatomical area, histological origin as well as clinical behavior (rate of recurrence, frequency, and malignant potential; **Table 1**). **Table 1** depicts the classification of the cysts of the oral cavity.

2. Cysts of the oral bone and periodontal tissue

2.1 Odontogenic cysts of inflammatory origin

Radicular necrotic cyst (RC) is the most common cyst of the oral cavity which is caused by the loss of pulp of the tooth (biological barrier) due to carious lesions or dental trauma. There is the presence of pulp necrosis and the cyst is derived from the cellular remnants of the "Malassez." This can preside to form inflammatory radicular necrotic cyst which can either be periradicular or periapical. Initially, the granuloma forms, and after which it gives rise to a cyst whose epithelium demonstrates odontogenic CK19 in the superficial cell layers and co-expresses CK5 in the cyst lining. Residual radicular cysts are a unique variant of the radicular cyst which develops from apical granulomas or residual fragments of RC.

Collateral inflammatory cysts (Juvenile paradental cyst and Paradental cyst) have overlapping histological features with radicular cysts. Their etiology is also considered inflammatory or meta-traumatic. It is present on the lateral surface of a tooth which is vital. It occurs as a result of a chronic inflammatory process in the periodontal pocket. In a young patient, the juvenile paradental cyst is seen in the root area of the mandibular molars whereas it is present distally to a lower wisdom tooth in adults. These lesions are considered the same unit, regardless of the localization. The histological features of these cysts cannot be distinguished from those of the inflammatory radicular cysts but this appearance emphasizes the origin from the remains of the Mallasez.

It becomes important to differentiate these cysts from the other radiolucent jaw lesions, such as unicystic ameloblastoma, keratocystic odontogenic tumor, dentigerous cysts, and LPC. A combination of immunohistochemical markers such as CK10, CK13, CK17, PCNA, UEA, and perlecan can help in the differential diagnosis.

2.2 Odontogenic cysts of developmental origin

Dentigerous cysts surround the crown of a tooth that has not migrated into the oral cavity. They are named follicular, germinal, and eruptive cysts. There is an accumulation of pathological fluid in the layers of the reduced enamel epithelium or between it and the crown of an unerupted tooth. CK5, CK6, and CK19 are present while CK7 is absent in this type of cyst.

Periodontal tissues (parodontal cysts and Botryoid cysts) form a single nosological group named "cyst of the periodontal tissue" because they are of dental origin and the periodontal tissue is contiguous to the teeth and bone. The cysts which affect the periodontal tissue are gingival cysts which are frequently present in adults and periodontal cysts (lateral parodontal cyst and its variant; botryoid cyst). The periodontal cysts are unicystic with a differential diagnosis of ameloblastoma. Two or three layers of flattened cells mimicking a squamous epithelium are present along with areas of nodular type thickening and clear cells rich in glycogen. The lateral parodontal cysts (LPC) have a multilocular variant defined as "Botryoid cyst." They arise from the remnants of Serres incorporated into the periodontal tissue or from the reduced enamel epithelium of the follicle which expands to occupy a space in the periodontal ligament during the eruptive phase producing a paradontal cyst, while a gingival cyst may form due to a portion remaining in the gum after the eruption. CK13 and CK17 are expressed in the surface layers of the lateral parodontal cyst, whereas perlecan and UEA are present on the cell border of the whole layer. LPC is negative for CK10.

Botryoid odontogenic cyst is a rare pathological multilocular cyst that may or may not have close proximity to a root of a tooth. This is considered a variant of lateral parodontal cyst and it is derived from more groups of converging cellular debris of Serres. It has also been considered to represent a variant of glandular odontogenic cyst due to the presence of mucous cells and the columnar cells. Presence of CK18 and CK13 which is specific for rests of Serres, show the origin from the odontogenic tissues. CD56 and calreatin help in differentiating ameloblastoma from BOC as these markers are absent in the latter.

Gingival cysts of infants are also known as Newborn gingival cysts, Dental lamina cysts, or Bohn's nodules. They are present in newborns and develop from the remains of the dental lamina. Presence of squamous epithelium lining with areas of parakeratosis and keratin-filled cavities.

2.3 Non odontogenic cysts

Epstein's Pearl are also known as Mid palatal raphe non-odontogenic cysts of infants. They have similar histological and clinical features to gingival cysts. They arise from non-odontogenic epithelial remnants after medican palatal fusion.

Nasopalatine duct cysts are formed by the proliferation of epithelial remnants that are organized in clusters or cords and are present in the incisive canal of the maxilla. These remnants cause the formation of the cyst with the presence of a squamous ciliated epithelium layer.

2.4 Cysts of the globulomaxillary area

These cysts display constant clinical and radiological features, however, they do not present the same histological features always. Various histological features such as stratified squamous (odontogenic), parakeratinic (orthokeratocystic), or cylindrical respiratory (non-odontogenic) epithelium have been described in these cysts. In this group of cysts, we can always include intraosseous cysts that develop between the roots of the lateral incisior and the canine teeth which causes divergence. Moreover, cysts originating from the respiratory epithelium remained trapped in the globule maxillary site and parodontal cyst. It is possible to find neoplastic cysts in this site.

2.5 Cysts with malignant variants with neoplastic characteristics

Orthokeratinized odontogenic cysts are characterized by a keratinized lining epithelium. The term keratocystic odontogenic tumor (KCOT) is preferred when the epithelium displays significant parakeratosis or orthokeratosis and presents more aggressively with a tendency to recur. Whereas, these two cysts show a different pattern of expression of CKs: OOC expresses CK1, CK2, CK10, and loricrin, while KCOT expresses CK4, CK10, CK13, CK16, CK17, and CK19, similar to the dental lamina. The differential immunohistochemical expression of CD-56, CD-105, and calreatin help in distinguishing these cysts from ameloblastoma from a clinical view point.

Calcifying odontogenic cyst (COC) have three entities, simple intraosseous COC, extra osseous peripheral COC, and the malignant form calcifying cystic odontogenic tumor. Radiologically, they show cystic imaging with small scattered areas of calcification which often resembles an odontoma. They have a peculiar histological pattern with their epithelial lining consisting of a basal layer of columnar cells and an overlying epithelium, which is thick and vacuolated. Furthermore, groups of eosinophilic cells with non-stainable cellular structures are visible in the epithelial lining, connective tissue capsule, or both. These cells are referred to as "ghost cells" and are considered dystrophic cells with aberrant keratinization or apoptotic cells with intracellular calcification. These particular cells are present in different pathological entities such a craniopharyngioma, odontoma, pilomatrixoma, ameloblastic fibroma, and some visceral tumors. They lose the cytoskeletal components and become CK1013 negative as they accumulate some substances during the differentiation process. While, CK14 is expressed in the basal layer, CK10/13 are present in the upper layer of the cyst. P63 expression is present in all layers of COC examined.

Glandular odontogenic cyst (GOC) contain acidophilic cuboidal or columnar cells arranged in glandular structures with papillary growth and projections into cyst-like spaces. This cyst can be differentiated by mucoepidermoid carcinoma based on the diverse immunohistochemical expression of mammary serine protease inhibitor (MASPIN) as well as Ki67 and P63 tumor markers.

Cysts of the maxillary sinus have three types of primary cysts, the first type is the true cysts which are due to an occlusion of the excretory ducts of the sinus mucous glands. The second type is mucoceles which are formed from the non-external drainage of normal mucous and the third type is secondary mucoceles. They are formed as a result of post-radical sinus surgery and probably due to residues of sinus mucosa forming a new mucocele in a closed compartment. Pseudocysts are also present, they are formed between the inner surface of the bone wall and the connective tissue layer while the sinus mucosa remains on the outside. These cysts may be formed due to allergies, inflammation of the maxillary sinus and mucosal odontogenic inflammation. Sometimes, the secondary odontogenic cysts develop in the bone base of maxilla and invade the maxillary sinus. These cysts are particularly "intrusive sinus oral cysts."

3. Pseudocysts present in the oral cavity

Solitary bone pseudocysts (SBP) are devoid of any epithelium lining. They have a traumatic origin hence they are also known as bone pseudocysts or bone traumatic pseudocysts, whereas aneurysmal bone cysts (ABP) are blood-filled sinusoidal or cavernous spaces without cystic epithelium. The pathology of this cyst is similar to ABP. A trauma could lead to a bone hemorrhage and the clot may not be re-canalized which eventually leaves the cavity devoid of content and may present as continuous micro-hemorrhages. This causes a local reaction of macrophages or vascular dilation. The ubiquitous protease USP-6 which is mapped on chromosoma 16q22 are used as a diagnostic tool for ABPs.

3.1 Soft tissue non-odontogenic cysts

Nasolabial cysts are considered as one of the soft tissue non-odontogenic cysts. The concept that it is considered a fissural cyst is because it is related to the globule-maxillary cyst and its peripheral form is no longer valid. Histologically, it consists of a cyst that is lined by a bi-layered epithelium with a cuboidal basal layer and sometimes pseudo-stratified with goblet cells along with areas of squamous metaplasia. CK7 and CK19 are present in all layers whereas CK5 and CK6 are expressed only in the basal layer. The mucin in the goblet cells is positive for MUC-2 and MUC-5 AC. It is a developmental non-odontogenic cyst that originates from the lower portion of the naso-lacrimal duct.

Dermoid and epidermoid congenital cysts are positive for CK10. They are derived from embryonic pluripotential cells trapped which was trapped during the early weeks of intrauterine life and subsequently develop into one or into all three layers—ectoderm, mesoderm, and endoderm. They are present in the floor of the mouth, tongue, parotid gland, and mandible.

Salivary cysts and pseudocysts are soft tissue cysts. While salivary retention cysts are considered as a pseudo-cyst. Histologically, oncocyte-like cells and pseudo-stratified columnar epithelium are present. The Ranula represents a mucocele on the floor of the mouth. It is formed due to salivary accumulation in the sublingual or the submaxillary gland which is followed by a rupture and extravasation of saliva in the surrounding connective. The presence of an epithelial coating is not there. Ranulas are located above the mylohyoid muscle which is known as the simple type or can grow downwards forming an hourglass shape which is known as the complex type.

Salivary duct cysts represent less than 10% of all salivary gland disorders, especially in the major salivary glands. Sialocyst is another name given to the salivary duct cyst (SDC). Salivary gland cysts can be either ephemeral or persistent. It is caused due to ductal obstruction that leads to cystic dilation of salivary ducts. Different terminologies have been given to these lesions; although, "salivary duct cyst (SDC)" is the most adequate by virtue of its origin being related to the epithelial lining of salivary gland ducts. SDCs typically occur in the major salivary glands with 80% occurring in the parotid and minimal cases are reported in the submandibular and sublingual glands. They present as dome-shaped, sessile, slow-growing, unilateral, asymptomatic, and compressible nodules in adult patients [2]. They are fluctuant to palpation but usually painless and if a sialolith is present then it may feel firmer. Secondary infection may present as mucus or pus from dilated ductal orifices when palpated. Blue tinge due to the Tyndall effect is present. They do not typically wax or wane over time, whereas its occurrence in minor salivary glands is rare and occurs more commonly in the sixth decade of life. Symptoms generally involve eating there was no pain or increase in the size of swelling. Intra-oral examination depicts a painless, mobile, non-compressible, soft, nodular, solitary swelling along with a soft brownish cystic sac filled with slimy gel-like material (**Figure 1**). Majority of the swellings range from 1 to 3 cm. Hematoxylin & Eosin (H&E) stained sections demonstrate a dilated salivary gland duct with intraluminal mucous plug (**Figures 2** and **3**) with dense chronic inflammatory infiltrate composed chiefly of lymphocytes around the dilated duct [3, 4]. Salivary

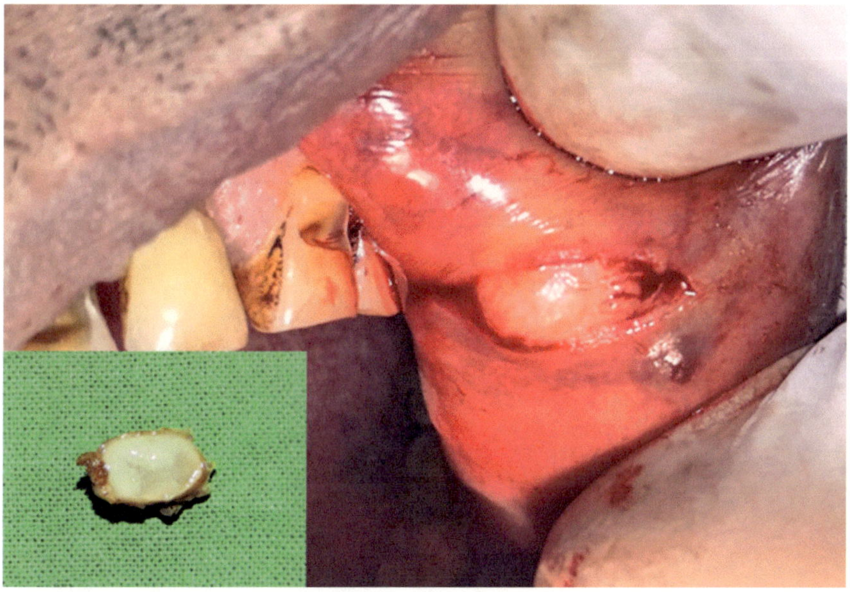

Figure 1.
Clinical image shows surgical exposure of salivary duct cyst in the left buccal mucosa and gross specimen showing cystic sac filled with slimy gel-like material (inset).

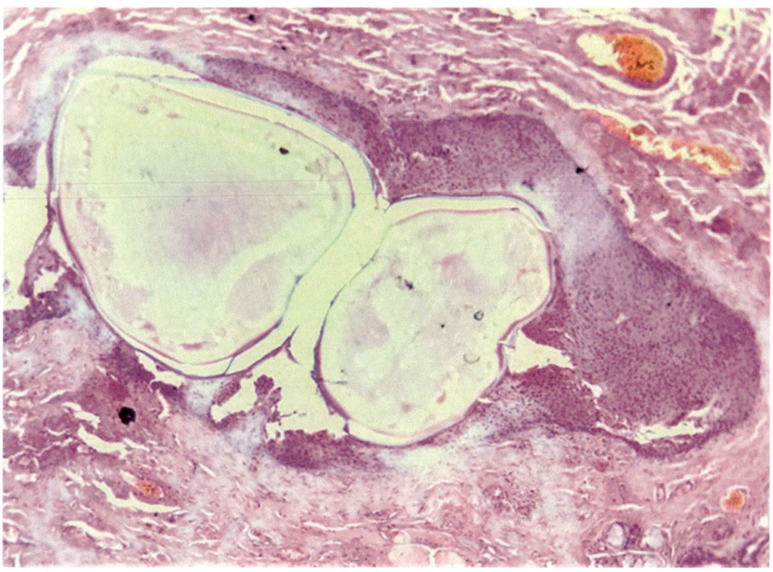

Figure 2.
Histopathological image showing cystically dilated salivary gland duct with intraluminal mucous plug and squamous metaplasia of the lining epithelium (H&E stain; ×100 magnification).

duct cysts may be congenital or acquired in origin. However, studies show that the vast majority of the cases are acquired and occur following obstruction in the duct. The exact factors that cause the obstruction are usually unknown, some suggestions include the involvement of mucus plugs, calculi, or postoperative or postinflammatory structures. Salivary secretion reduces with an increase in the age which may lead to

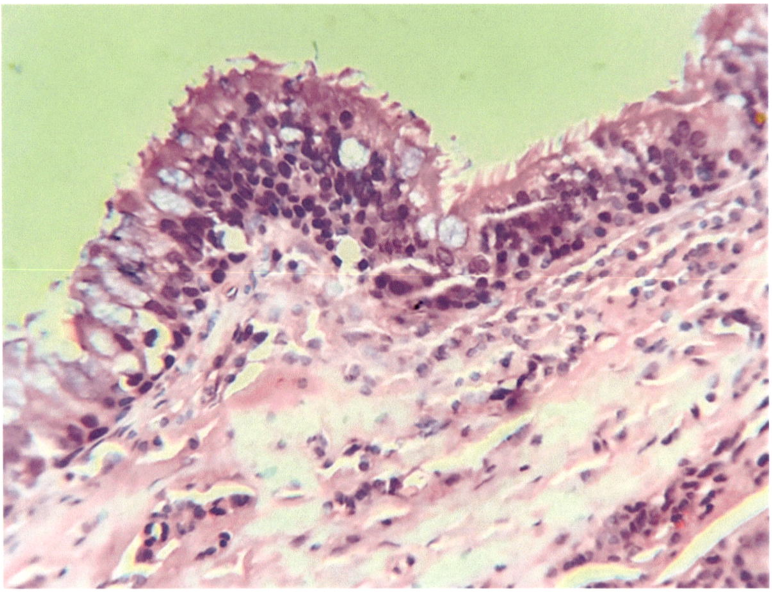

Figure 3.
Histopathological image revealed cystic lining exhibiting ciliated, mucous, and oncocytoid metaplasia (H&E stain; ×400 magnification).

the formation of a mucous plug. This has detrimental effects as it blocks the salivary gland ducts that eventually result in dilation of the duct and the intraluminal pressure increases. Another study suggests that restriction of the duct is frequently reported to be associated with mouth wash which includes hydrogen peroxide, fragrant mouth washes, and toothpaste that control tartar accumulation. Luminal pressure marginally increases due to a continuous flow of saliva as a result of recreation. This invariably leads to ductal dilation.

Cysts in the salivary ducts often present themselves as an asymptomatic, unilateral swelling that usually occurs in sites that are less prone to trauma. They are evenly distributed between the contiguous area of the buccal mucosa, lower lip mucosa, mandibular vestibule, the floor of the mouth, hard and soft palate, as well as minor salivary glands with a size range of 0.8–10 cm in size [5]. They are rarely present in the major salivary glands and if involved, are usually found in the superficial lobe of the parotid with no involvement of the facial nerve. Salivary duct cysts may affect children to older adults, mostly those over 30–40 years of age. SDCs affect the male and female population equally.

Salivary gland cysts can often be an early manifestation of a salivary gland tumor, therefore diagnosis and early treatment interventions play an important role in the prognosis of this lesion. Presence of epithelial alterations, such as metaplasias and focal papillary proliferations observed, are comparable to similar changes seen in odontogenic cysts and maybe an early markers of tumor manifestation [6]. On rare occasions, these cysts can progress and develop into benign and malignant neoplasms such as adenocarcinoma and mucoepidermoid carcinoma from the lining of a salivary duct cyst.

Primary diagnostic interventions involve imaging and histopathology. Imaging helps with determining the extent of the involvement, the borders, and the core content. Internal blood flow is absent in color Doppler while CT reports the cyst as a well-circumscribed lesion with low-density areas. On MRI, these lesions appear as high signal areas and no enhancement is observed upon administration of gadolinium while ultrasonography demonstrates a posterior acoustic enhancement lesion with imperceptible walls. Finally, sialography permits only indirect visualization of the cyst, evaluated by the displacement of the ducts around them [7].

Histologically, these lesions appear unilocular along with a ductal epithelium that may be cuboidal or columnar in conjunction with a completely, or partially lined squamous epithelium. Occasionally, oncocytic metaplasia is present. The lesions composed of oncocytic cells range from oncocytic metaplasia, and hyperplasia to benign and malignant neoplasms, including oncocytomas and oncocytic carcinomas [8].

SDCs may present clinical-pathological characteristics similar to those of salivary gland neoplasms, making diagnosis difficult and subject to errors in treatment. Pleomorphic adenoma, cystoadenoma, and low-grade mucoepidermoid carcinoma may present in a similar manner to that of SDCs. Salivary duct cysts comprise 0.5–10% of all salivary gland cysts and ideally arise from the salivary duct as non-neoplastic lesions and a majority of these lesions are between 1 and 3 cm in dimension. Since these cysts demonstrate an epithelial cystic lining histopathologically, they are considered to be a “true cyst.” These cysts tend to develop post-obstruction because of the calculi, mucus plugs, trauma, or post-inflammatory scarring. In pediatric patients, the most common pathology lesions involving the parotid gland are benign neoplasms that are not limited to sialocele, lymphoepithelial cyst, first branchial cleft cyst (BCC), and a vascular or lymphatic malformation. Salivary duct cysts can be easily histopathologically differentiated from branchial cleft cysts by the presence of their epithelial lining since the former have epithelium lining of duct cells similar to intercalated, striated, or excretory duct cells whereas the latter is lined with squamous or respiratory epithelium. SDCs are extremely rare and should not be overlooked as part of the differential for any cystic salivary gland lesion since they easily and very quickly progress into a larger lesion in a few months. Sometimes, there might resemble a lymphatic malformation such as chyle-filled cysts lined with endothelium that can be macrocystic or microcystic. And these lesions can appear identical on radiographs and both display high signal intensity on T2-weighted MRI. However, these can be distinguished via MRI and STIR images since SDCs tend to be well-circumscribed masses while lymphatic malformations can be infiltrative and permeate across fat planes [9].

One of the differential diagnoses for SDCs is papillary cystadenoma lymphomatosum (Warthin Tumor). In this, there is the presence of lymphoid stroma in the cyst wall and multiple papillary infoldings with a bilayer of columnar and oncocytic epithelial lining. The second differential diagnosis is gingival cyst of the adult. These transpire only on the gingiva which has no minor salivary glands. The third differential diagnosis is cystadenoma, low-grade mucoepidermoid carcinoma (LG-MEC). Cystadenoma presents often as a well-circumscribed or encapsulated neoplasm together with a collection of the proliferation of ducts. These cysts often occur in the parotid gland and their histological variants include papillary cystadenoma, papillary oncocytic cystadenoma, and papillary mucinous cystadenoma. SDCs may present clinical-pathological characteristics similar to those of mucocele. Clinically, both represents an asymptomatic nodule, but salivary duct cysts are rare in appearance comparing mucocele. In the latter, the presence of true salivary gland duct epithelial lining is absent and instead, this is mimicked by epithelioid macrophages at the periphery of the extravasated mucin. Mucocele is present in the lower lip mucosa and a younger age group contrary to SDCs.

The treatment option for salivary duct cysts includes cryosurgery, carbon dioxide laser surgery, and conservative surgical excision. Because of the fact that benign tumors of the salivary glands are able to clinically mimic salivary duct cysts, excision is extremely necessary. Complete surgical excision along with the feeding minor salivary gland is curative. In this method, iatrogenic intraoperative damage may occur to the neighboring salivary gland parenchyma which would contribute to the development of postoperative mucocele. Then partial or total removal of the feeding major salivary glands may be needed. Chlorhexidine mouthwash and oral antibiotics are provided for secondarily infected SDCs. Sialagogues are also provided which may help in decreasing the risk of salivary stasis within dilated ducts by stimulating salivary flow.

In conclusion, intraoral salivary duct cysts are reactive ductal ectasia that develops secondary to intraluminal obstruction that may require clinical attention when it reaches a particular size. Although the SDCs is considered a rare condition in the oral cavity, it is important to include this lesion in the differential diagnosis of lesions that affect the buccal mucosa and may sometimes transform into a malignant lesion such as adenocarcinoma and mucoepidermoid carcinoma from the lining of a salivary duct cyst along with an association of a latent Epstein–Barr virus infection. With an increase in the aging population, SDC should be considered as one of the differential diagnoses in geriatric patients.

Conflict of interest

The authors declare no conflict of interest.

Author details

Saurabh R. Nagar[1,2,3]*, Gabriela Fernandes[4,5], Shivani Bansal[6], Rajiv S. Desai[6] and Diya Jayanth Kamdar[7]

1 Department of Pathology, Advanced Centre for Treatment, Research and Education in Cancer, Tata Memorial Centre, Mumbai, India

2 Homi Bhabha National Institute, Mumbai, India

3 Department of Oral Pathology and Microbiology, Government Dental College and Hospital, Mumbai, Maharashtra, India

4 Department of Periodontics and Endodontics, SUNY Buffalo, Buffalo, New York, USA

5 Department of Oral Biology, SUNY Buffalo, Buffalo, New York, USA

6 Department of Oral Pathology and Microbiology, Nair Hospital Dental College, Mumbai, India

7 Faculty of Dental Sciences, Bangalore, Karnataka, India

*Address all correspondence to: saurabh.nagar90@gmail.com

IntechOpen

© 2022 The Author(s). Licensee IntechOpen. This chapter is distributed under the terms of the Creative Commons Attribution License (http://creativecommons.org/licenses/by/3.0), which permits unrestricted use, distribution, and reproduction in any medium, provided the original work is properly cited.

References

[1] Antoniades D, Epivatianos A, Markopoulos A, et al. Coexistence of mucous retention cyst and basal cell adenoma arising from the lining epithelium of the cyst. Medical Principles and Practice. 2009;**18**(3):248-252

[2] Work WP. Cysts and congenital lesions of the parotid gland. Otolaryngologic Clinics of North America. 1977;**10**(2):339-343

[3] Batsakis JG, Raymond AK. Sialocysts of the parotid glands. The Annals of Otology, Rhinology, and Laryngology. 1989;**98**(6):487-489

[4] Chi AC, Lambert PR 3rd, Richardson MS, Neville BW. Oral mucoceles: A clinicopathologic review of 1,824 cases, including unusual variants. Journal of Oral and Maxillofacial Surgery. 2011;**69**:1086-1093

[5] Hruban RH, Pitman MB, Klimstra DS. American Registry of Pathology, Armed Forces Institute of Pathology (US). Tumors of the Pancreas. Washington, DC: American Registry of Pathology in collaboration with the Armed Forces Institute of Pathology; 2007. p. 422

[6] Hayashida AM, Zerbinatti DC, Balducci I, et al. Mucus extravasation and retention phenomena: A 24-year study. BMC Oral Health. 2010;**10**:15

[7] Seifert G. Mucoepidermoid carcinoma in a salivary duct cyst of the parotid gland. Contribution to the development of tumours in salivary gland cysts. Pathology, Research and Practice. 1996;**192**:1211-1217

[8] Eversole LR. Oral sialocysts. Archives of Otolaryngology – Head & Neck Surgery. 1987;**113**:51-56

[9] Stojanov IJ, Malik UA, Woo SB. Intraoral salivary duct cyst: Clinical and histopathologic features of 177 cases. Head and Neck Pathology. 2017 Dec 1;**11**(4):469-476

Section 3

Teledentistry

Chapter 14

Perspective Chapter: Teledentistry and Distance Learning – Access to Oral Health State during COVID-19

Shaimaa Hussein Rafat Kotb

Abstract

Background: COVID-19 virus is the most interesting pandemic in the last two years because of its life-threatening conditions. The American Dental Association defines dental emergencies as potentially life-threatening that require immediate treatment to stop ongoing tissue bleeding or alleviate severe pain or infection. Children and adolescents frequently have traumatic dental injuries (TDIs) damaging permanent teeth. Crown fractures and luxations of these teeth are the most common forms of dental trauma. A Favorable outcome requires accurate diagnosis, treatment planning, and follow-up care. Telemedicine/Teledentistry refers to the remote delivery of clinical care through electronic communications. Dental's virtual consultation is a convenient way to connect with patients from the comfort of their homes to show support and interest in teeth.

Keywords: COVID19, traumatic dental injuries, telemedicine, teledentistry, dental's virtual consultation

1. Introduction

COVID-19 is a member of the coronavirus family. In Wuhan, China, the first instances were reported between December 2019 and January 2020. All viruses include DNA or RNA nucleic acids encased in a protein coat. Additionally, some viruses have lipid and protein complexes around them. Coronaviruses have a 30 kb, nonsegmental, positive-sense RNA genome with a high rate of mutation and recombination. Coronaviruses cause upper and lower respiratory infections. Rapid COVID-19 transmission by droplets, coughing and sneezing from symptomatic and asymptomatic individuals prior to the start of symptoms. These infectious droplets are capable of traveling up to 2 meters before settling on surfaces. Typically, droplets do not exceed 2 meters in height and do not adhere to the air. In favorable environmental conditions, the virus can remain active on surfaces for days, but conventional disinfectants such as sodium hypochlorite and hydrogen peroxide can eliminate it in less than one minute [1].

The SARS-CoV-2 virus can be spread by inhalation or by contacting contaminated surfaces prior to touching the nose, mouth, and eyes. Some persons may exhibit super spreading behavior despite the fact that they may stay infectious as long as symptoms persist and even after achieving clinical recovery. The incubation time for SARS-CoV-2 infection is estimated to be 14 days following exposure, with the majority of patients developing symptoms within four to five days. A SARS-CoV-2 infection can affect anyone of any age, but the majority of those infected are middle-aged and elderly. Important clinical symptoms include fever, dry cough, tiredness, sore throat, rhinorrhea, conjunctivitis headache, myalgia, dyspnea, nausea, vomiting, and diarrhea. On the basis of this symptom, there are no clinical criteria that distinguish COVID-19 from other upper/lower airway viral infections. Under some situations, COVID-19 can cause pneumonia, lung failure, and death within the first week [2].

Among the many mechanisms of COVID-19 transmission include coughing and sneezing, direct contact with virus-infected surfaces, and inhalation of aerosols. Due of the disease's rapid contagiousness, folks avoided public settings, particularly hospitals. On persons with probable COVID-19 infection, infection control and public health authorities must be applied. Minor illnesses that can be successfully isolated can be properly treated at home. In order to prevent the transmission of illness, individuals should be encouraged to wash their hands after having contact with unwell persons. Although asymptomatic individuals seldom use facemasks, social isolation is recommended in all places where the illness is common [3, 4].

Dentistry is the profession mostly affected by the global COVID-19 pandemic. Future workplaces will be forced to follow a clinical protocol to avoid the emergence of new illnesses and the spread of viruses. The patient's oral secretions, contaminated materials, and dental unit surfaces may serve as possible sources of infection for the dentist, the assistant, and the patient during routine clinical practice. Saliva and blood droplets generated on surfaces, as well as aerosol inhalation from spinning machinery and ultrasound handpieces, offer considerable danger to current and future occupants. To prevent infections, dental practitioners must use disinfectants and personal protective equipment (PPE). The rapid spread of SARS-CoV-2 has forced adjustments to preventative and restorative dental practices. In dentistry, COVID-19 preventive measures include telephone and clinical triage supported by a questionnaire on recent symptoms and movements, body temperature measurement, oral rinses with 1 percent hydrogen peroxide, and the use of appropriate PPEs [5].

The maximum number of COVID-19 cases and fatality rate will be registered globally in January 2021. During the first phase of the lockdown, which covered March and April of 2020, all dental services save for emergency care were suspended. During the disastrous pandemic, a telephone triage system was implemented to keep in contact with patients in need of immediate dental care and to invite them to an in-person appointment. The goal is to reduce the possibility of viral transmission by eliminating unnecessary hospital foot traffic and imposing social distance constraints. The American Dental Association (ADA) guidelines for patients with a cured COVID-19 infection, plan to reschedule dental treatment at least 72 h after the resolution of symptoms, or 7 days after the onset of initial symptoms, such as fever controlled without antipyretics and spontaneous improvement of breathing, set the required recovery period for infected patients to 30 days prior to non-deferrable dental care [6].

During COVID-19, emergency dental treatment was expected to adhere to newly established criteria. On June 19, 2020, the program will no longer provide Urgent Dental Care and will begin promoting the reintroduction of elective services. With the second wave of COVID-19 infections and another lockout, the service is now well-organized, and a treatment strategy has been created to ensure patient safety and efficacy. During a pandemic, a dental hospital has adequate dental chairs and personnel to meet the dental needs of a significant number of patients, even if not all patients are required to attend. To lower the risk of COVID-19 transmission, dentistry must undergo significant modifications. According to these standards, there are adequate UDC hubs, allowing patients' emergency circumstances to be addressed near their homes, hence decreasing the virus's spread [7].

Throughout the length of the pandemic, telephone triage has been an integral part of dentistry, ensuring that those in greatest need receive emergency care first. It was urged that frightened patients and those with swollen faces send photographs to an NHS email address, as well as call in ambiguous cases. The sharing of photographs aided in assessing whether a patient should be referred or asked to have a clinical evaluation. Practitioners may provide information on analgesics and how to use them in non-emergency situations, in addition to prescribing antibiotics as necessary [8].

The American Dental Association (ADA) and the Centers for Disease Control and Prevention (CDC) recommend eliminating waiting room reading and reducing appointment overlap. Except as otherwise specified, the minimum distance between patients must be 2 meters (6 feet) in each direction. It is advised, for the health and safety of patients, that they wait in their car, if feasible, or nearby the dental clinic, and that they are notified through phone call or text message when it is their turn. Despite the fact that pediatric dentistry is involved, those accompanying young patients are urged to limit their presence in the clinic and wear a protective mask in the waiting area. Based on our most thorough understanding of the situation, healthcare personnel, especially dentists, hygienists, and dental assistants, must comply with stringent clothing and safety equipment regulations. Caps, protective glasses, surgical masks or N95, and disposable gowns are recognised as crucial guidelines for the prevention of disease transmission [9].

2. Dental Treatment Recommendations for the COVID-19 Era

Hand hygiene is considered the first step in preventing the spread of the virus; WHO guidelines require meticulous handwashing before and after any contact with the patient, as well as the use of a rubber dam for containment and protection from oral fluids; it decreases the number of particles in the aerosol by 70% and significantly reduces the risk of cross-infection. If installation is impractical, Carisolv and an excavator should be provided as alternatives. During clinical procedures, high-speed spinning equipment, such as the turbine and the contra-angle, must be equipped with an anti-retraction device to prevent unintended inhalation of dirt and fluids by medical personnel. Meng et al. suggest minimizing the use of high-speed rotating devices; if this is not possible, patients requiring dental procedures including the use of such equipment should be booked for the day's final session. Moreover, they advise eschewing intraoral radiography in favor of orthopantomography or computed tomography (CT) if absolutely necessary [10].

Due to the risk of exposure to the COVID-19 virus, emergency dental care was difficult to give during the pandemic, making the operation high risk. Therefore, patient consent is necessary prior to make therapy decisions. Extractions must take precedence over restorative operations when infections endanger the airway. For the sake of patient and physician safety, digital follow-up should be prioritized above frequent

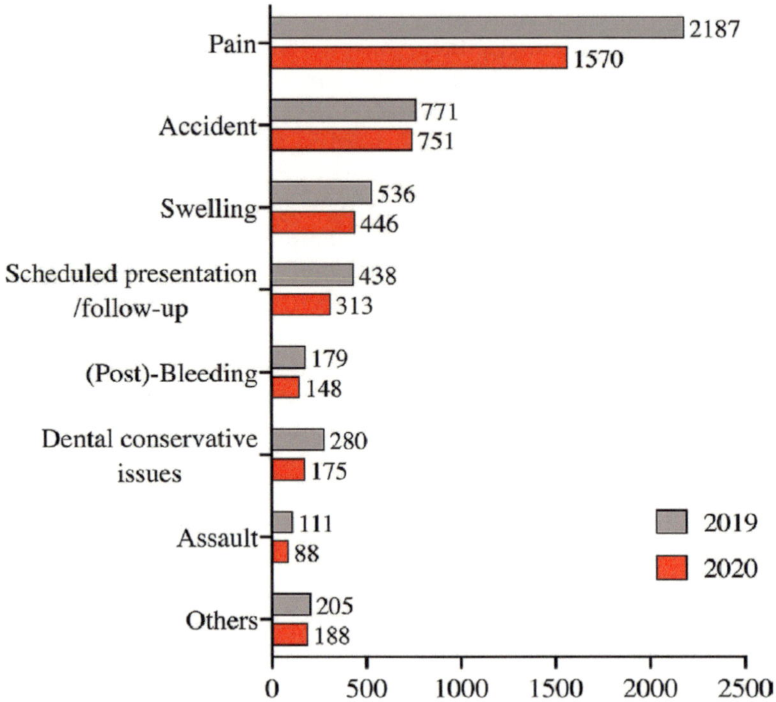

Figure 1.
Bar chart shows the distribution of patient-side reasons for presentation in dental and maxillofacial emergency services in comparison to the years 2019 (grey) and 2020 (red) [12].

patient appointments (such as video conferences). The vast majority of outpatient consultations are currently conducted by telephone [11].

The American Dental Association as part of its emergency recommendations, has incorporated urgent dental care, which focuses on the management of conditions needing immediate attention to alleviate severe pain and/or infection risk. Urgent dental care focuses on disorders requiring minimally invasive treatment, including severe tooth pain due to pulpal inflammation, pericoronitis or third-molar discomfort, surgical post-operative osteitis, and dry socket dressing changes. Abscess or localized bacterial infection resulting in localized pain and edoema. Tooth fracture produces localized pain or soft tissue damage. Trauma to the teeth with avulsion/ luxation (**Figure 1**) [13].

Permanent tooth traumatic dental injuries (TDIs) are a frequent reason why children and adolescents require immediate dental care. The most frequent types of dental injuries are crown fractures and tooth luxations. If just tooth structural abnormalities are seen, emergency physicians should evaluate the TDI, manage the patient's pain, and send them to a dentist; however, if bone involvement is present, they should refer the patient to an OMFS department. In instances of luxation or avulsion, they must move or replant the permanent teeth quickly and refer the patient to a dentist. In the event of an avulsed tooth, they must be familiar with the required abilities or storage media. Due to immature teeth and facial development throughout adolescence, therapies for these younger age groups may differ from those for adults. These Guidelines aim to improve the care of fractured teeth and decrease trauma-related complications. Frequent trauma to the dentoalveolar region causes tooth

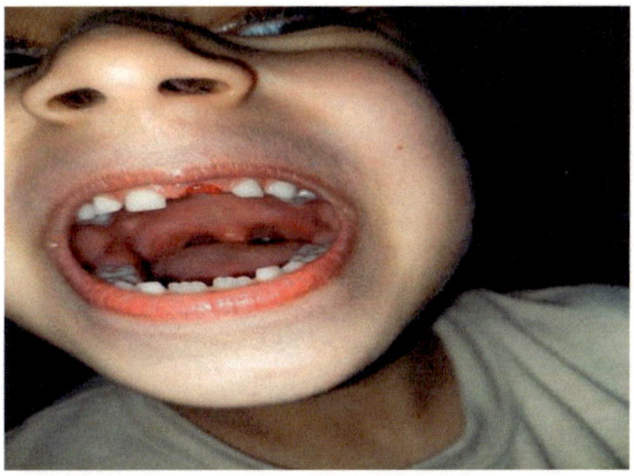

Figure 2.
Using clinical photograph in time of covid 19 for consultation.

breakage and displacement, bone-crushing and/or fracture, and soft tissue injuries including contusions, abrasions, and lacerations. When concussion or subluxation injuries and mature root development occur simultaneously in teeth, the risk of pulp necrosis and infection is significantly enhanced (**Figure 2**) [14, 15].

Crown fractures that do not expose the pulp in teeth with lateral luxation significantly increase the risk of necrosis and infection of the pulp, which can be fatal. Dental injury diagnosis relies heavily on radiographs. Tooth root and bone fractures are frequently overlooked when a single radiograph is used. When the clinical symptoms of more serious harm have subsided weeks after a traumatic occurrence, a person may also seek counseling. Therefore, dentists must employ clinical discretion while weighing the advantages and disadvantages of each form of radiography. CBCT improves the visualisation of TDIs, namely root fractures, crown/root fractures, and lateral luxations [16].

This recommendation might be revised based on the progression of the COVID-19 pandemic. Dentists must utilise their professional discretion when determining whether a patient requires urgent or emergency care. The tooth's prognosis is dependent on how quickly dental trauma treatment is delivered. Clinicians must thus understand the appropriate diagnosis and initial therapy for TDI. Avulsion is the most severe kind of documented dental trauma. The loss of an avulsed tooth has both physiological and psychological repercussions (e.g., on phonetics, chewing, and the integrity of supporting structures) (e.g., phonetics, mastication, integrity of supporting tissues). Appropriate first aid care can minimize negative psychological impacts, discomfort, tooth loss, protracted rehabilitation, and expensive costs. The International Association of Dental Traumatology suggests treating avulsed teeth with cautious storage and preservation until replantation is practicable, quick replantation if possible, splinting, and endodontic therapy as a follow-up. The success of reimplantation is dependent on the right storage of the tooth, the extra-alveolar period, the necessary drugs, the patient's dental cleanliness and overall health, as well as the kind of retention used and the time between endodontic operations [17].

When a permanent tooth was knocked out, expert treatment was "very necessary." In order to minimize unnecessary suffering, it is essential that parents get detailed advice on how to successfully handle acute symptoms. Root fractures and luxation injuries including avulsion and lateral intrusion can produce excruciating pain. In this circumstance, analgesics are recommended. Occasionally, it may be necessary to apply pressure (e.g., with a cloth) to stop bleeding or to replant or preserve avulsed teeth in cold milk until a dentist can be seen [18].

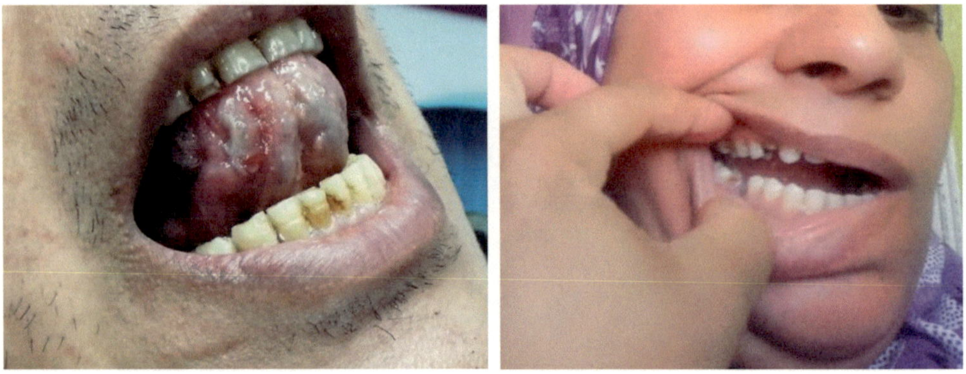

Figure 3.
Clinical photograph sends via email in covid 19 for consultation & prescribe pain killer.

Managing oral complications and decreasing the risk of COVID-19 spread to employees and patients. Remote consultation (e.g., telephone, pictures, or video conferencing) can assist medical professionals in developing a definitive diagnosis and treatment plan following an acute injury. Throughout the length of the pandemic, telephone triage has been a vital component of dentistry, ensuring that those in greatest need receive emergency treatment first. In addition to documenting the medical history of a patient, this strategy encourages talks with the patient's parents or caregivers to prepare them for what to anticipate and mask-free encounters. An efficient remote consultation may also reduce face-to-face time in the clinic, maximizing the potential use of the facility and reducing the need for Personal Protective Equipment. When feasible, problematic events should be reported to senior coworkers (**Figure 3**) [19, 20].

Telemedicine is the creative delivery of remote health care using electronic communications and the use of communication and information technologies to offer therapeutic services from a distance. In the 1970s, the World Health Organization (WHO) developed the term to describe the authorised exchange of medical information for the diagnosis, treatment, and prevention of disease and injury through information and communication technologies, with the goal of enhancing patients' health status. Telemedicine cannot be regarded as a unique medical specialty; rather, it is viewed as a tool for healthcare practitioners to disperse conventional medical practice outside the boundaries of traditional medical practice [21].

Applications and services for telemedicine include email, two-way video, wireless tools, smartphones, and further communication technologies. Telemedicine involves group treatment, nurse contacts, teaching and training, tele visits with community health experts, and medical image transfer. Telehealth, in contrast to telemedicine, provides a larger range of remote healthcare services that are not often limited to the clinical context. These services, known as remote nonclinical services, consist of training, medical education, and administrative meetings. The two primary types of telemedicine are store-and-forward telemedicine and real-time telemedicine. Store-and-forward telemedicine does not need communication partners to concurrently transfer data. It is possible to gather, organise, and store data. Data are sent as often as possible to the desired destination for diagnosis or analysis. In addition to the patient's information and medical history, images of skin lesions or electrocardiograms are sent to a physician in the linked area. Real-time telemedicine, like videoconferencing, needs simultaneous communication between the healthcare provider and the patient [22].

Lienert et al. [23] discovered that telemedical services were beneficial in circumstances requiring dental trauma at a Swiss telemedical center, and they provided crucial support when a specialized dentist was unavailable. MD et al. discovered that teledentistry provides distant, cost-effective professional dental consultations for rural Australians [24]. Utilizing teledentistry for expert consultations, diagnosis, treatment planning, referral and coordination, and continuity of care will provide decision support and allow dentists to transmit patient-specific context information. In place of dental charts and written explanations, actual images of dental problems will be utilised to fulfill second opinions, preauthorization, and other online insurance needs extremely quickly. Teledentistry will also provide the opportunity to improve current dental education teaching methodologies and provide new chances to dental students and practitioners [25].

Teledentistry is not a new field of study. The definition of teledentistry is "the remote diagnosis and suggestion of treatment using videoconferencing technology." It is an alternative to the standard delivery of dental treatment. The utility of teledentistry in rural and isolated places cannot be overstated. In rural and urban areas with access to specialized navigation, its use is of the highest relevance and value. Teledentistry is a revolutionary aspect of patient treatment that is gaining popularity and importance fast. Incalculable benefits would accrue to patients of a primary care physician who utilizes the tremendous knowledge accessible via teleconsultation. The exchange of information will result in enhanced patient care, and the capacity to engage more effectively with colleagues will increase comprehension of treatment goals [25].

In rare instances, telemedicine for the first visit was permitted with limits. After an initial telemedicine consultation, face-to-face contact was often necessary. With the development and extensive deployment of COVID-19 in 2020, the Japanese Ministry of Health, Labour, and Welfare (MHLW) has relaxed prohibitions on the use of telemedicine and dental telemedicine during the first consultation in restricted and exceptional circumstances. The MHLW has suggested discontinuing dental telemedicine for first consultations once the COVID-19 epidemic in Japan is under control. Due to the COVID-19 pandemic, we analysed the interim authorization of dental telemedicine in Japan in 2020 [26].

Teledentistry's limitations and constraints must be understood. The most prevalent technical concerns were Internet access and sound quality. All telemedicine mistakes may be categorised as technical, organizational, or severe. Universities and colleges must include telemedicine in their curricula and offer training for doctors. Telemedicine allows physicians to participate in continuing education programs without leaving their existing roles. Teledentistry may thus be used to optimise and lower the cost of dental treatment. Additionally, teledentistry is often used during the anamnesis phase of patient evaluation [27].

Internet is the basis of modern teledentistry systems since it is current, rapid, and capable of delivering vast amounts of data. Recent teledentistry technology and remote consultation methods exist only on the Internet. Today, almost every dentist clinic is outfitted with intra-oral cameras, digital cameras, and Internet-connected computers, allowing for the rapid examination of teledental possibilities. Teledentistry is a novel part of patient care that is rapidly rising in popularity and significance. Practitioners who want to include teledentistry in their practices must educate themselves on the legal, technological, and ethical obstacles posed by this burgeoning field. Dentists are required to take initiative and adapt to the digital world. They must understand not only how the digital transformation of healthcare will affect their practices, but also how they and their patients may benefit from the expansion of teledentistry. Implementing teledentistry in professional dental education is a realistic and effective strategy for fostering teledental skills [28].

Virtual consultations are a simple method to communicate with your dentist from the comfort of your home in COVID-19 situations. We would want to assist you with any oral issues you may have during the Circuit Breaker. Clinical diagnosis is NOT the aim of the virtual consultation with the dentist. Therefore, a virtual consultation cannot substitute a physical examination for clinical diagnosis. It enables dental office teams to deliver individualized care and diagnostics when on-site visits are impractical or forbidden. During this appointment, a dentist may decide whether you are having a dental emergency and recommend treatment. Due to the benefits of virtual consultation, it is not necessary to take time off from work to see the dentist. Eliminate disease transmission risks and decrease wait times. Evaluate the need for an urgent/emergency visit. Explore several treatment options [29].

Telemedicine is a fascinating new development that improves the quality of medical and health care services as a whole. Practitioners who want to include teledentistry into their practices must educate themselves on the legal, technological, and ethical concerns this emerging subject presents. Dentists are required to familiarize themselves with the electronic environment. They must first understand not only how their practices will be affected by the digital transformation of healthcare, but also how they and their patients may benefit from the expansion of teledentistry [30].

Before you may treat a patient referred to you through teledentistry, you must establish a doctor-patient relationship and get an adequate medical history. If you are considering incorporating teledentistry into your practice, you must assess the criteria below. Before beginning teledentistry therapy, authorization must be acquired from the patient. Before giving treatment through teledentistry, a suitable medical history is required. Thirdly, any dental records generated through teledentistry must comply with the same retention rules as those generated during in-person dental visits. You must adhere to your state's e-prescribing requirements if you prescribe medications through teledentistry. Dentists who practice teledentistry are required to take every care to ensure the security of their systems, data collecting, and processing of all types of collected data. For example, data encryption, password protection, and user access logs may contribute to avoiding the misuse of the information of the majority of persons and, ultimately, protecting patient privacy [31].

The significance of teledentistry is investigated. Numerous subspecialties of teledentistry, such as teleconsultation, telediagnosis, telemonitoring, and teletriage, perform essential dental practice-related tasks. Teleconsultation reduces the number of non-urgent patient referrals, hence alleviating the strain on already overburdened healthcare systems. Telediagnosis permits the remote diagnosis of oral problems via the transmission of patient data, intraoral imaging, and radiographic pictures. Due to the pandemic, teletriage prioritizes patients in urgent need of dental treatment based on a remote evaluation of their oral health, hence eliminating the need for non-essential travel [32].

Teledentistry is advantageous for both dentists and patients. Teledentistry is helpful for internet-based dental education and training for dentists since it minimizes patient expenditures and remote self-education. Dentists feel that teledentistry may provide novel means of maintaining regular dental practice under non-pandemic settings. Future teledentistry will provide appointment schedule simplification so that new patients may be assessed in two ways. The first stage will consist of obtaining the patient's medical history and consent, while the second will comprise an in-person examination, diagnosis, and treatment. The frequency of hospital/clinic admissions would decrease, hence decreasing the spread of COVID-19 [33].

Similarly, to telemedicine, teledentistry has developed as a viable alternative for a number of dental specialties, including endodontics, orthodontics, oral surgery, and pediatric dentistry. Acceptable for identifying children with a reduced risk of developing dental caries. The accurate diagnosis of oral disorders, such as oral cancer, may be difficult in diagnostic dentistry, particularly in low-income regions with limited access to specialized dental treatment. Teledentistry may thus satisfy this requirement and enhance treatment quality [34].

Covid-19 has advocated the use of teledentistry and telemedicine during the current epidemic, a move that has been favorably accepted by both patients and medical professionals. Dentists may integrate teledentistry into conventional dental practice by educating themselves and their staff in this technology field. Teledentistry is a fantastic way to supplement the current insufficient dental system and aid those in need. This project's clinical mailbox for teledentistry was developed to be as user-friendly, time-efficient, and easy as possible in order to overcome these obstacles. Using email templates with links to each digital information booklet allows clinicians to easily personalize each patient's contact by excluding unnecessary details [35].

Teledental care provides obvious benefits for limiting the spread of COVID-19 among younger patients. Some dentists at private dental clinics exploit dental telemedicine to recruit patients. It is seen as a unique strategy that might help improve access to medical and dental treatment. Utilizing "Attend Anywhere" virtual video conferencing software might enable video consultations to minimize patient foot traffic and aid physicians in managing patient backlogs caused by the cessation of elective services. This necessitates the availability of enough rooms to provide privacy. The current COVID-19 epidemic has prompted dentists to explore alternatives to direct clinical examination for the delivery of healthcare. Virtual dental consultation is distinct from teledentistry, one of the few remote patient treatments and monitoring approaches that do not involve the transmission of the COVID-19 virus [32].

The Internet plays a key role in facilitating good communication between dentists and patients, a need in contemporary society. Despite the limits that prevent individuals from physically meeting, invest in active contact through email, social media, the telephone, and video chat. A new aim is to feel comfortable and protected when obtaining medical advice or services. Thus, we are better able to interact with and connect with the global community [36].

Teledentistry's clinical uses include patient record keeping, diagnostics, and clinical decision-making. Teledentistry helps impoverished individuals to get dental treatment. In addition to its therapeutic benefits, teledentistry may be useful in eradicating inequities and fostering equitable access to oral health care. The technology used in teledentistry permits the rapid transmission of photos, data, and papers and gives practitioners access to this information [25, 37].

Despite the vast number of specialties that may benefit from teledentistry and the variety of applications, there are still restrictions on the transmission and use of information technology. Digital photographs may be useful for recognizing obvious issues, but they have their limitations. Photos provide a two-dimensional depiction of three-dimensional objects, which may diminish diagnostic accuracy. Teledentistry requires the use of high-quality pictures, which are unavailable at all remote clinics and facilities. The expensive expense of teledentistry for both governments and people is a serious barrier. Teledentistry is a fast-expanding subject with enormous promise, but it is still in its infancy, and greater focus must be made on the distribution of money and grants for more clinical research to offer more data and establish the position of teledentistry in the delivery of oral healthcare [33].

3. Conclusion

Dentistry forms an important part of our healthcare system, which has become severely compromised during the current pandemic of COVID-19. Teledentistry can be used to successfully record a patient's chief complaint and medical history and to assign the number of missing and filled teeth at acceptable levels. However, teledentistry tends to overestimate the number of decayed teeth. The need of the hour is to incorporate teledentistry into routine dental practice. If not fully replaced, at least teledentistry can complement the existing compromised dental system during the current pandemic.

Recommendations

For oral screening, teledentistry may be similar to face-to-face technology, especially for school-based programmes, caries assessment, referrals, and teleconsultations. Several studies comparing teledentistry to traditional clinical evaluation revealed that teledentistry is less sensitive. Therefore, the validity of teledentistry and telemedicine in dental specialties requires further research.

Funding

This research received no external funding.

Conflicts of interest

The authors declare no conflict of any interest.

Author details

Shaimaa Hussein Rafat Kotb
Alazhar University, Faculty of Dentistry, Oral Medicine and Periodontology Department, Assuit branch, Egypt

*Address all correspondence to: shaymarafat.dental@gmail.com

IntechOpen

© 2022 The Author(s). Licensee IntechOpen. This chapter is distributed under the terms of the Creative Commons Attribution License (http://creativecommons.org/licenses/by/3.0), which permits unrestricted use, distribution, and reproduction in any medium, provided the original work is properly cited. (cc) BY

References

[1] WHO. Coronavirus disease (COVID-19): Variants of SARS-COV-2 2021 [cited 2021]. 2021. Available from: https://www.who.int/emergencies/diseases/novel-coronavirus-2019/question-and-answers-hub/q-a-detail/coronavirus-disease-%28covid-19%29-variants-of-sars-cov-2?gclid=Cj0KCQjwyYKUBhDJARIsAMj9lkEJo4-9j5Ujff-46JiL2ZMFBNNMTQbPHoP8pl_6Mdsl4rWcvMjGba0aAoz7EALw_wcB

[2] Kampf G, Todt D, Pfaender S, Steinmann E. Persistence of coronaviruses on inanimate surfaces and their inactivation with biocidal agents. The Journal of Hospital Infection. 2020;**104**(3):246-251

[3] Kilic AU, Kara F, Alp E, Doganay M. New threat: 2019 novel Coronavirus infection and infection control perspective in Turkey. North Clinics of Istanbul. 2020;**7**(2):95-98

[4] Adhikari SP, Meng S, Wu YJ, Mao YP, Ye RX, Wang QZ, et al. Epidemiology, causes, clinical manifestation and diagnosis, prevention and control of coronavirus disease (COVID-19) during the early outbreak period: A scoping review. Infectious Diseases of Poverty. 2020;**9**(1):29

[5] Luzzi V, Ierardo G, Bossù M, Polimeni A. Paediatric oral health during and after the COVID-19 pandemic. International Journal of Paediatric Dentistry. 2021;**31**(1):20-26

[6] Villani FA, Aiuto R, Paglia L, Re D. COVID-19 and dentistry: Prevention in dental practice, a literature review. International Journal of Environmental Research and Public Health. 2020;**17**(12):4609

[7] Ostrc T, Pavlović K, Fidler A. Urgent dental care on a national level during the COVID-19 epidemic. Clinincal and Experimental Dental Research. 2021;**7**(3):271-278

[8] Ball M, Akintola D, Harrington Z, Djemal S. Emergency dental care triage during the COVID-19 pandemic. British Dental Journal. 2021;**29**:1-5

[9] Yang Y, Soh HY, Cai ZG, Peng X, Zhang Y, Guo CB. Experience of diagnosing and managing patients in oral maxillofacial surgery during the prevention and control period of the new coronavirus pneumonia. The Chinese Journal of Dental Research. 2020;**23**(1):57-62

[10] Peng X, Xu X, Li Y, Cheng L, Zhou X, Ren B. Transmission routes of 2019-nCoV and controls in dental practice. International Journal of Oral Science. 2020;**12**(1):9

[11] Jiang CM, Duangthip D, Auychai P, Chiba M, Folayan MO, Hamama HHH, et al. Changes in oral health policies and guidelines during the COVID-19 pandemic. Frontiers in Oral Health. 2021;**2**:668444

[12] Thiem D, Polsak M-T, Römer P, Gielisch M, Blatt S, Al-Nawas B, et al. The impact of the COVID-19 pandemic on the dental-maxillofacial emergency service of a German university hospital in the year 2020. Clinical Oral Investigations. 2021;**26**:385-395

[13] WHO. WHO Coronavirus (COVID-19) Dashboard. 2021. Available from: https://covid19.who.int/

[14] American Dental Association. ADA Develops Guidance on Dental

Emergency, Nonemergency Care 2020. 2020. Available from: https://www.ada.org/en/publications/ada-news/2020-archive/march/ada-develops-guidance-on-dental-emergencynonemergency-care

[15] Yeng T, O. Sullivan AJ, Shulruf B. Medical doctors' knowledge of dental trauma management: A review. Dental Traumatology. 2020;**36**(2):100-107

[16] Moule A, Cohenca N. Emergency assessment and treatment planning for traumatic dental injuries. Australian Dental Journal. 2016;**61**(Suppl. 1):21-38

[17] Cohenca N, Silberman A. Contemporary imaging for the diagnosis and treatment of traumatic dental injuries: A review. Dental Traumatology. 2017;**33**(5):321-328

[18] Frujeri Mde L, Costa ED Jr. Effect of a single dental health education on the management of permanent avulsed teeth by different groups of professionals. Dental Traumatology. 2009;**25**(3):262-271

[19] Pagliarin CL, Zenkner CL, Barletta FB. Knowledge of physical education teachers about emergency management of tooth avulsion. Stoma. 2011;**17**(33):32-42

[20] Levin L, Day PF, Hicks L, O, Connell A, Fouad AF, Bourguignon C, et al. International Association of Dental Traumatology guidelines for the management of traumatic dental injuries: General introduction. Dental Traumatology. 2020;**36**(4):309-313

[21] Schmeler MR, Schein RM, McCue M, Betz K. Telerehabilitation clinical and vocational applications for assistive technology: Research, opportunities, and challenges. International Journal of Telerehabilitation. 2009;**1**(1):59-72

[22] Mars M. Telemedicine and advances in urban and rural healthcare delivery in Africa. Progress in Cardiovascular Diseases. 2013;**56**(3):326-335

[23] Lienert N, Zitzmann NU, Filippi A, Weiger R, Krastl G. Teledental consultations related to trauma in a Swiss telemedical center: A retrospective survey. Dental Traumatology. 2010;**26**(3):223-227

[24] Snow MD, Canale E, Quail G. Teledentistry permits distant, cost-effective specialist dental consultations for rural Australians. Journal of Telemedicine and Telecare. 2000;**6**(1):216

[25] Jampani ND, Nutalapati R, Dontula BS, Boyapati R. Applications of teledentistry: A literature review and update. Journal of International Society of Preventive and Community Dentistry. 2011;**1**(2):37-44

[26] Monaghesh E, Hajizadeh A. The role of telehealth during COVID-19 outbreak: A systematic review based on current evidence. BMC Public Health. 2020;**20**(1):1193

[27] Younai FS, Messadi DV. E-mail-based oral medicine consultation. Journal of the California Dental Association. 2000;**28**(2):144-151

[28] Bauer JC, Brown WT. The digital transformation of oral health care. Teledentistry and electronic commerce. Journal of the American Dental Association (1939). 2001;**132**(2):204-209

[29] Crummey A, Graham A, Besi E. Virtual consultations for oral surgery patients. BMC Oral Health. 2022;**22**(1):83

[30] Dar-Odeh N, Babkair H, Alnazzawi A, Abu-Hammad S, Abu-Hammad A, Abu-Hammad O.

Utilizationofteledentistryinantimicrobial prescribing and diagnosis of infectious diseases during COVID-19 lockdown. European Journal of Dentistry. 2020;**14**(1):S20-S26

[31] Ghai S. Teledentistry during COVID-19 pandemic. Diabetes and Metabolic Syndrome: Clinical Research and Reviews. 2020;**14**(5):933-935

[32] Subhan R, Ismail WA, Musharraf S, Khan M, Hafeez R, Alam MK. Teledentistry as a supportive tool for dentists in Pakistan. BioMed Research International. 2021;**2021**:875

[33] Sharma H, Suprabha BS, Rao A. Teledentistry and its applications in paediatric dentistry: A literature review. Pediatric Dental Journal. 2021;**31**(3):203-215

[34] Estai M, Bunt SM, Kanagasingam Y, Kruger E, Tennant M. A resource reallocation model for school dental screening: Taking advantage of teledentistry in low-risk areas. International Dental Journal. 2018;**68**(4):262-268

[35] Patel T, Wong J. The role of real-time interactive video consultations in dental practice during the recovery and restoration phase of the COVID-19 outbreak. British Dental Journal. 2020;**229**(3):196-200

[36] Ha JF, Longnecker N. Doctor-patient communication: A review. The Ochsner Journal. 2010;**10**(1):38-43

[37] Wallace CK, Schofield CE, Burbridge LAL, O'Donnell KL. Role of teledentistry in paediatric dentistry. British Dental Journal. 2021:1-6